ECG ROUNDS

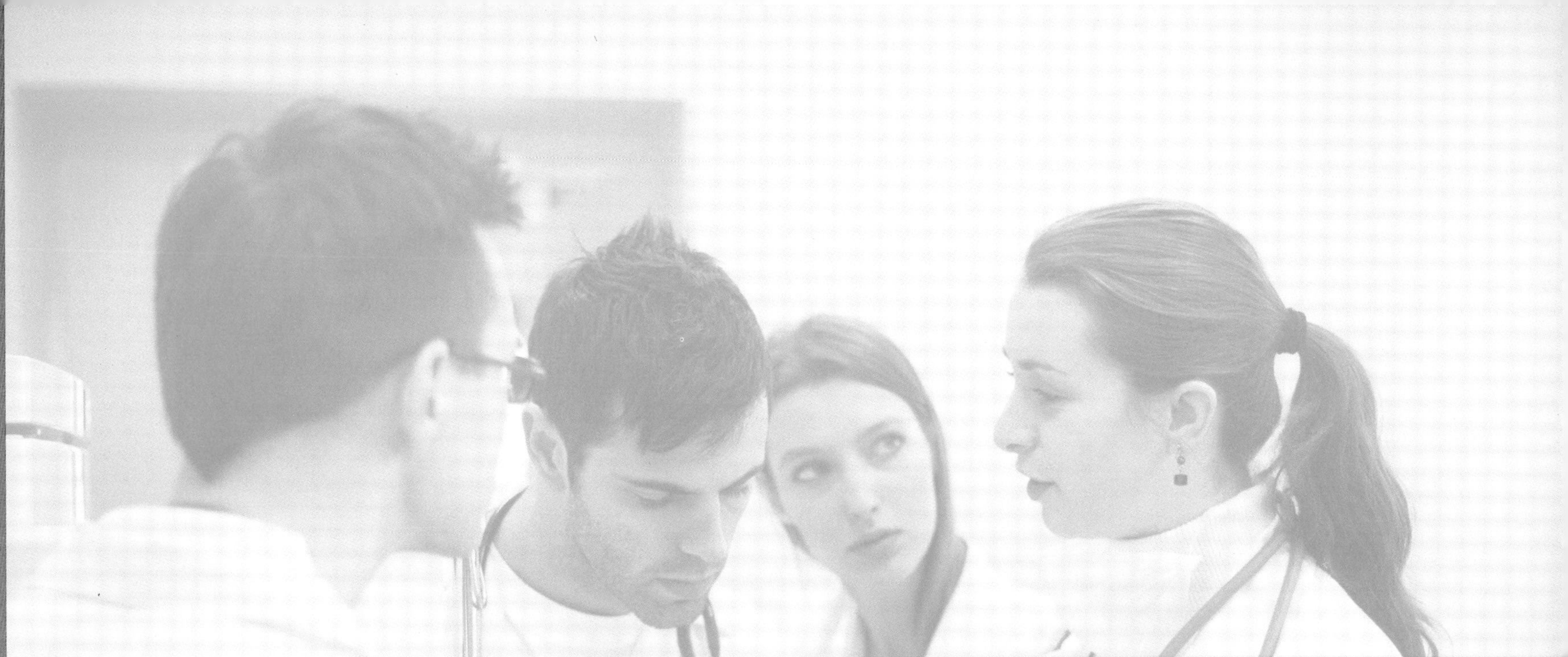

ECG ROUNDS

Thomas S. Metkus, Jr, MD
Fellow in Cardiovascular Medicine
Department of Cardiology
The Johns Hopkins Hospital
Baltimore, Maryland

Mc Graw Hill Education | Medical

New York Chicago San Francisco Athens London Madrid
Mexico City Milan New Delhi Singapore Sydney Toronto

ECG Rounds

1 2 3 4 5 6 7 8 9 0 QLM/QLM 18 17 16 15 14 13

ISBN 978-0-07-180763-0
MHID 0-07-180763-2

This book was set in Minion Pro by Thomson Digital.
The editors were Christine Diedrich and Christina M. Thomas.
The production supervisor was Richard Ruzycka.
The illustration manager was Armen Ovsepyan.
Project management was provided by Shaminder Pal Singh, Thomson Digital.
The designer was Eve Siegel; the cover designer was Mary McKeon.
Cover credit: © MIKA/CORBIS; inset, istockphoto.com
Quad Graphics/Leominster was printer and binder.

This book is printed on acid-free paper.

Library of Congress Cataloging-in-Publication Data

Metkus, Thomas S., Jr.
ECG rounds / Thomas S. Metkus, Jr.
p. ; cm.
ISBN-13: 978-0-07-180763-0 (softcover : alk. paper)
ISBN-10: 0-07-180763-2 (softcover : alk. paper)
I. Title.
[DNLM: 1. Cardiovascular Diseases—diagnosis—Case Reports. 2. Cardiovascular Diseases—diagnosis—Examination Questions. 3. Electrocardiography—Case Reports. 4. Electrocardiography—Examination Questions. 5. Image Interpretation, Computer-Assisted—Case Reports. 6. Image Interpretation, Computer-Assisted—Examination Questions. WG 18.2]
RC683.5.E5
616.1'207547—dc23

2013011826

CONTENTS BY DIFFICULTY LEVEL

CONTENTS BY SUBJECT MATTER

Tracings arranged by subject matter

CONTRIBUTORS

Glenn A. Hirsch, MD, MHS, FACC
Adjunct Assistant Professor of Medicine
Division of Cardiology
Johns Hopkins University School of Medicine
Associate Professor of Medicine
Division of Cardiovascular Medicine
Department of Medicine
University of Louisville
Louisville, Kentucky

Jonathan W. Waks, MD
Clinical Cardiology Fellow
Division of Cardiovascular Disease
Beth Israel Deaconess Medical Center
Clinical Fellow in Medicine
Harvard Medical School
Boston, Massachusetts

Matthew I. Tomey, MD
Chief Fellow
Department of Cardiology
The Mount Sinai Hospital
New York, New York

Yee-Ping Sun, MD
Division of Cardiology
Department of Medicine
Clinical Cardiology Fellow
Columbia University Medical Center
New York-Presbyterian Hospital
New York, New York

Sammy Zakaria, MD, MPH
Assistant Professor of Medicine
Division of Cardiology
Johns Hopkins University School of Medicine
Baltimore, Maryland

Ramon A. Partida, MD
Fellow in Cardiovascular Medicine
Division of Cardiology
Massachusetts General Hospital
Harvard Medical School
Boston, Massachusetts

Dipan A. Desai, DO
Clinical Associate
Division of Cardiology
Johns Hopkins University School of Medicine
Johns Hopkins Bayview Medical Center
Baltimore, Maryland

Samuel C. Volo, MD
Cardiology Fellow
Division of Cardiology
New York-Presbyterian Hospital Weill Cornell Medical Center
New York, New York

Dedication

To my parents: you are my first role models both as physicians and as people.

To mentors too numerous to list here, in particular Drs. Joseph Loscalzo, Steve Schulman, and the late Ken Baughman: thank you!!

For Kate and for Hailey: it's all for you, always.

FOREWORD

Over the past 25 years I have rounded with countless numbers of wonderful house staff in the Coronary Care Unit. In the CCU and the wards, the electrocardiogram tells a story for each patient. From acute coronary syndrome, cardiomyopathy, hypertrophy, and electrolyte and drug toxicities, the electrocardiogram helps us link a patient's symptoms and exam findings with a diagnosis. Asking a house officer to not only describe the electrocardiogram, but interpret the findings is a particularly effective method of bedside teaching. I find that this method of electrocardiographic teaching helps house officers and students learn and remember important electrocardiographic findings. This book brings bedside electrocardiographic teaching to these pages. Everyone who enjoys clinical care will enjoy these ECG-based cases.

Steven Schulman, MD

PREFACE

On several occasions during residency, a junior colleague approached me with some variation of the following request: "I'm starting a cardiology rotation soon, and I feel uncomfortable reading ECGs ... can you recommend a resource?" I have spent a lot of time since then considering the mechanism by which residents and students learn the art and science of ECG interpretation.

First, what are the ECG abnormalities that most physicians should be comfortable recognizing, or, put differently, "what do I need to know?" Second, in what context is this information best delivered? I was taught to read ECGs in a fairly haphazard fashion using several different exercises. A faculty member would host the occasional workshop or lecture (during which I would invariably embarrass myself!). A random assortment of ECG tracings would invariably appear on in-service, shelf, and board examinations. Much learning necessarily happened in the context of clinical care—myself and fellow interns intently studying the ECGs of our patients, often in the wee hours of the morning and without senior staff guidance. Finally, many of us have had the privileged experience of a truly gifted clinical teacher reading an ECG with us on morning rounds, skillfully linking ECG abnormalities to the patient in the bed in front of us.

It is this final method of learning that this book attempts to replicate. I endeavor to present a set of tracings, which, taken together, demonstrate most abnormalities that a generalist physician trainee would "need to know." Each tracing is followed by clinical questions meant to reinforce electrocardiographic concepts and simulate the experience of rounding with a master clinician teaching in the Socratic Method. At the conclusion of the book, I hope you will have been exposed to a wide array of ECG abnormalities relevant to your current practice.

Practical interpretation, cogitation, and cognition are the focus rather than memorizing vast arrays of criteria. You can choose to interpret the tracings by level of difficulty, by teaching topic, or sequentially as presented (see Table of Contents). I assume a basic knowledge of the skills of ECG interpretation, which will be reviewed only briefly; readers are referred to several excellent texts for a more in-depth review of basic interpretation skills and the physiology of the ECG. Likewise, this book is not a comprehensive reference text for ECG criteria, and readers are referred to several excellent texts for this purpose.

I hope you find this book useful and enjoyable. Interpreting ECGs connects us to our roots as medical physiologists, clinicians, and teachers, and I hope that sense of joy and purpose shows through in this work.

Warm regards,

TM

Disclaimer: The cases presented herein are fictional and created by the authors solely for illustrative teaching purposes alone. Any resemblance of cases to actual patients in any context is purely coincidental. This book does not purport to offer medical advice nor management guidance on specific cases. As always, all ECG interpretation and clinical decisions rendered in the context of patient care are solely at the discretion of the treating physician.

ECG ROUNDS

INTRODUCTION: A focused step-wise guide to ECG interpretation

Reading an ECG is like juggling fire while riding a unicycle: performing the fundamentals systematically, the same way, every time, will prevent you from getting burned. Presented here is the authors' approach to reading an ECG. It is less important to follow 1 particular approach; rather, choose 1 validated approach that works for you and apply it the same way, every time, to every tracing.

Step 1: Rate

Recall that each "little box" on the time axis of a tracing is 0.04 seconds in duration, with each "big box" comprising 5 little boxes and equal to 0.2 seconds. Thus, calculate the rate as 300 divided by the number of big boxes between complexes (300/1 = rate of 300; 300/2 = rate of 150; etc). Alternatively (more accurate and more difficult math), calculate the rate as 1500 divided by the number of little boxes between complexes (1500/5 = rate of 300; 1500/17 = rate of 88; etc).

The above methods are accurate only if the rhythm is regular. A second approach to calculate rate is to recall that the rhythm strip is 10 seconds in duration. Count the number of complexes present in the rhythm strip and multiply by 6, yielding the rate. This method is accurate whether the rhythm is regular or irregular.

Using your choice of these methods, calculate the atrial rate (P waves) and the ventricular rate (QRS complexes).

Step 2: Rhythm analysis

First, search for atrial activity. Are there P waves? The best place to find P waves is in the inferior leads (II, III, and aVF) and V1.

Second, are the P waves sinus P waves or nonsinus P waves? Sinus P waves should be upright in the inferior leads and biphasic in lead V1. If the atrial activity is not a sinus P wave, what is it? Atrial flutter? Atrial tachycardia? Is there no organized atrial activity suggesting atrial fibrillation?

Finally, what is the relationship between the atrial activity and the ventricular activity? Does the atrial activity precede the ventricular activity with a constant interval? Does the atrial activity follow the ventricular activity, suggesting retrograde conduction? Are the atrial and ventricular depolarizations independent of each other? Is A-V block present?

Step 3: Axis

Consider first if the axis is normal or not. Recall that lead I is located at 0 degrees, lead II at +60 degrees, and lead aVF at +90 degrees:

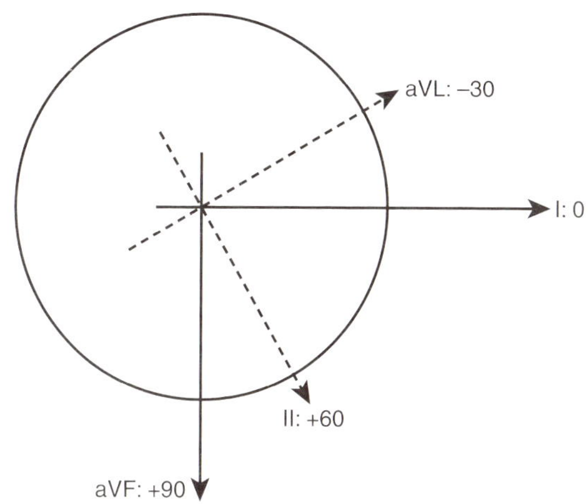

If the QRS complex is more positive than negative in leads I, II, and aVF, the axis is normal, defined as axis between +100 and –30 degrees.

If the QRS complex is positive in aVF but predominantly negative in lead I, a rightward axis is present.

If the QRS complex is negative in aVF but positive in lead I, assess lead II. If the QRS complex is positive in lead II, a normal axis is present. If the QRS complex is more negative than positive in lead II, a leftward axis is present.

One can be more sophisticated and can calculate the axis exactly by finding the lead in which the QRS complex is isoelectric: the axis must be 90 degrees to this lead.

Step 4: Intervals

Assess the PR interval: is it normal, prolonged, or shortened?

Assess the QRS width: is it narrow or widened? If widened, is the morphology for a diagnosis of bundle branch block or conduction delay present?

Assess the QT interval: is it prolonged or shortened? Is the morphology consistent with a particular diagnosis?

We will review criteria for the above diagnoses in the context of the tracings to come.

Step 5: Chamber enlargement and hypertrophy

As the next step in ECG interpretation, evaluate sequentially the left atrium, the right atrium, the left ventricle, and the right ventricle for chamber abnormality, enlargement, or hypertrophy. We will review criteria for each of these diagnoses in the context of tracings to come.

Step 6: Ischemia and infarction

Reading for ischemia and infarction as well as related abnormalities of ST segments and T waves requires evaluating the presence of Q waves, ST-segment changes, and T-wave abnormalities in groups of leads.

Recall that:

Leads II, II, and aVF represent the inferior aspect of the heart.
Leads I, aVL, V5, and V6 represent the lateral aspect of the heart.
Leads V1 and V2 represent the septum.
Leads V3 through V5 represent the anterior wall of the heart.

In addition, infarction of the posterior wall of the heart can manifest electrocardiographically as reciprocal anterior changes. ST-segment elevation in lead V1, usually associated with inferior infarction, can suggest right ventricular infarction.

Ischemic changes should be regional; therefore, look sequentially for Q waves, ST-segment depression, ST-segment elevation, and T-wave changes (inverted? pseudo-normalized? peaked? hyperacute?) in the inferior leads, septal leads, anterior leads, and lateral leads.

Identify any reciprocal changes. Abnormalities spanning the distribution of more than 1 coronary artery could be due to global ischemia (such as those occurring in aortic stenosis, tachycardia, or anemia), multivessel disease, or secondary to disorders such as pericardial disease. ST-segment abnormalities with morphology that appears atypical for ischemia may be due to early repolarization, ventricular hypertrophy, electrolyte disturbances, or other disorders that we will review.

Step 7: Additional findings

Look for additional findings depending on your clinical suspicion. Additional waves seen in some clinical disorders include epsilon waves, U waves, or the J waves of Osborn.

Step 8: Synthesize

William Osler famously noted that, along with the 4 classic physical examination maneuvers of inspection, percussion, palpation, and auscultation, a fifth maneuver was perhaps the most critical: cogitation. Re-stated, it is important to gather the data, but one must also consider what it means in the clinical context. So, after careful assessment of the tracing, take time to consider the clinical history and the findings together, opining on their relation to each other. What is the impact of your findings on diagnosis and treatment?

Section I

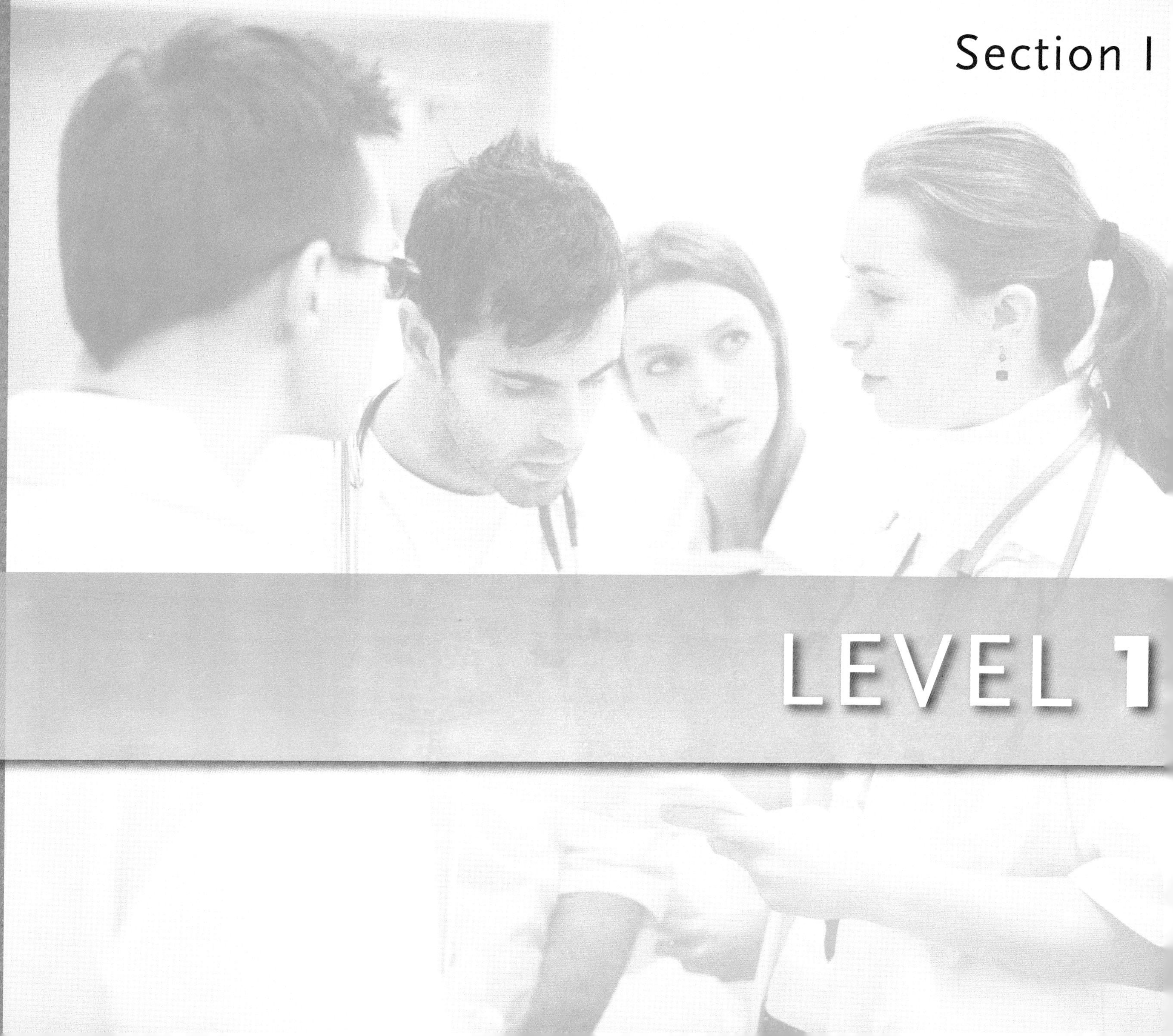

LEVEL 1

Case #1. A 47-year-old man presenting for preoperative evaluation prior to knee arthroscopy.

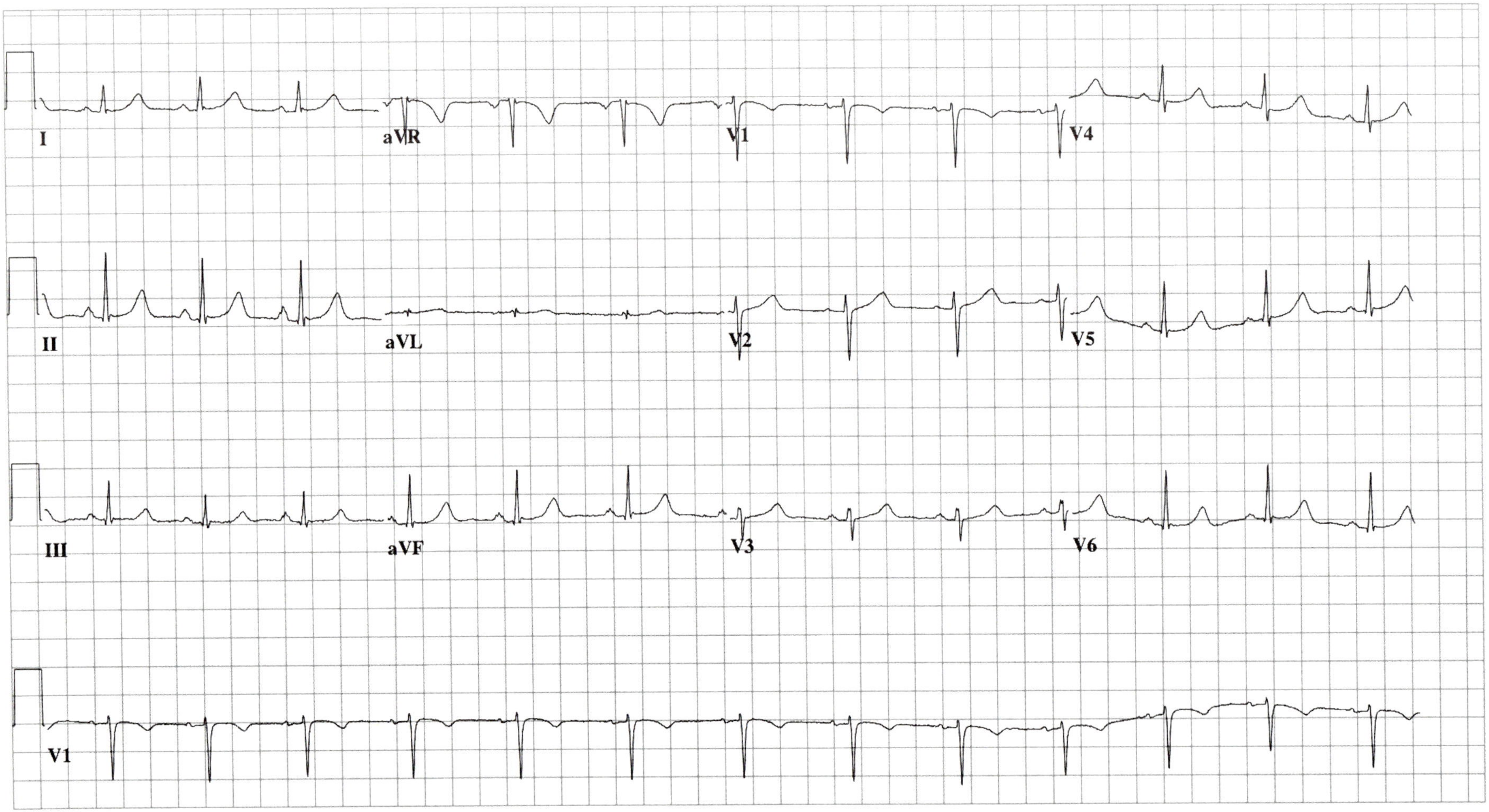

QUESTIONS

1-1. What are the ECG findings?

1-2. What ECG findings would concern you during a preoperative evaluation?

83
P2-4AC
15.0 cm MI 0.9
Gen TIs 1.1
[2d] G78/71 d
FA4/P90
HAR/FS|0
3
2.5

ANSWERS

1-1. What are the ECG findings?

This tracing demonstrates sinus rhythm at a rate of about 80 beats/min. The axis and intervals are normal. There is no evidence of chamber enlargement, hypertrophy, or ischemia. This is a normal ECG.

1-2. What ECG findings would concern you during a preoperative evaluation?

The preoperative ECG should first be assessed for any unstable cardiac conditions that would preclude elective surgery. These include active ischemia, ventricular tachycardia, or uncontrolled atrial arrhythmias such as rapid atrial fibrillation. Other findings of importance may include the presence of Q waves in a coronary distribution suggesting occult coronary disease and prior myocardial infarction, and chamber enlargement possibly suggesting occult valvular disease.

Case #2. An asymptomatic 56-year-old gentleman presents for routine follow-up.

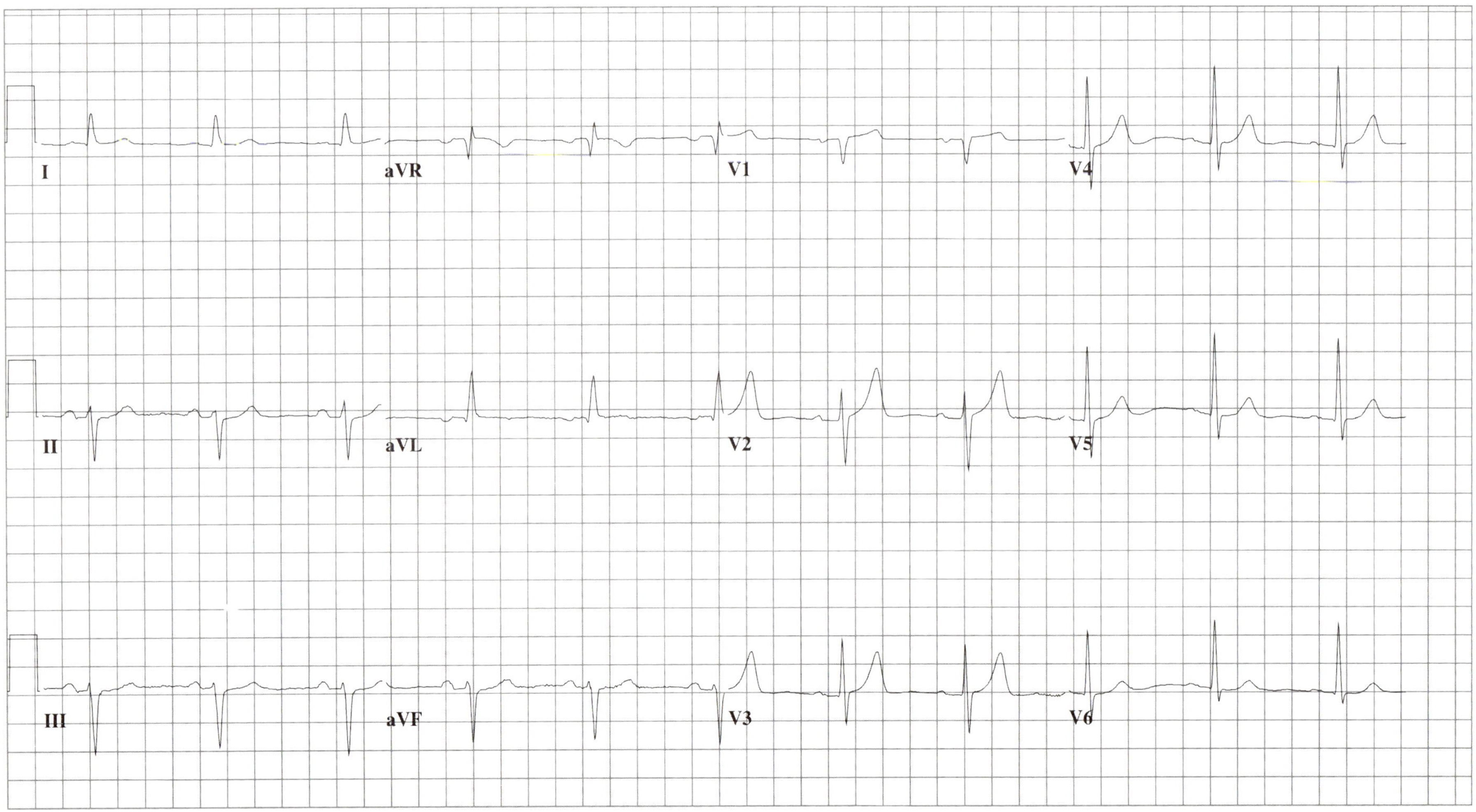

QUESTIONS

2-1. What abnormalities are present on the ECG?

2-2. What is the differential diagnosis for left-axis deviation?

83
15.0 cm MI 0.9
P2-4AC
Gen TIs 1.1
[2d] G78/71 d
FA4/P90
HAR/FSI0
[C] G50/0.80 kHz
FA5/F1/B
TDI
Amplitude (V)
S-T
S-T
interval
2.5
3
3.5

ANSWERS

2-1. What abnormalities are present on the ECG?

There is sinus rhythm at 66 beats/min. The axis is deviated leftward, evidenced by the positive QRS complex in lead I and the negative QRS complex in leads II and aVF. This left-axis deviation is associated with small q waves and large R waves in leads I and aVL, and small r waves and large S waves in the inferior leads. There is no evidence of left ventricular hypertrophy or other chamber abnormalities. There are no pathologic Q waves suggesting prior infarction, and no ST-segment or T-wave abnormalities. The presence of leftward axis deviation in the absence of left ventricular hypertrophy or prior infarction with this pattern of qR complexes in leads I and aVL and rS complexes in the inferior leads is consistent with left anterior hemiblock, also known as left anterior fascicular block. Recall that the His bundle bifurcates into the left and right bundle branches. The left bundle branch further branches into the left anterior fascicle and the left posterior fascicle. Block in the left anterior fascicle is more common than block in the left posterior fascicle. Hypertension, ischemic heart disease, cardiomyopathy, and degenerative conduction system disease of the elderly (Lev's syndrome) are all associated with left anterior hemiblock. The QRS duration is normal when left anterior hemiblock alone is present, although a delayed intrinsicoid deflection (the duration between the onset of the QRS and the peak of the R wave) of greater than 45 milliseconds should be observed in lead aVL as is present in this case.

2-2. What is the differential diagnosis for left-axis deviation?

Left-axis deviation can be associated with left anterior hemiblock (as in this case), left ventricular hypertrophy, prior myocardial infarction, Wolff-Parkinson-White syndrome, and atrial septal defect.

Case #3. A 43-year-old asymptomatic man.

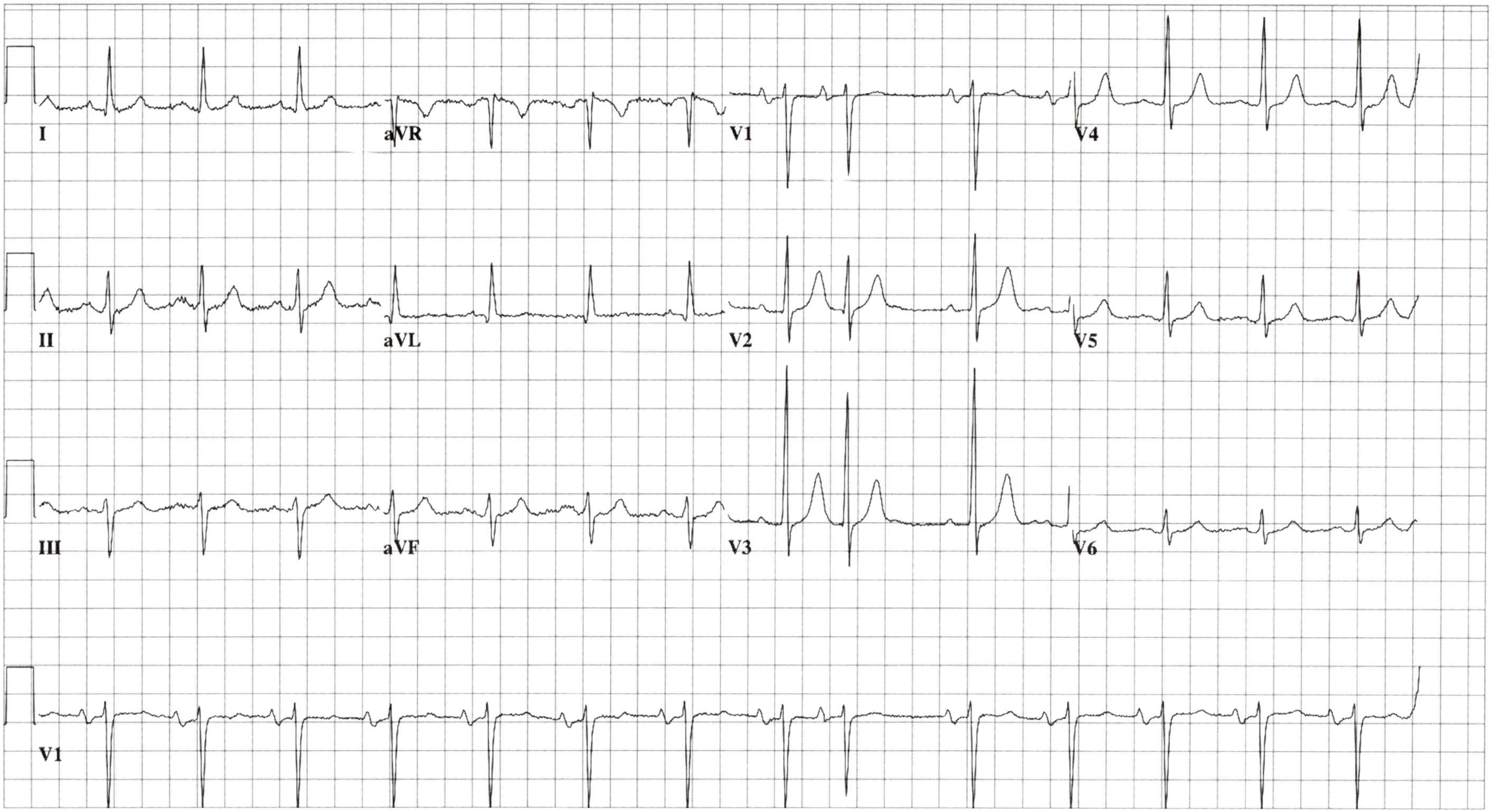

QUESTIONS

3-1. What abnormalities are present?

3-2. What would you do next?

83
P2-4AC
15.0 cm MI 0.9
Gen TIs 1.1
[2d] G78/71 d
FA4/P90
HAR/FS0
[C] G50/0.80 kHz
FA5/F1/8
TDI
Amplitude (V)
S-T
interval
2.5
3
Time (s)

ANSWERS

3-1. What abnormalities are present?

Sinus rhythm is present at approximately 85 beats/min. The axis is normal as are the intervals. There is no evidence of chamber enlargement, hypertrophy, or ischemia. The ninth P–QRS complex occurs earlier than expected, and the P wave has a slightly different morphology than the other P waves. This beat represents a premature atrial contraction. The P–P interval (amount of time between P waves) following the ectopic beat is longer than the sinus P–P interval, a compensatory pause. Overall, this ECG can be classified as a normal ECG, as a single premature atrial beat is not pathologic.

3-2. What would you do next?

If no symptoms are present, no further action is indicated. Frequent premature atrial contractions can sometimes occur as a manifestation of hyperthyroidism, electrolyte abnormalities, or medication toxicity, none of which are supported by this history. β-Blockers can be prescribed for symptomatic atrial ectopy, but in this case, no further treatment is necessary.

Case #4. A 65-year-old woman complaining of 3 hours of severe epigastric "bloating."

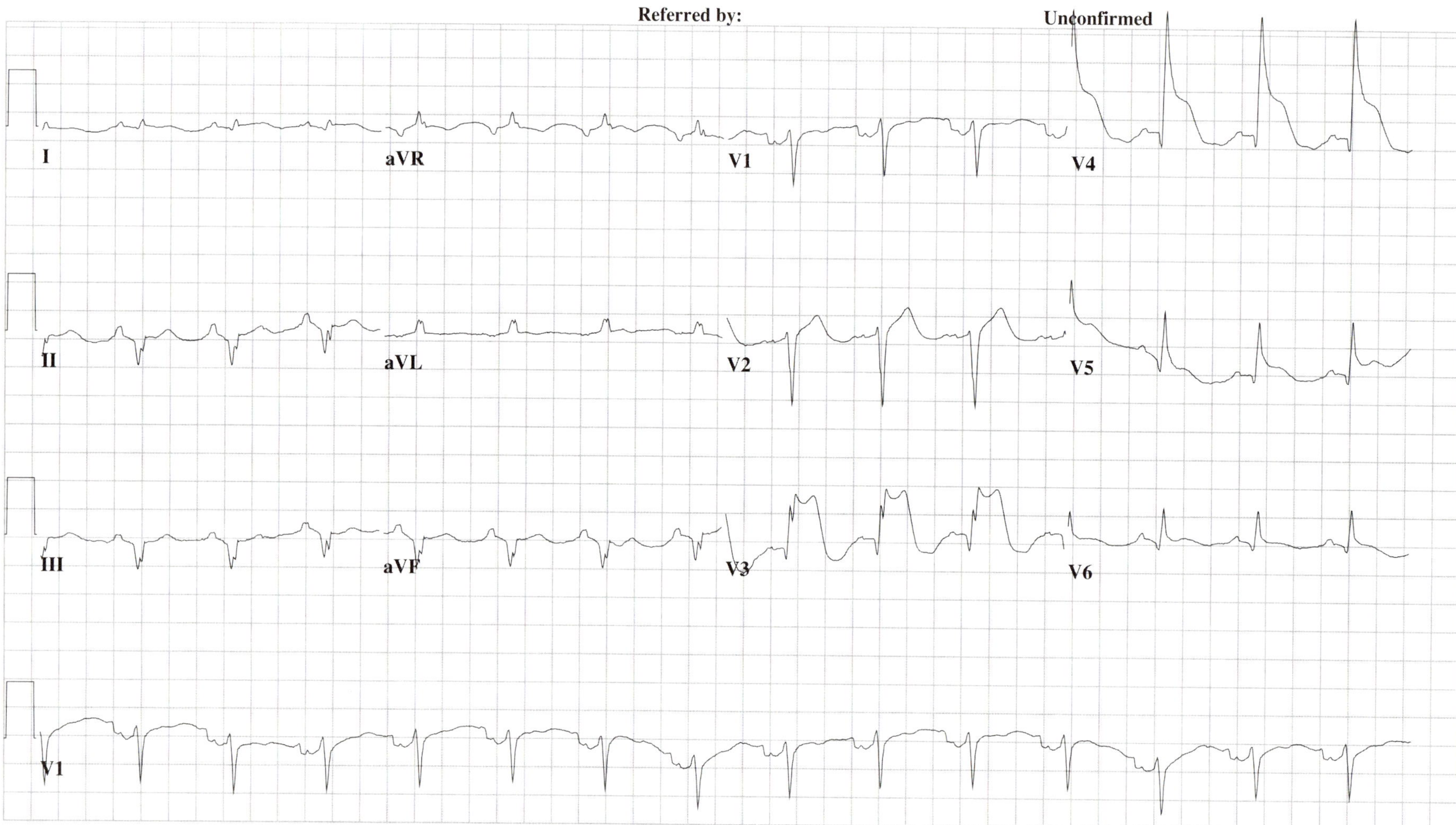

QUESTIONS

4-1. What abnormalities are present?

4-2. What is the cause of her abdominal symptoms?

4-3. Which coronary artery is most likely affected?

83
P2-4AC
15.0 cm MI 0.9
Gen TIs 1.1
[2d] G78/71 d
FA4/P90
HAR/FSI0
[C] G50/0.80 kHz
FA5/F1/8
TDI
S-T
S-T
Interval
2.5
3
Time (s)
3.5
Amplitude (V)

ANSWERS

4-1. What abnormalities are present?

Baseline artifact is present in lead V1. There is sinus rhythm at a rate of approximately 90 beats/min. The axis is leftward. Intervals are normal. There are broad, deep Q waves present in leads II, III, and aVF consistent with inferior myocardial infarction of undetermined age. In addition, there are Q waves and striking ST-segment elevation in the anterior leads V3, V4, and V5 consistent with acute myocardial injury and infarction in this territory.

4-2. What is the cause of her abdominal symptoms?

Patients with myocardial infarction can present with a range of symptoms, from typical substernal chest discomfort to other more atypical symptoms. Dyspnea, abdominal pain, neck or jaw discomfort, nausea and vomiting, and arm pain can all signify myocardial infarction. Older patients and patients with diabetes often present with atypical symptoms. This patient's abdominal discomfort was the presenting feature of her myocardial infarction.

4-3. Which coronary artery is most likely affected?

The ischemic changes including ST-segment elevation and Q-wave formation in leads V2 through V4 are present in the anterior leads and most likely represent occlusion of the left anterior descending coronary artery.

Case #5. A 68-year-old male with a history of diet-controlled diabetes and well-controlled hypertension presents for follow-up.

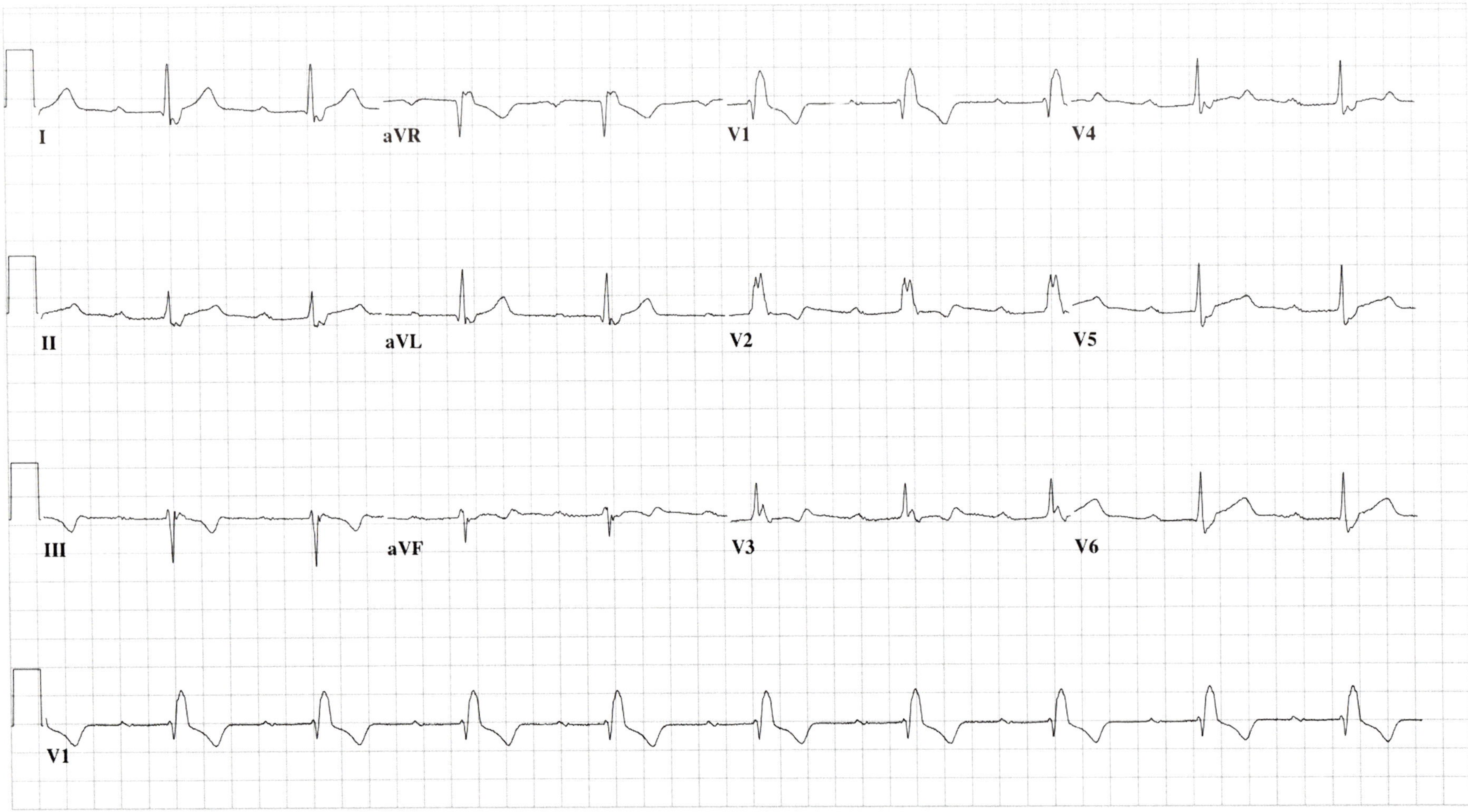

QUESTIONS

5-1. Interpret this ECG. What abnormalities are present on this tracing?

5-2. Explain why the QRS complex has this particular morphology.

83
P2-4AC
15.0 cm MI 0.9
Gen TIs 1.1
[2d] G78/71 d
FA4/P90
HAR/FS0
[C] G50/0.80 kHz
FA5/F1/B
TDI
S-T
interval
2.5
3
3.5
Time (s)
Amplitude (V)

ANSWERS

5-1. Interpret this ECG. What abnormalities are present on this tracing?

This tracing demonstrates sinus bradycardia with a heart rate of 56 beats/min. The axis is normal. The PR interval is prolonged to 360 milliseconds and the QRS duration is prolonged to approximately 150 milliseconds with a right bundle branch block (rSR′ pattern with a wide terminal R′ wave in lead V1; RS wave with a wide and slurred terminal S wave in leads I, aVL, V5, and V6). The QT interval is normal. There are T-wave inversions in leads V1 to V3 (the leads with terminal R′ waves) that are secondary to the right bundle branch block.

5-1. Explain why the QRS complex has this particular morphology.

Right bundle branch block causes delayed activation of the right ventricle because activation of the entire ventricular myocardium proceeds via the left bundle branch and thereafter through ventricular myocardium. The first portion of the QRS complex is unaffected because initial septal activation normally proceeds via part of the left bundle branch. On the surface ECG, this is manifest as a normal r wave in lead V1 and a normal q wave in leads V5 to V6 (normal septal activation is in the left to right direction). This septal activation is followed by the S wave in lead V1 and R waves in leads I, aVL, and V6 because the normal left ventricular activation vector points toward the left-sided leads. Finally, there is delayed depolarization of the right ventricle (a rightward structure), which corresponds to the wide terminal R′ wave in rightward leads such as V1, and the wide terminal S wave in leftward leads such as I, aVL, and V6.

Case #6. A 74-year-old gentleman with distant history of myocardial infarction presents for routine follow-up.

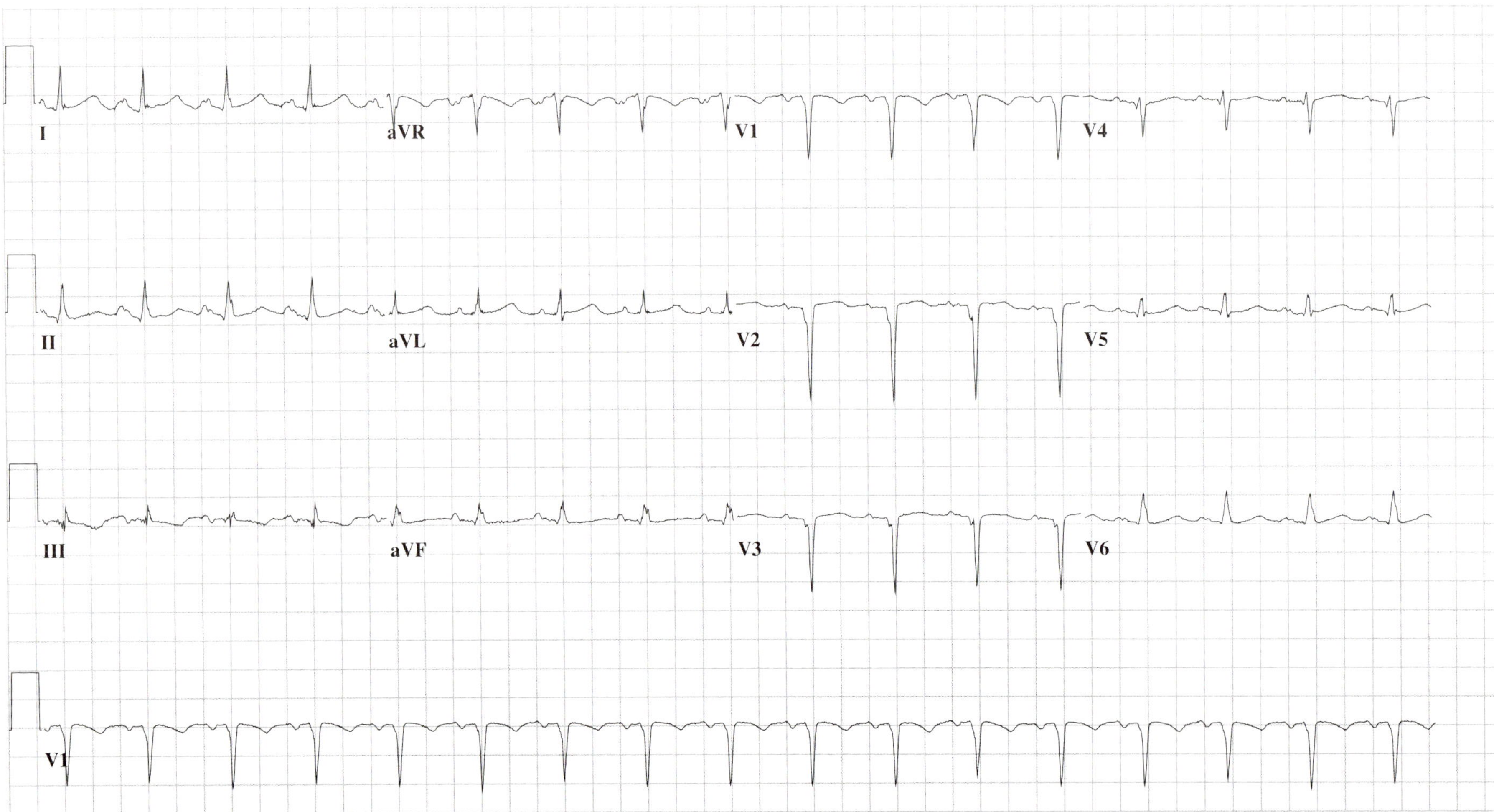

QUESTIONS

6-1. What abnormalities are present on this tracing?

6-2. Which coronary artery was the most likely culprit for the patient's prior myocardial infarction? What would an echocardiogram demonstrate?

83
P2-4AC
15.0 cm MI 0.9
Gen TIs 1.1
[2d] G78/71 d
FA4/P90
HAR/FS|0
[C] G50/0.80 kHz
FA5/F1/8
TDI
S-T
S-T
interval
2.5
3
3.5
Amplitude (V)

ANSWERS

6-1. What abnormalities are present on this tracing?

There is borderline sinus tachycardia at just approximately 100 beats/min. The QT interval is slightly prolonged. There is left atrial abnormality based on the presence of a broad, notched P wave with breadth greater than 120 milliseconds in lead II. Pathologic Q waves are present in leads V1, V2, V3, and V4 consistent with anteroseptal infarction of an indeterminate age. There is associated poor R-wave progression across the precordium, with S-wave amplitude greater than R-wave amplitude through V4, which is abnormal.

6-2. Which coronary artery was the most likely culprit for the patient's prior myocardial infarction? What would an echocardiogram demonstrate?

Q waves in the septal and anterior leads suggest prior infarction of the left anterior descending artery. An echocardiogram may demonstrate abnormal motion in the anterior wall of the left ventricle with either impaired or no contraction of the infarcted myocardium.

Case #7. A 63-year-old lifelong smoker presents with dyspnea and diffuse wheezes.

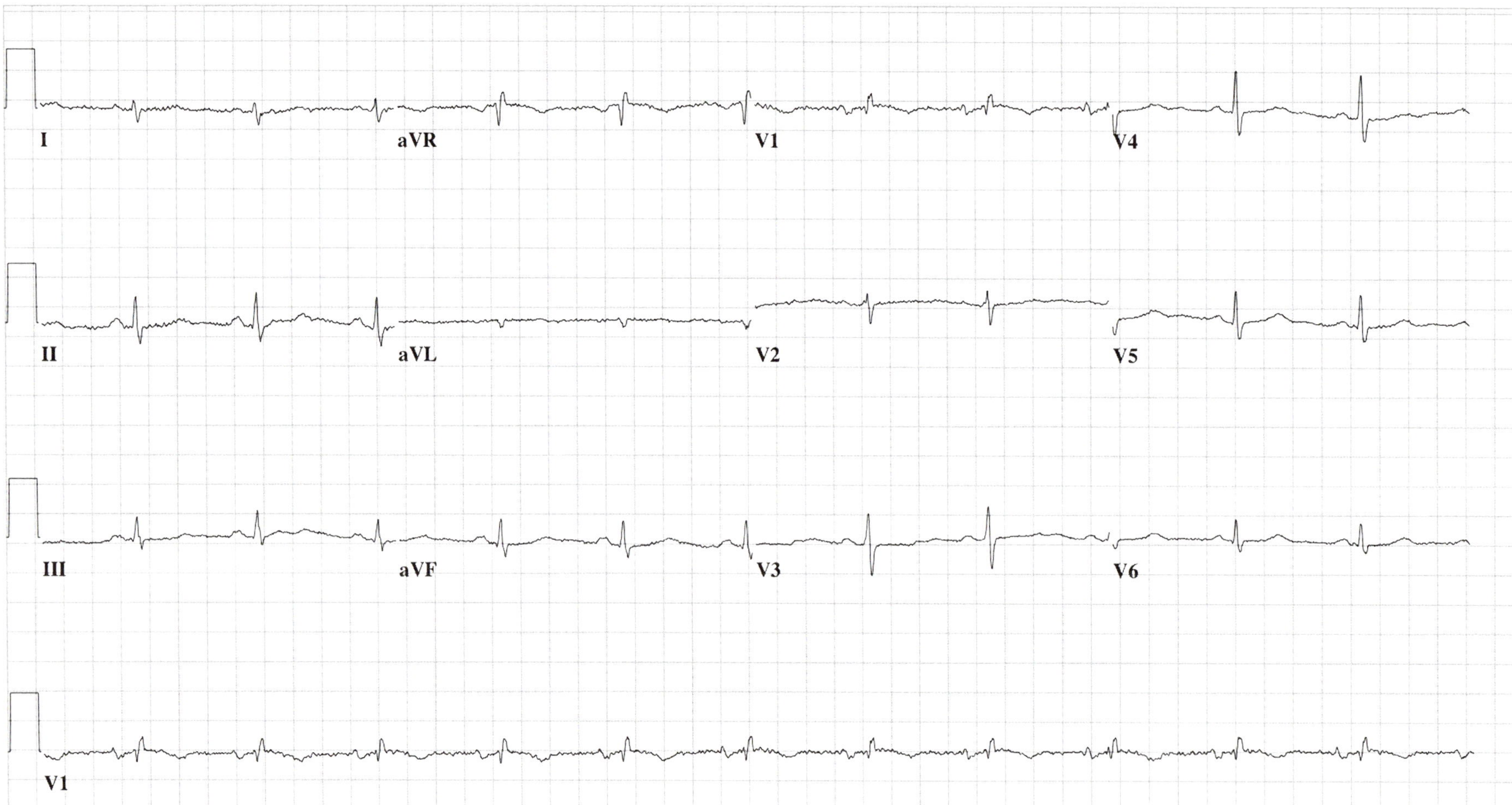

QUESTIONS

7-1. What does the ECG demonstrate?

7-2. What would you expect to find on physical examination?

83
P2-4AC
15.0 cm MI 0.9
Gen TIs 1.1
[2d] G78/71 d
FA4/P90
HAR/FSI0
[C] G50/0.80 kHz
FA5/F1/8
TDI
Amplitude (V)
S-T
interval
3
2.5

ANSWERS

7-1. What does the ECG demonstrate?

The rhythm is sinus at 75 beats/min. The axis is rightward with a tall R wave in V1 and RSR′ pattern with normal QRS duration (right ventricular conduction delay). In addition, the voltage is borderline-low, not quite meeting the criteria for low voltage (less than 5 mm in all limb leads, and 10 mm in all precordial leads). The findings of rightward axis, tall R wave in lead V1, right ventricular conduction delay, and borderline low voltage are typical of patients with chronic obstructive pulmonary disease (COPD). The rightward axis and RV conduction delay may be due to change in the intrathoracic position of the heart as well as right ventricular pressure overload from intrinsic lung disease. The low voltage typically results from the pulmonary hyperinflation, which interposes air-filled lung between the cardiac conduction system and the electrodes on the skin.

7-2. What would you expect to find on physical examination?

Patients with COPD typically have a quiet precordium due to hyperinflation and "barrel chest" anatomy, which impedes transmission of heart sounds to the stethoscope. Wheezes can also be present. Other findings may include Hoover's sign, an inward retraction of the subxiphoid angle on inspiration due to diaphragm flattening, or a tracheal tug, which is due to downward motion of the trachea from lung hyperinflation.

Case #8. A 44-year-old obese woman presents with fever and right upper quadrant abdominal pain that began after a meal at a fast-food restaurant.

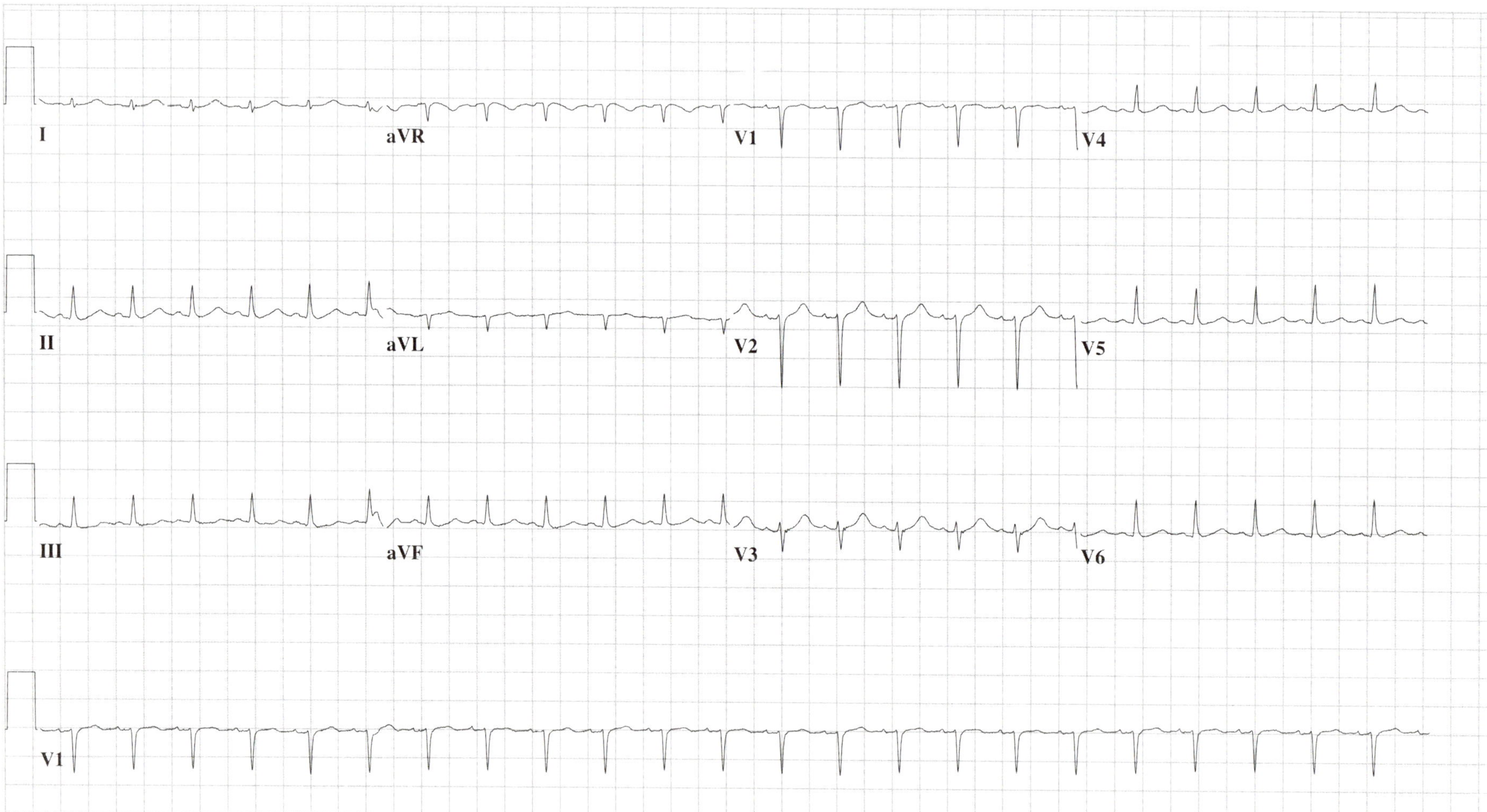

QUESTIONS

8-1. What abnormalities are present on this ECG?

8-2. How is this arrhythmia managed?

83
P2-4AC
15.0 cm MI 0.9
Gen TIs 1.1
[2d] G78/71 d
FA4/P90
HAR/FSI0
[C] G50/0.80 kHz
FA5/F1/8
TDI
S-T
interval
2.5
3
Time (s)
3.5
Amplitude (V)

ANSWERS

8-1. What abnormalities are present on this ECG?

There is a regular narrow complex tachycardia at approximately 140 beats/min. There is a P wave that precedes each QRS complex, and a QRS complex after each P wave. The RP interval (distance from an R wave to the following P wave) is more than one-half the RR interval (distance between R waves). Thus, we can classify this arrhythmia as a "long RP tachycardia." The long RP tachycardias include sinus tachycardia, atrial tachycardia, and atypical AVRT with an accessory pathway that has slow retrograde conduction. The P-wave morphology in this case suggests sinus rhythm—P waves are upright in leads I, II, V5, and V6. Thus, the diagnosis is sinus tachycardia, precipitated by fever and abdominal pain. In addition to the sinus tachycardia, the remainder of the tracing reveals borderline low voltage of the QRS complexes, not quite meeting criteria for diagnosis. This finding may be secondary to obesity. The rest of the ECG is essentially normal.

8-2. How is this arrhythmia managed?

The treatment of sinus tachycardia is to identify and correct the underlying cause. In this patient presenting with suspected acute cholecystitis, the underlying causes may include fever, pain, a systemic inflammatory response, and volume depletion.

Case #9. A 54-year-old gentleman presents with chest discomfort. He had rhinorrhea and cough 1 week ago.

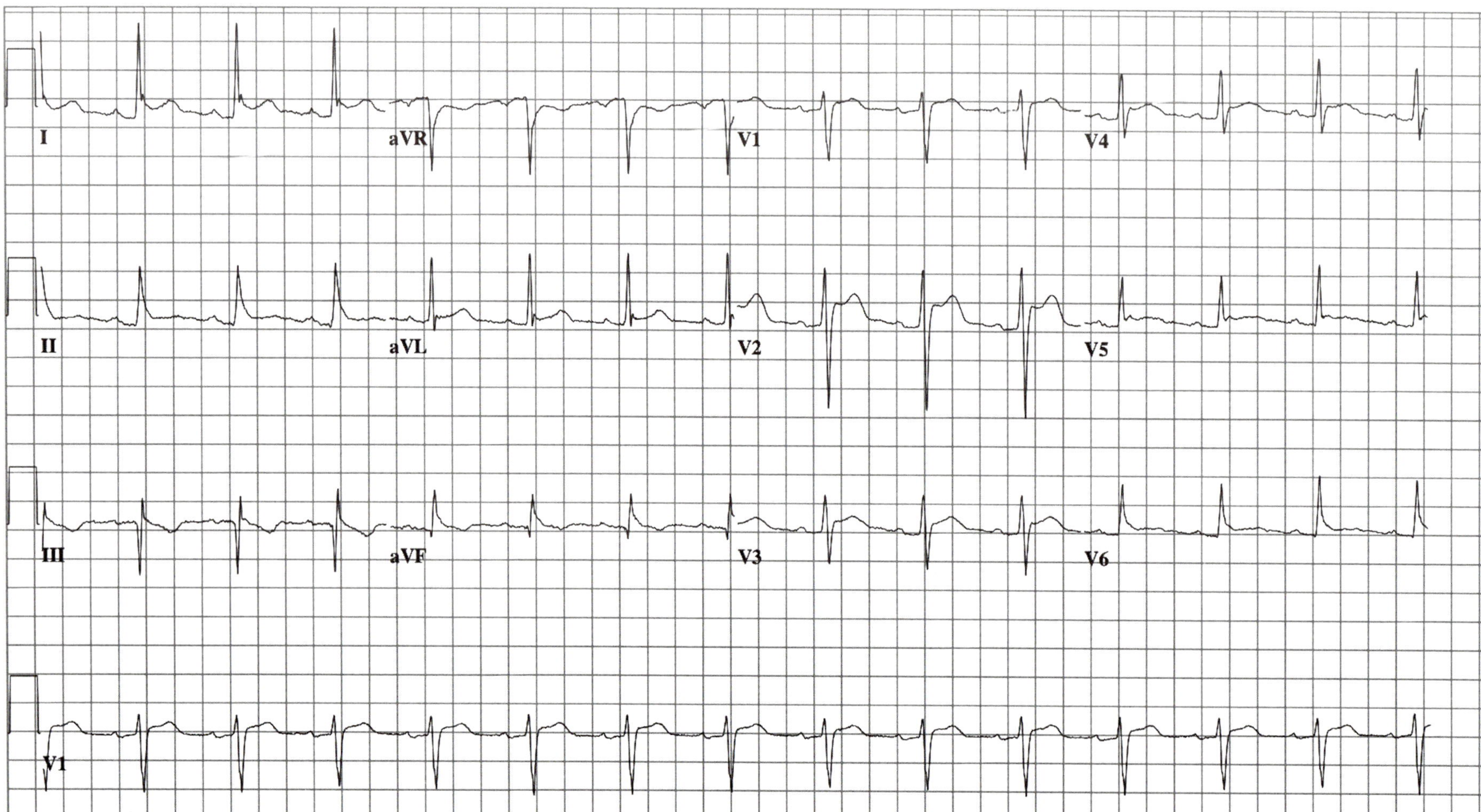

QUESTIONS

9-1. What are the abnormalities?

9-2. What do you expect to find on physical examination?

83
15.0 cm MI 0.9
P2-4AC
Gen TIs 1.1
[2d] G78/71 d
FA4/P90
HAR/FS|0
[C] G50/0.80 kHz
FA5/F1/B
TDI
S-T
interval
2.5
3
Time (s)
3.5
Amplitude (V)

ANSWERS

9-1. What are the abnormalities?

This tracing demonstrates sinus rhythm at 90 beats/min. There is a normal QRS axis. The intervals are normal. ST-segment elevation is noted in the inferior leads, lateral leads, septal leads, and anterior leads. The global nature of the ST-segment elevation, not in a single coronary distribution, suggests pericarditis as the cause. Other causes of ST-segment elevation besides pericarditis and ischemia include ventricular aneurysm, early repolarization, bundle branch blocks, left ventricular hypertrophy, and Brugada syndrome. In addition to the ST-segment elevation, PR-segment depression is visible in lead I. This suggests a current of atrial injury. Assess also the morphology of the ST-segment elevation: in this tracing, the ST segments are concave upward. One could imagine sitting on these ST segments without sliding off. In contrast, the ST elevation of ischemia is classically concave downward.

9-2. What do you expect to find on physical examination?

A pericardial friction rub should be sought; rubs can be transient, and serial examinations are useful. Often, leaning the patient forward and listening at the sternal border in end-expiration with the patient's breath held can bring out a soft rub. Rubs can have three components representing atrial systole, ventricular systole, and ventricular diastole. Findings of pericardial effusion such as an enlarged area of cardiac dullness and Ewart's sign of dullness in the left mid lung zone may be present. If there is associated effusion and tamponade, elevated neck veins and a pulsus paradoxus may be present.

Case #10. A 56-year-old woman with word-finding difficulty and hand weakness.

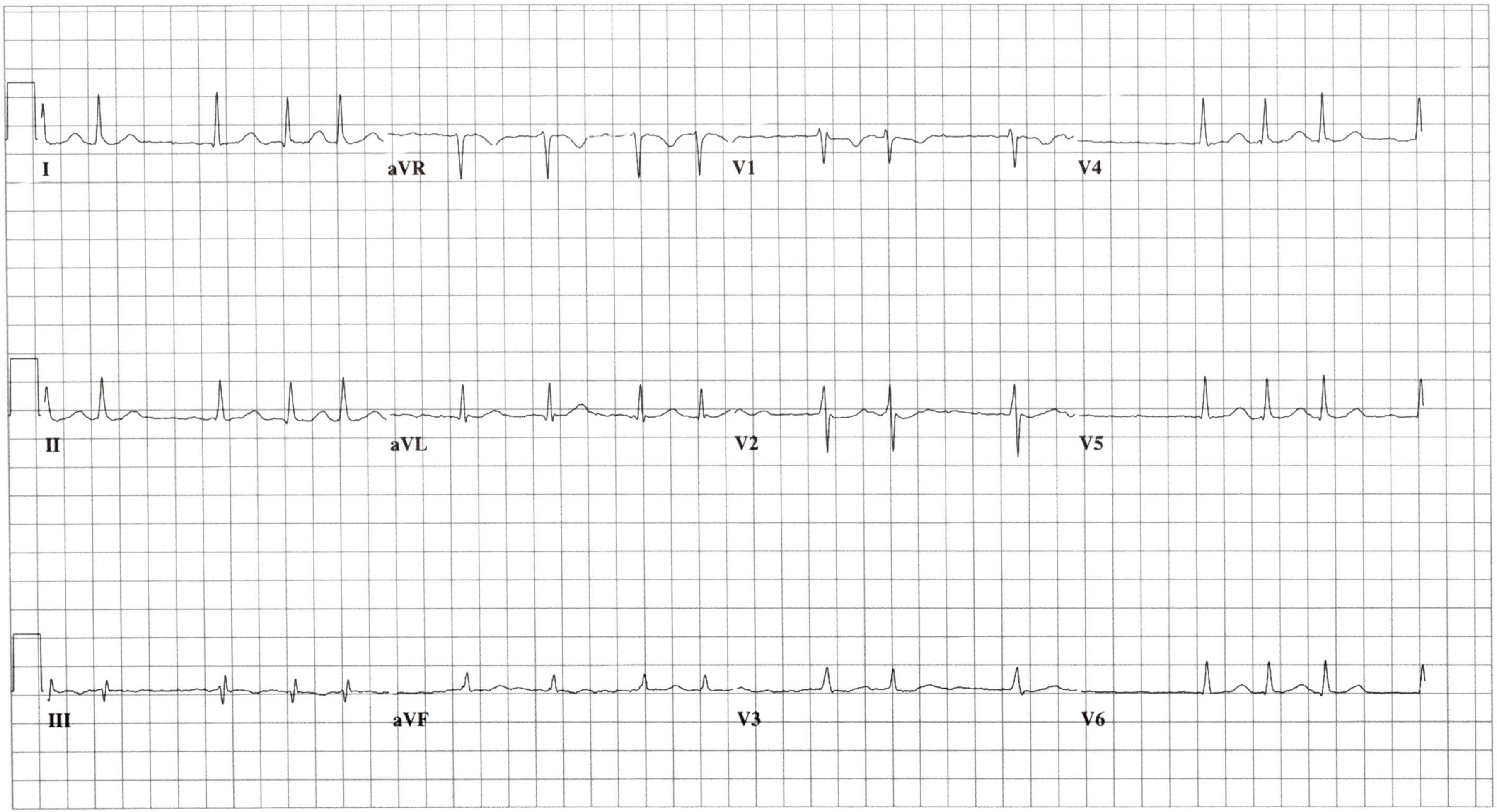

QUESTIONS

10-1. What is the rhythm?

10-2. What is the cause of her symptoms?

10-3. What would you do next?

83
P2-4AC
15.0 cm MI 0.9
Gen TIs 1.1
[2d] G78/71 d
FA4/P90
HAR/FS0
[C] G50/0.80 kHz
FA5/F1/8
TDI
3
2.5

ANSWERS

10-1. What is the rhythm?

The rhythm is irregularly irregular at a rate of approximately 90 beats/min. There is no clear atrial activity; thus, the diagnosis is atrial fibrillation. Other findings include a normal axis, normal intervals, no evidence of chamber enlargement or hypertrophy, and nonspecific ST-T wave abnormalities (inversions and flattening) in leads V1 and V2.

10-2. What is the cause of her symptoms?

The symptoms are consistent with cerebral ischemia and would be classified as transient ischemic attack or stroke, depending on the duration. Atrial fibrillation is a major stroke risk factor, as the fibrillating atria no longer contract regularly, leading to stasis of blood with subsequent thrombus formation, particularly in the left atrial appendage.

10-3. What would you do next?

Typical workup for stroke includes urgent noncontrast head CT to exclude a hemorrhagic etiology. In this case, we suspect thrombotic disease due to atrial fibrillation. If the stroke onset is recent and symptoms are not improving, thrombolytic therapy could be considered in consultation with a neurologist. In the long term, the patient will need oral anticoagulation.

Case #11. A 42-year-old gentleman presents with palpitations.

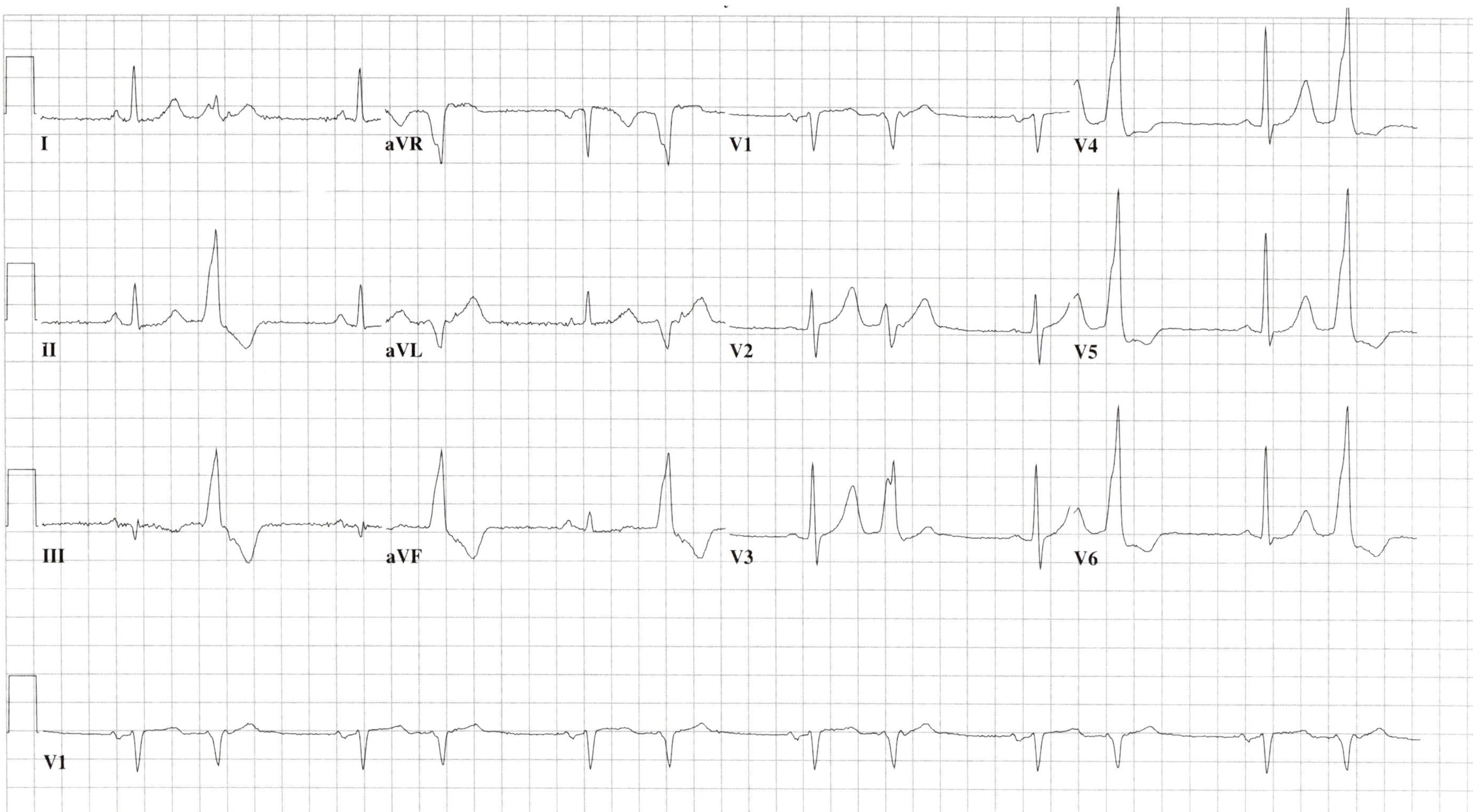

QUESTIONS

11-1. What does the ECG show?

11-2. How should his palpitations be managed?

83
P2-4AC
15.0 cm MI 0.9
Gen TIs 1.1
[2d] G78/71 d
FA4/P90
HAR/FSI0
[C] G50/0.80 kHz
FA5/F1/B
TDI
S-T
Interval
2.5
3
Time (s)
3.5

ANSWERS

11-1. What does the ECG show?

Sinus rhythm is present alternating with premature ventricular contractions (PVCs). When every other beat is a PVC, a pattern of "ventricular bigeminy" is present (if every third beat were a PVC, "ventricular trigeminy" could be diagnosed). The sinus beats are otherwise normal with no evidence of chamber enlargement and no ischemia. The PVCs have a morphology similar to that of a left bundle branch block in the precordial leads, suggesting origin in the right ventricle. Examining the inferior leads II, III, and aVF, the PVCs have positive polarity, suggesting depolarization is moving from superior to inferior. These findings suggest that the origin of the PVC localizes to the right ventricular outflow tract, which is a common site of origin for such ectopy.

11-2. How should his palpitations be managed?

If asymptomatic, no treatment may be necessary, although some patients having extremely high numbers of PVCs can develop a PVC-induced cardiomyopathy. If symptomatic, β-blockers can sometimes be effective in suppressing PVCs. Rarely, other antiarrhythmic agents can be used. For ectopy originating in the right ventricular outflow tract, calcium channel blockers may be effective for suppression. Finally, ablation therapy for symptomatic PVCs originating in the right ventricular outflow tract can be curative.[1]

---

[1]Ng GA. Treating patients with ventricular ectopic beats. *Heart* 2006; 92: 1707-1712.

Case #12. A 47-year-old man with chest pain and shock.

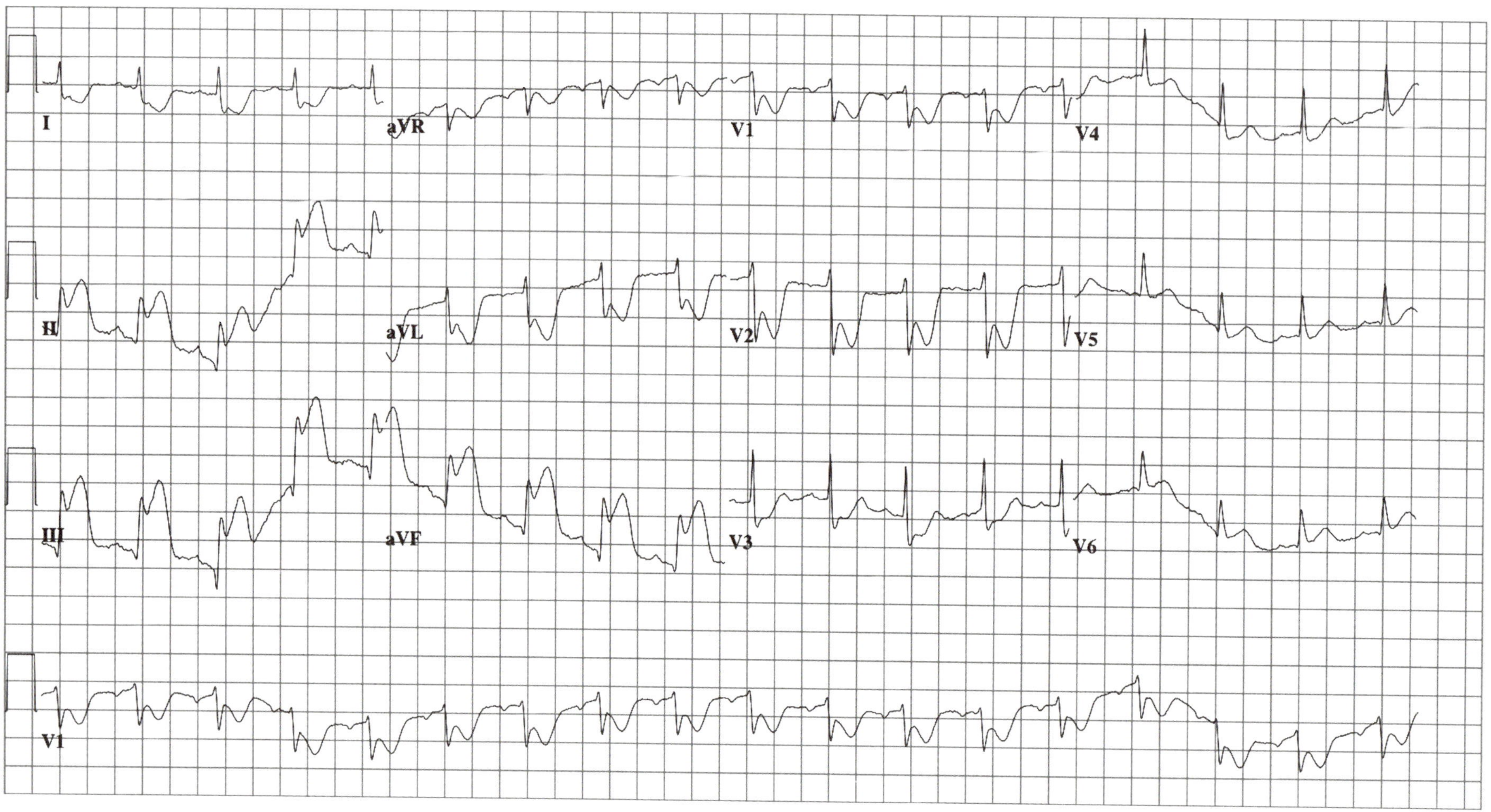

QUESTIONS

12-1. What is the diagnosis?

12-2. What is the distribution of ischemia?

83
P2-4AC
15.0 cm MI 0.9
Gen TIs 1.1
[2d] G78/71 d
FA4/P90
HAR/FSI0
[C] G50/0.80 kHz
FA5/F1/B
TDI
S-T
interval
3
2.5
Time (s)
3.5

ANSWERS

12-1. What is the diagnosis?

Prominent baseline artifact is present, which is common in critically ill patients. Despite this, interpretation is possible. Sinus tachycardia is present at a rate of 100 beats/min. The axis and intervals are normal, and there is no evidence of chamber enlargement or hypertrophy. There are ST-segment elevations in the inferior leads II, III, and aVF. There are only tiny, nonpathologic Q waves present in those leads with upright T waves. Significant ST-segment depression is present in leads I and aVL as well as leads V1 through V3.

12-2. What is the distribution of ischemia?

The ST-segment elevations in leads II, III, and aVF correspond to ischemia of the inferior wall of the left ventricle. Inferior wall ischemia is typically due to occlusion of either the right coronary artery or the left circumflex coronary artery. Recall that lead III is oriented more rightward at +120 degrees and lead II is oriented more leftward at +60 degrees. Hence, when an inferior infarction is present, a larger amount of ST-segment elevation in lead III compared to lead II, as is seen in this tracing, suggests occlusion of the right coronary artery as opposed to the left circumflex.[1] This anatomy also explains the significant ST-segment depression in leads I and aVL as "reciprocal depression" reflecting the ST-segment elevation inferiorly.

The right coronary artery also supplies the posterior wall of the heart in 70% of the population. The prominent ST depressions present in leads V1 to V3 represent posterior wall ischemia, or a "posterior STEMI." Thus, the distribution of ischemia in this tracing is best characterized as inferoposterior. Posterior ECG leads could be placed to confirm the posterior wall involvement.

---

[1]Zimetbaum PJ, Josephson ME. Use of the electrocardiogram in acute myocardial infarction. *New Engl J Med* 2003; 348: 933-940.

Case #13. An 80-year-old male presents with syncope. On examination, a late-peaking, crescendo-decrescendo systolic murmur is heard.

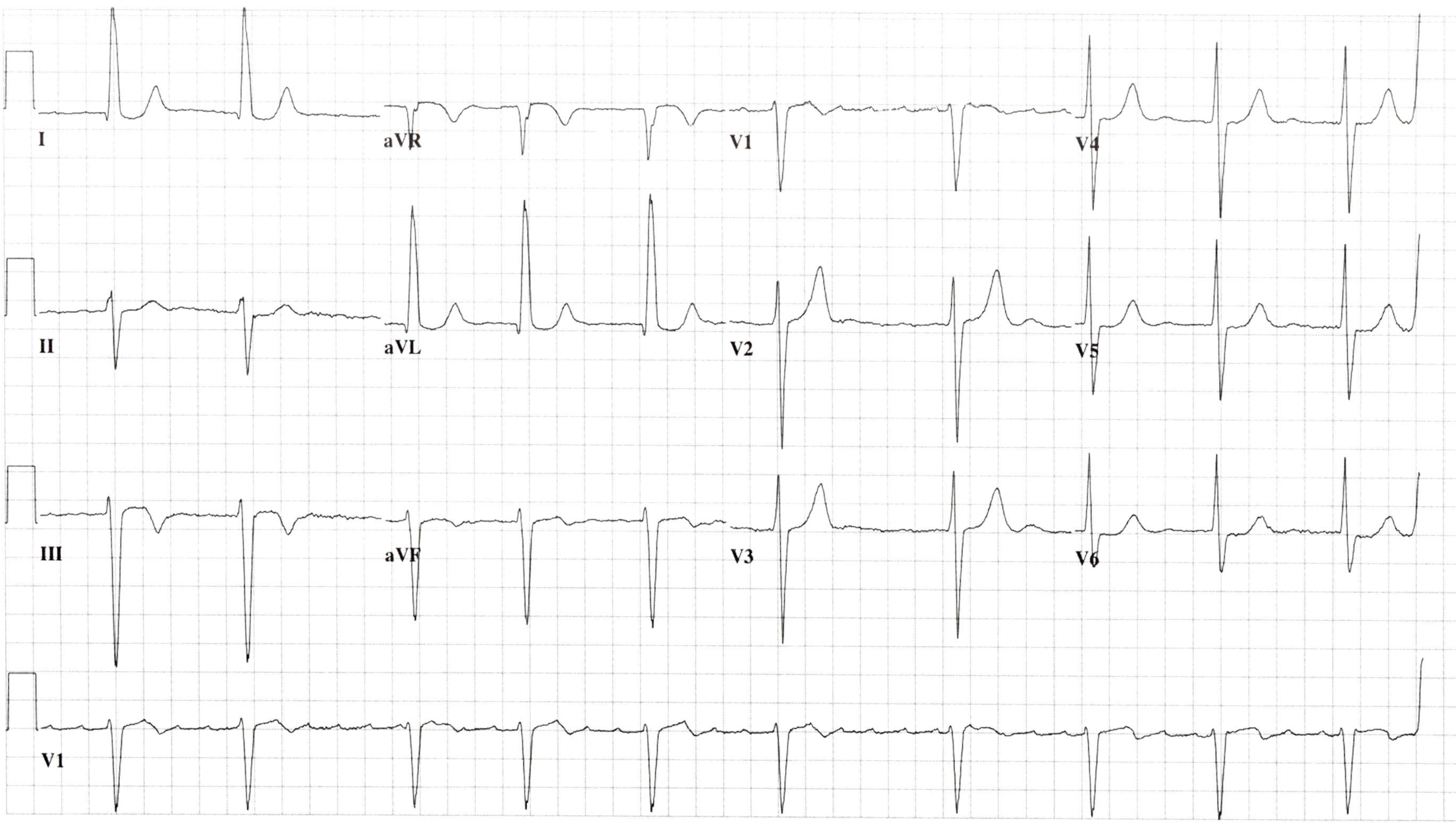

QUESTIONS

13-1. What abnormalities are present on this tracing?

13-2. What additional physical examination findings might you expect?

83
P2-4AC
15.0 cm MI 0.9
Gen TIs 1.1
[2d] G78/71 d
FA4/P90
HAR/FS|0
[C] G50/0.80 kHz
FA5/F1/8
TDI
S-T
S-T
interval
2.5
3
Time (s)
Amplitude (V)

ANSWERS

13-1. What abnormalities are present on this tracing?

The rate is approximately 60 beats/min. The rhythm is irregularly irregular with no clear atrial activity consistent with atrial fibrillation. There is left-axis deviation. The QRS interval is widened to greater than 128 milliseconds but does not meet morphologic criteria for a left bundle branch or right bundle branch block. This is best characterized as a nonspecific intraventricular conduction delay. Left ventricular hypertrophy is present, evidenced by magnitude of the R wave in lead aVL plus the magnitude of the S wave in lead V3 greater than 24 mV. Furthermore, in the presence of left-axis deviation, left ventricular hypertrophy is suggested by an R-wave magnitude greater than 13 mV in lead aVL and S-wave magnitude greater than 15 mV in lead III, both of which are present in this tracing. Finally, there is a positive wave after the T wave in V2 and V3 consistent with a U wave. Classically seen in hypokalemia, U waves are also associated with LVH and some forms of ischemic heart disease.

13-2. What additional physical examination findings might you expect?

This patient likely has aortic stenosis given the combination of a late-peaking systolic murmur and findings of left ventricular hypertrophy on the electrocardiogram. Other classic physical findings in patient with aortic stenosis include "pulsus parvus et tardus," or a delayed, weakened carotid pulse. A sustained apical impulse may be present, and one may palpate a thrill in the suprasternal area.

Case #14. A 64-year-old woman abruptly loses consciousness and is found to be pulseless. After successful defibrillation, the following ECG is recorded.

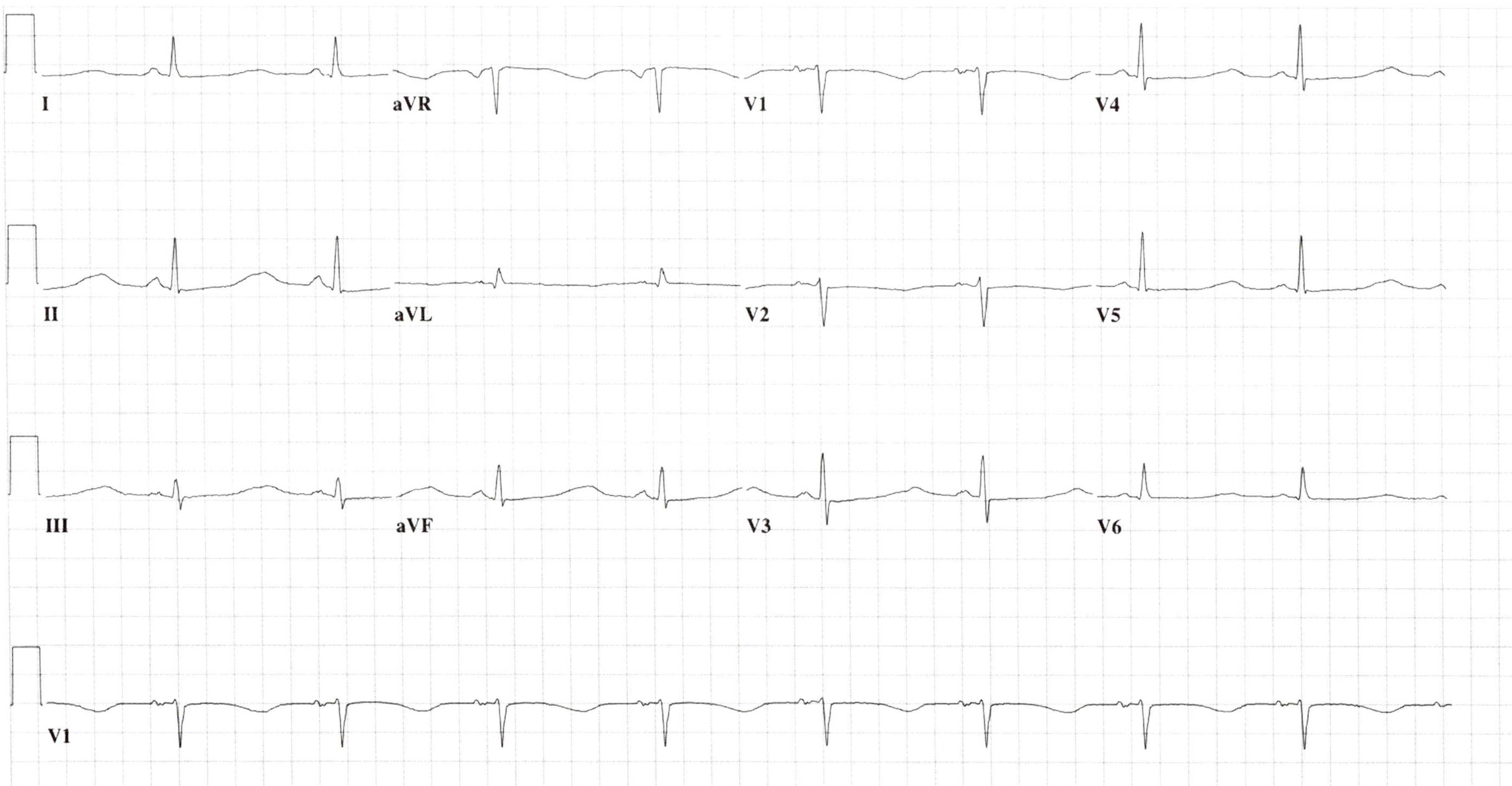

QUESTIONS

16-1. Interpret this ECG: what is the rhythm?

16-2. What is one possible reason she suffered a stroke?

83
P2-4AC
15.0 cm MI 0.9
Gen TIs 1.1
[2d] G78/71 d
FA4/P90
HAR/FS|0
[C] G50/0.80 kHz
FA5/F1/8
TDI
S-T
interval
QRS
interval
2.5
3

ANSWERS

16-1. Interpret this ECG: what is the rhythm?

The ventricular rate is 60 with a regular, paced rhythm. There is no discernible organized atrial activity underlying the paced rhythm, which is most consistent with atrial fibrillation. The axis is leftward, and the QRS has a left bundle configuration consistent with pacing from the right ventricular apex.

16-2. What is one possible reason she suffered a stroke?

Atrial fibrillation can cause stroke! This tracing and case illustrate that simply interpreting an ECG as "paced" is not a sufficient interpretation. Despite the pacing in the ventricles, the atria are still fibrillating. Thus, proper recognition of this atrial arrhythmia should mandate consideration of anticoagulation for stroke prevention.

Case #17. A healthy 26-year-old medical student has an ECG performed as part of his physical diagnosis class. He is asymptomatic.

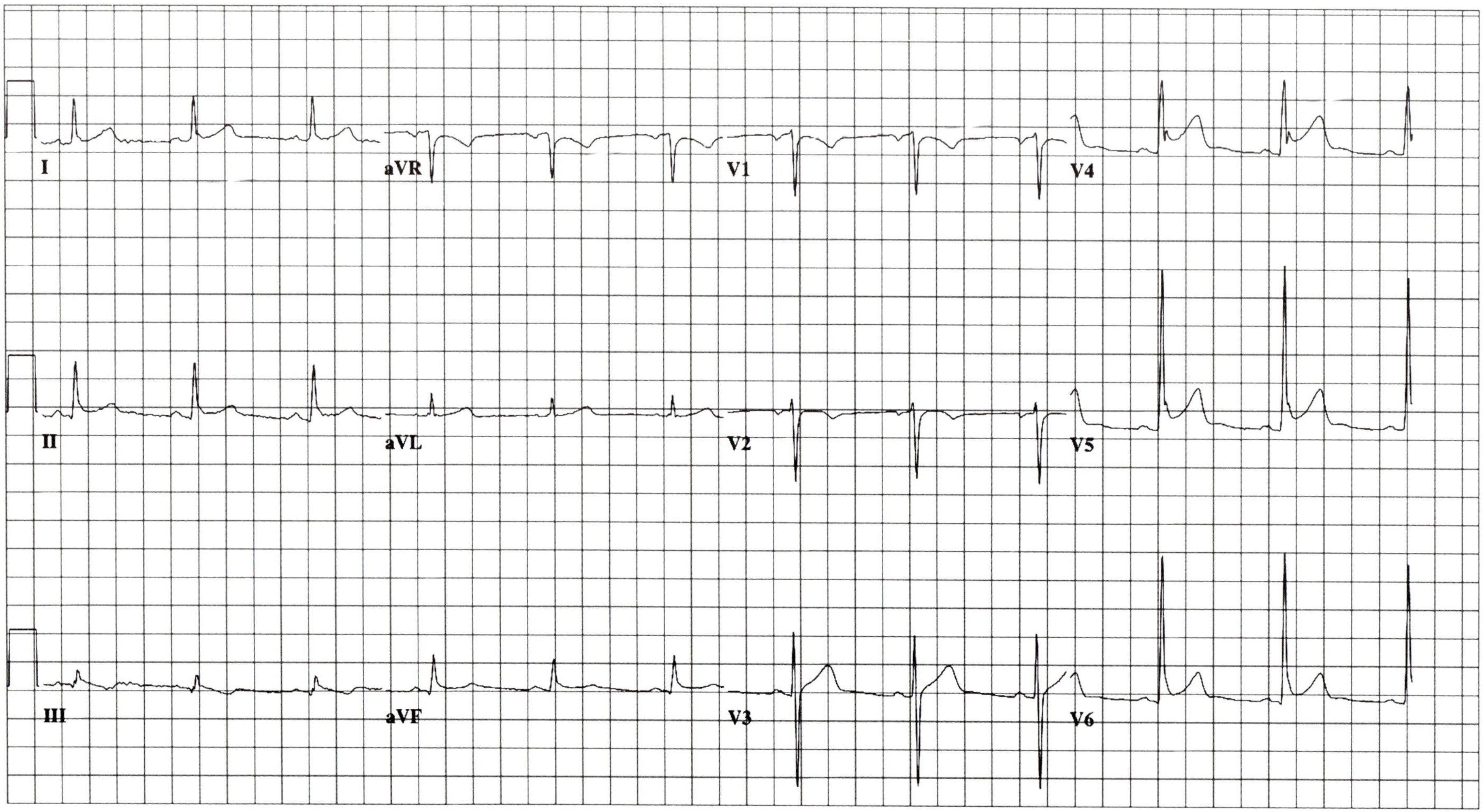

QUESTIONS

17-1. Interpret this ECG: what is your diagnosis?

17-2. Is further workup required?

83
P2-4AC
15.0 cm MI 0.9
Gen Tls 1.1
[2d] G78/71 d
FA4/P90
HAR/FSI0
[C] G50/0.80 kHz
FA5/F1/8
TDI
S-T
S-T
interval
2.5
3
Time (s)
3.5
Amplitude (V)

ANSWERS

17-1. Interpret this ECG: what is your diagnosis?

There is sinus rhythm at 60 beats/min, normal axis and intervals, and no evidence of chamber enlargement. There is ST-segment elevation most prominent in the precordial leads V4 through V6 with a "notched" J point (figure). The differential diagnosis of ST-segment elevation includes ischemia, ventricular aneurysm, pericarditis, electrolyte abnormalities, and repolarization abnormalities. The morphology of the ST segment here is consistent with an "early-repolarization" pattern that is common and overall normal in young, otherwise healthy people. There are some reports suggesting a small increase in sudden cardiac death risk, particularly if the J point is above the baseline by more than 1 mm in the inferior leads, but this association merits further study.[1]

ST-segment elevation with a notched J point (arrow) consistent with an early repolarization pattern.

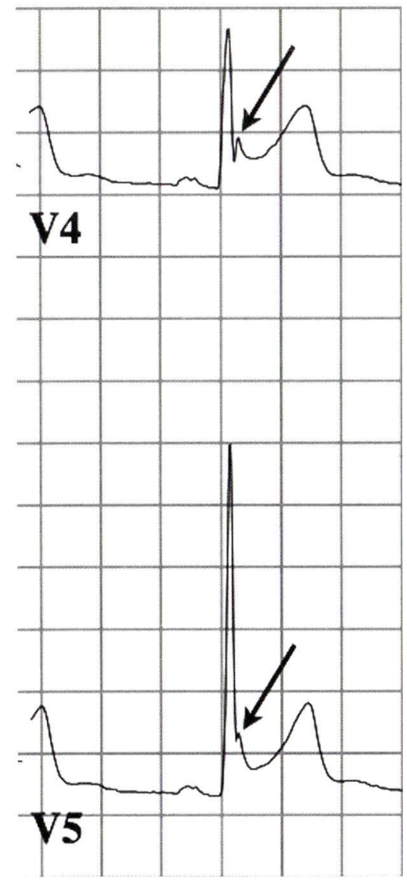

17-2. Is further workup required?

No further workup is required; this is an overall normal ECG.

[1]Haissaguerre M, Derval N, Sacher F, et al. Sudden cardiac arrest associated with early repolarization. *N Engl J Med* 2008; 358: 2016-2023.

Case #18. A 51-year-old gentleman presents to his primary care physician for a yearly physical exam. He is asymptomatic.

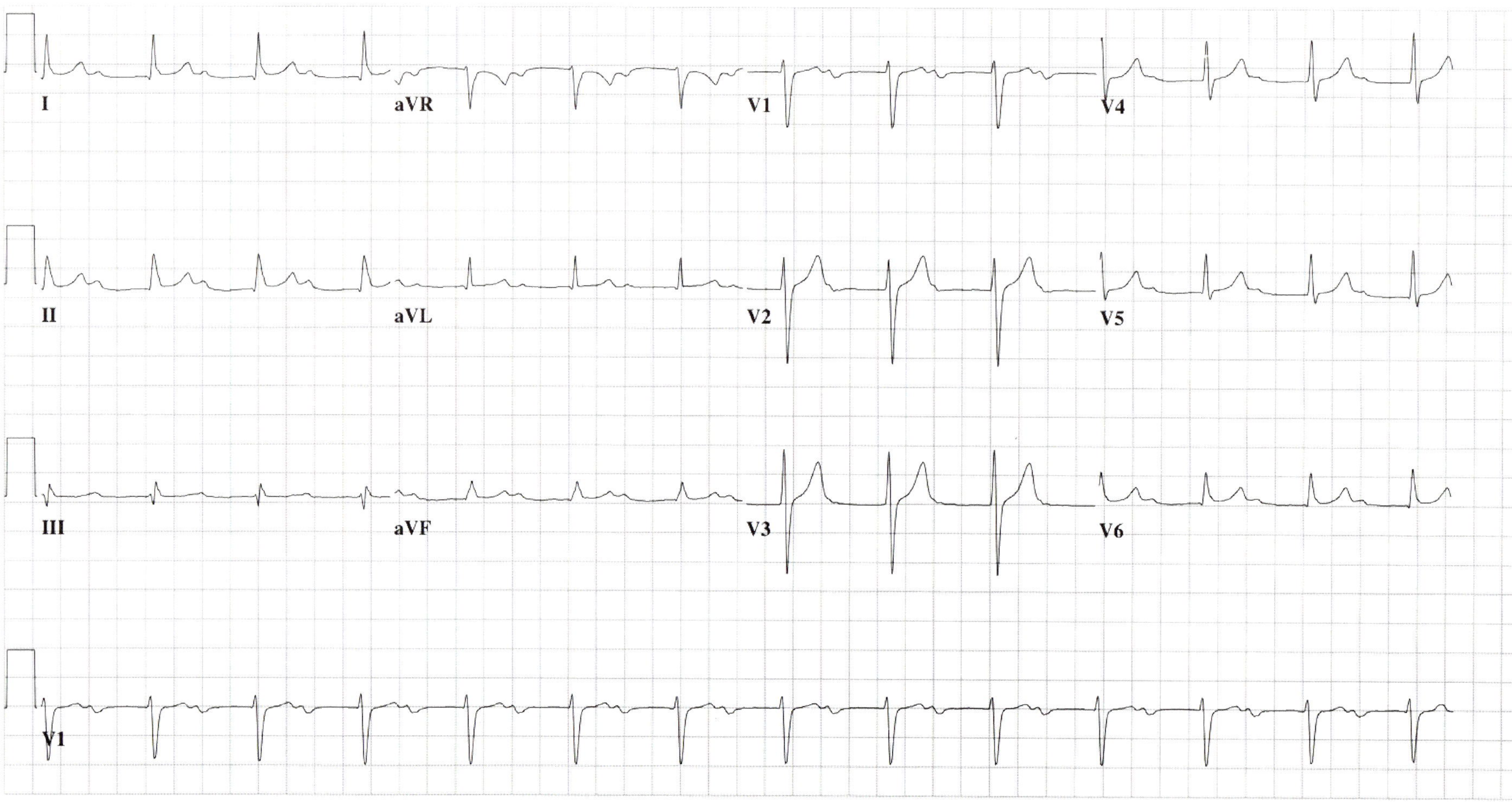

QUESTIONS

18-1. Interpret this ECG. What abnormalities are present on this tracing?

18-2. Where in the cardiac conduction system is there delayed conduction?

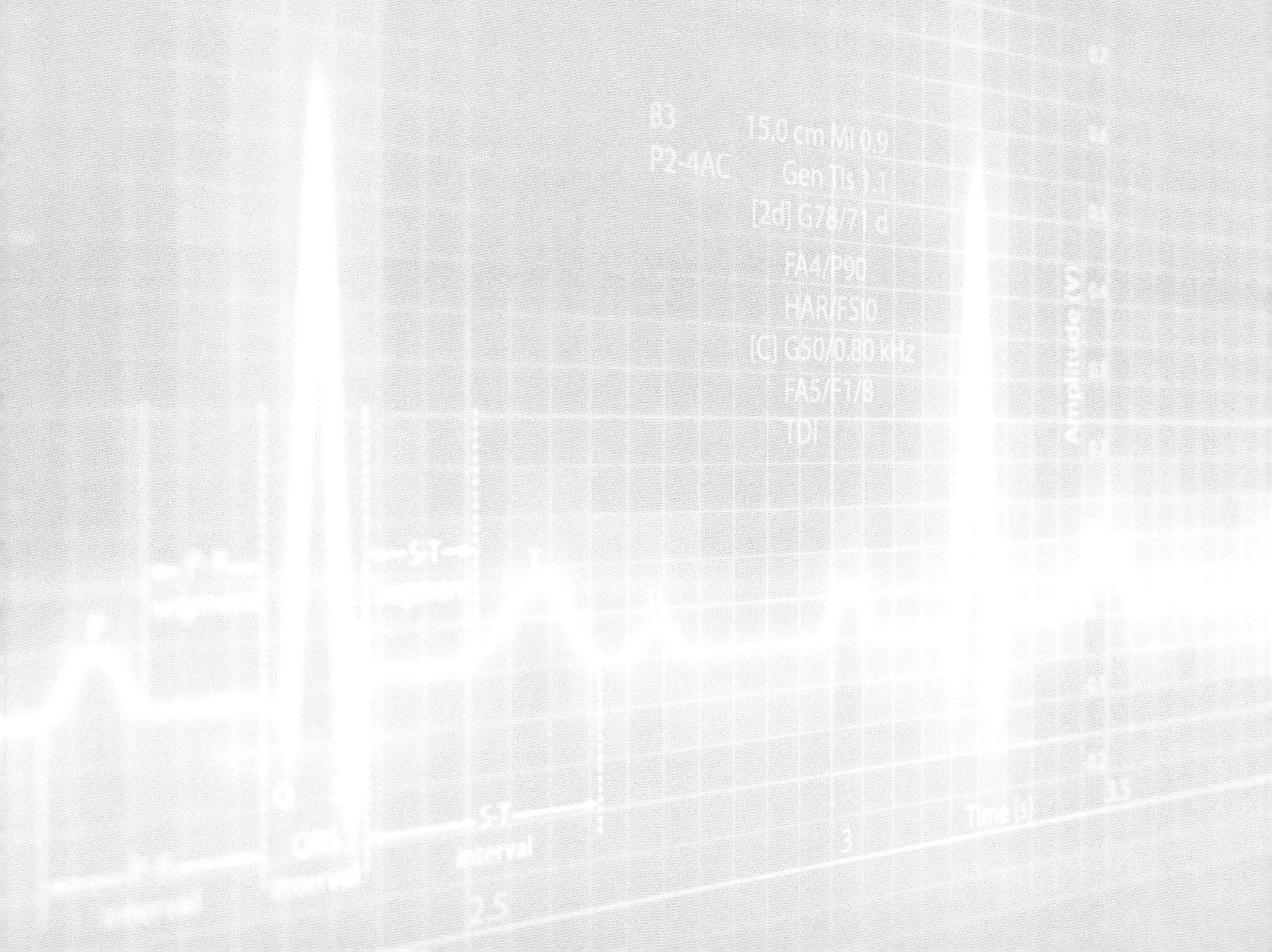
83
P2-4AC
15.0 cm MI 0.9
Gen TIs 1.1
[2d] G78/71 d
FA4/P90
HAR/FSI0
[C] G50/0.80 kHz
FA5/F1/8
TDI
Amplitude (V)
Time (s)
S-T
interval
2.5
3
3.5

ANSWERS

18-1. Interpret this ECG. What abnormalities are present on this tracing?

This tracing demonstrates normal sinus rhythm at a rate of 80 beats/min with a normal QRS axis. The PR interval is very prolonged to 400 milliseconds, and the P wave is partially fused with the preceding T wave, consistent with the diagnosis of AV conduction delay or "first-degree AV block." The QRS duration is normal at approximately 80 milliseconds, and the QT interval is normal. The P wave is biphasic in lead V1 with a prominent negative deflection that is >40 milliseconds long (1 small box) and approximately 1 mm deep (1 small box), diagnostic of left atrial abnormality.

18-2. Where in the cardiac conduction system is there delayed conduction?

The patient has marked AV conduction delay/first-degree AV block given the PR interval is greater than 200 milliseconds. The PR interval represents the summed delay between electrical depolarization of the atria and conduction through the AV node, bundle of His, bundle branches, and the Purkinje fibers just prior to ventricular depolarization at the start of the QRS complex. Physiologic delay at the AV node normally makes up the majority of the normal PR interval, but AV conduction delay/first-degree AV block can represent delayed conduction at any of the parts of the conduction system noted above.

Note that, although the term first-degree AV block is widely accepted, a more physiologically appropriate term for a PR interval greater than 200 milliseconds is "AV conduction delay" or simply "PR interval prolongation." A prolonged PR interval represents delayed conduction without true conduction "block."

Case #19. A 65-year-old man with hypertension and chronic kidney disease presents with presyncope.

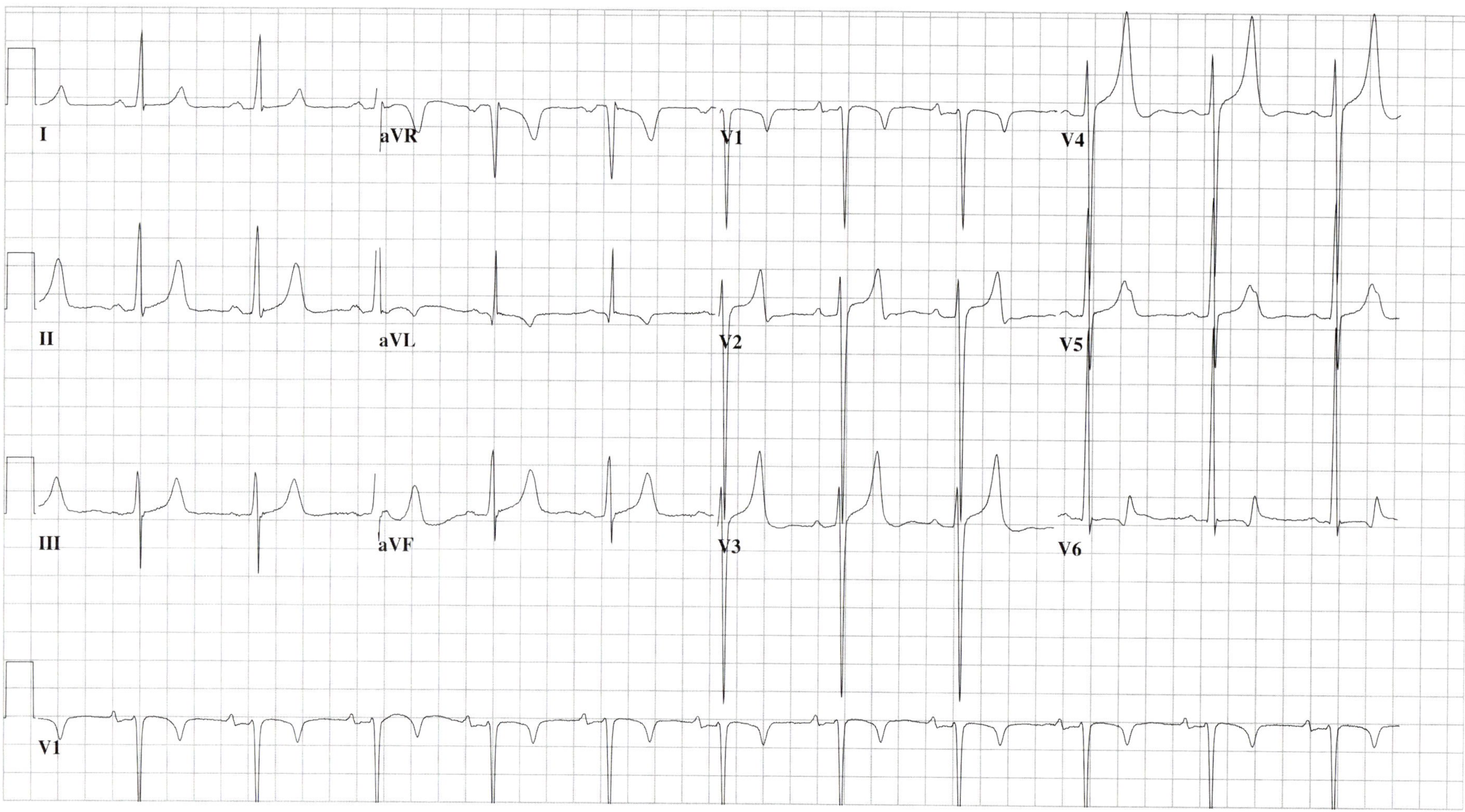

QUESTION

19-1. Interpret this tracing.

83
15.0 cm MI 0.9
P2-4AC
Gen Tls 1.1
[2d] G78/71 d
FA4/P90
HAR/FS|0
[C] G50/0.80 kHz
FA5/F1/8
TDI
Amplitude (V)
S-T
S-T
Interval
3
2.5
Time (s)
3.5

ANSWER

19-1. Interpret this tracing.

This ECG reveals sinus rhythm at a rate of approximately 70 beats/min. The QRS axis is normal. There is left ventricular hypertrophy present by voltage criteria with associated ST-segment and T-wave abnormalities in leads V6 and aVL, the so-called "strain pattern." Finally, the T waves are tall, pointed, and narrow based, particularly in leads V2 through V6. The T-wave abnormalities coupled with the clinical history suggest hyperkalemia.

Case #20. A 34-year-old woman presents with syncope. She has no medical history except for 3 miscarriages in the past.

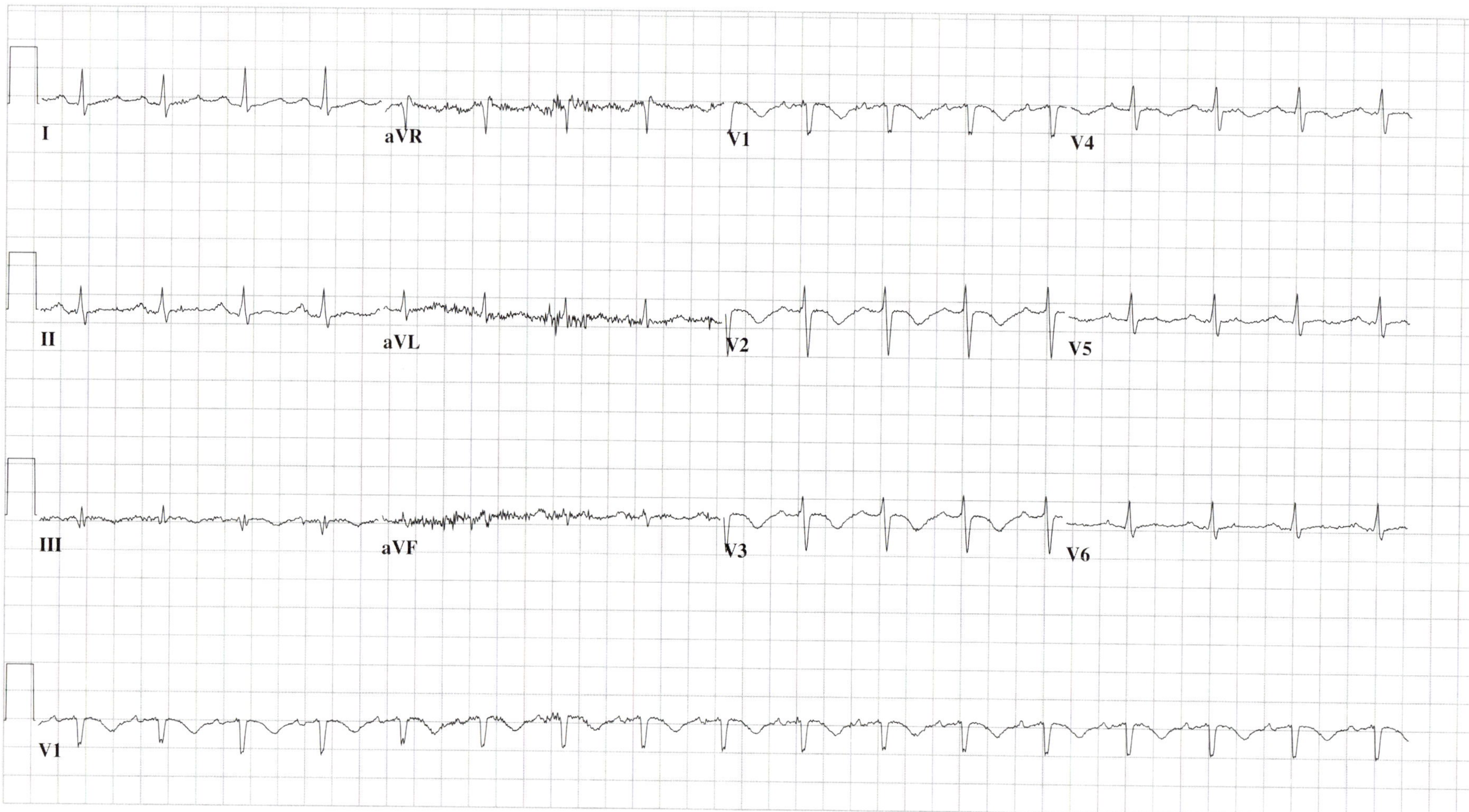

QUESTIONS

20-1. What abnormalities are present on this tracing?

20-2. What is the most likely diagnosis?

20-3. What ECG findings can be associated with this diagnosis? Which is the most common finding?

83
15.0 cm MI 0.9
P2-4AC
Gen Tls 1.1
[2d] G78/71 d
FA4/P90
HAR/FSI0
[C] G50/0.80 kHz
FA5/F1/8
TDI
Amplitude (V)
Time (s)
3
2.5

ANSWERS

20-1. What abnormalities are present on this tracing?

This tracing demonstrates sinus tachycardia at approximately 100 beats/min. There is a normal QRS axis of approximately 0 degrees. The QT interval is prolonged. There are T-wave inversions in leads V1, V2, V3, and V4. There is a small Q wave as well as T-wave inversion in lead III as well as an S wave in I. Baseline artifact is present.

20-2. What is the most likely diagnosis?

A pattern of "SI-QIII-TIII" can be caused by any disease process leading to acute right heart strain, including pneumothorax, pneumonia, or an exacerbation of reactive airways disease. The classic association, however, is that of pulmonary embolism, which is the most likely diagnosis in this young woman. Anteroseptal T-wave inversions are also consistent with this diagnosis. Her history of multiple miscarriages alludes to a thrombophilic state, namely, the antiphospholipid antibody syndrome. Large pulmonary embolism was subsequently demonstrated on computed tomographic pulmonary angiography.

20-3. What ECG findings can be associated with this diagnosis? Which is the most common abnormal finding?

The ECG is insensitive for the diagnosis of pulmonary embolism. While an SI-QIII-TIII pattern is the "classic" association, it is seen in a minority of cases. The most common abnormality seen is sinus tachycardia. Other ECG findings in pulmonary embolism may include a rightward axis, partial or complete right bundle branch block, right atrial abnormality, atrial ectopic beats and atrial arrhythmias, and anteroseptal ST-segment and T-wave changes.

Case #21. A 42-year-old gentleman status post radiofrequency ablation for paroxysmal atrial fibrillation.

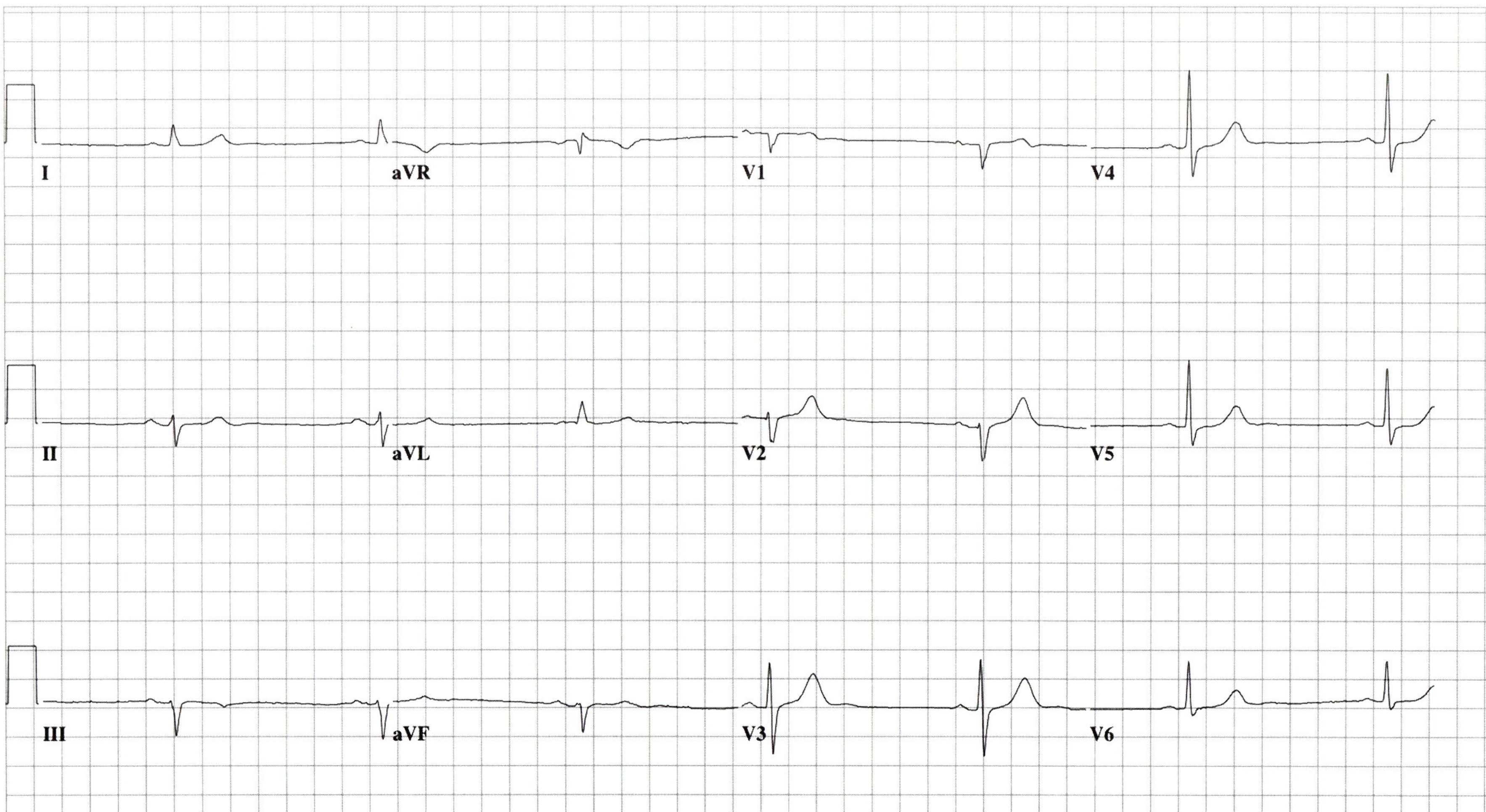

QUESTION

21-1. What abnormalities are present?

83
P2-4AC
15.0 cm MI 0.9
Gen TIs 1.1
[2d] G78/71 d
FA4/P90
HAR/FS10
[C] G50/0.80 kHz
FA5/F1/B
TDI
S-T
Interval
Time (s)
3
2.5

ANSWER

21-1. What abnormalities are present?

Sinus bradycardia is present at a rate of 42 beats/min. The PR interval is normal. Axis is leftward. Intervals are normal, and there is no evidence of ST-segment or T-wave abnormalities. Overall, the major finding is significant sinus bradycardia. Sinus bradycardia may be physiologic, as in a well-conditioned young athlete, or pathologic, as in a patient with sick sinus syndrome or after aggressive treatment with medications such as β-blockers.

Case #22. A 72-year-old woman with hypertension and mitral regurgitation is seen in follow-up.

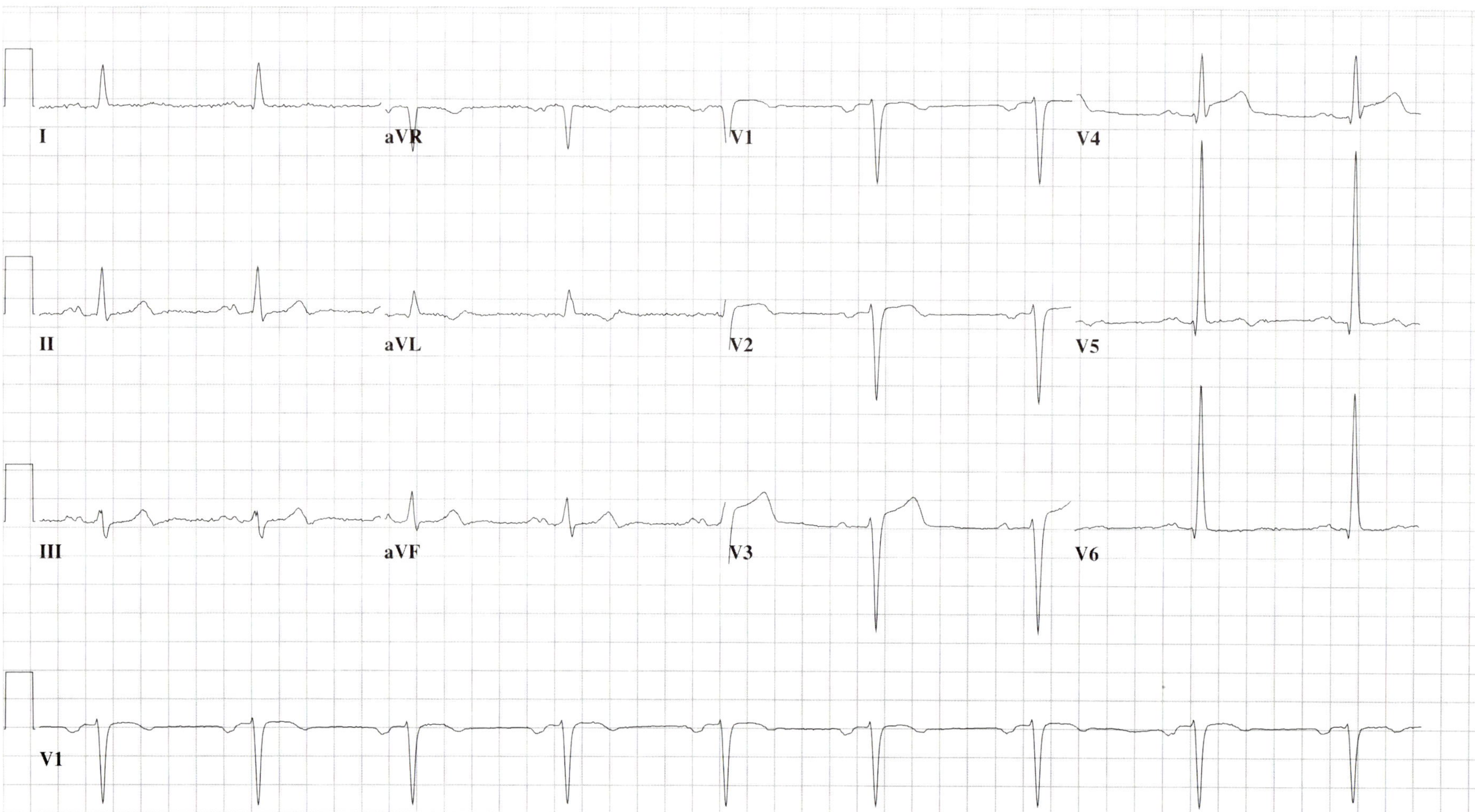

QUESTIONS

22-1. Interpret this ECG.

22-2. What are the likely causes of this ECG abnormality?

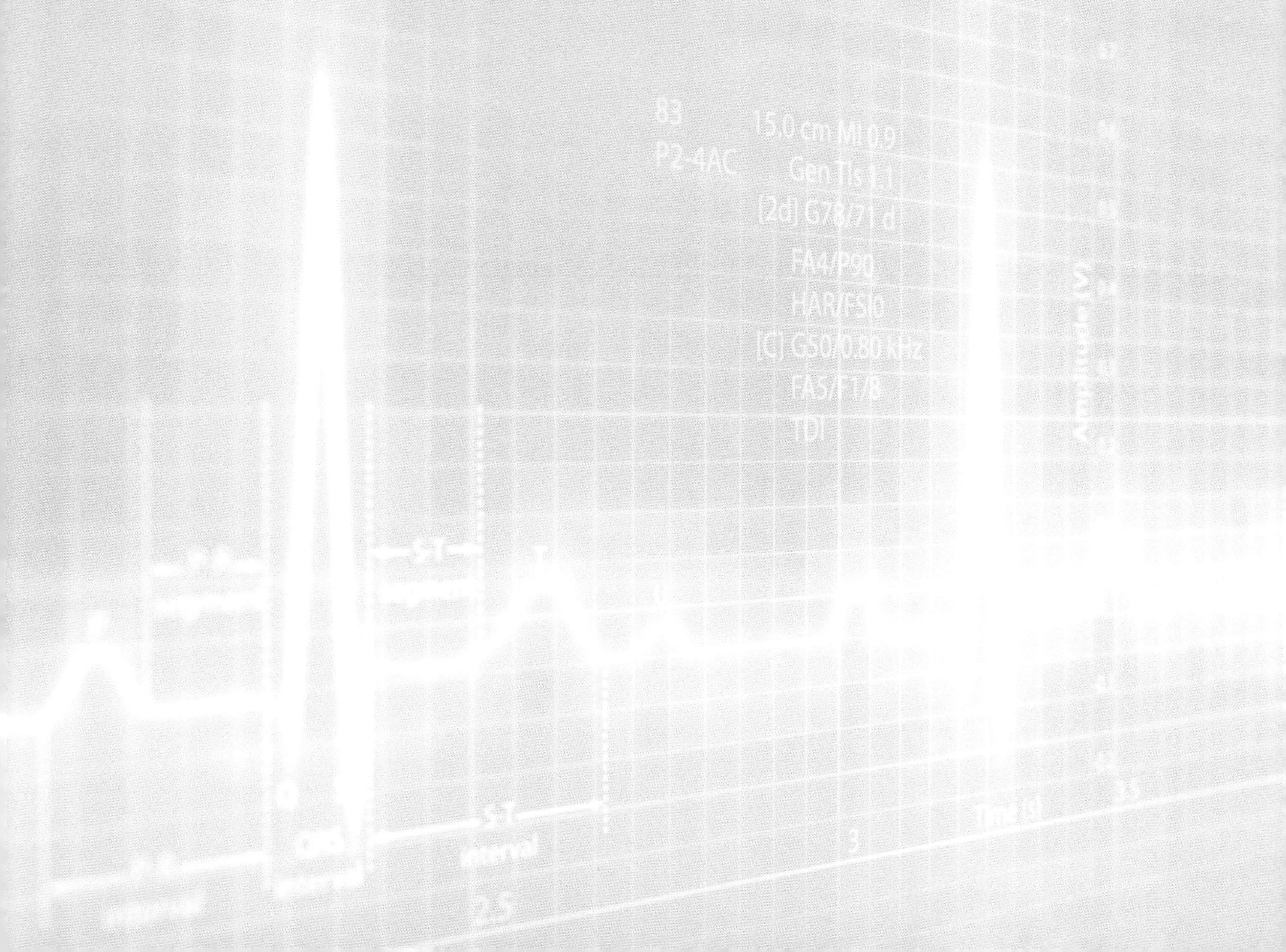
83
P2-4AC
15.0 cm MI 0.9
Gen TIs 1.1
[2d] G78/71 d
FA4/P90
HAR/FS|0
[C] G50/0.80 kHz
FA5/F1/8
TDI
S-T
T
S-T
interval
3
2.5
Time (s)
3.5
Amplitude (V)

ANSWERS

22-1. Interpret this ECG.

There is sinus bradycardia at a rate of 54 beats/min. The QRS axis is normal. First-degree AV block is present with a PR interval prolonged to greater than 200 milliseconds. There is left atrial abnormality—the P wave in lead II is broader than 120 milliseconds with prominent notching. In lead V1, the terminal negative deflection of the P wave subscribes greater than 1 mm^2 of area. Either of these criteria is diagnostic of left atrial abnormality. There is left ventricular hypertrophy as well on the basis of the R-wave amplitude in lead V5 added to the S-wave amplitude in lead V1 equaling greater than 35 mV.

22-2. What are the likely causes of this ECG abnormality?

This patient's left atrial abnormality and left ventricular hypertrophy are most likely due to decreased atrial and ventricular compliance from hypertension and atrial and ventricular volume overload secondary to mitral valve disease.

Case #23. A 68-year-old woman presents to her primary care physician. She has a history of remote myocardial infarction and congestive heart failure.

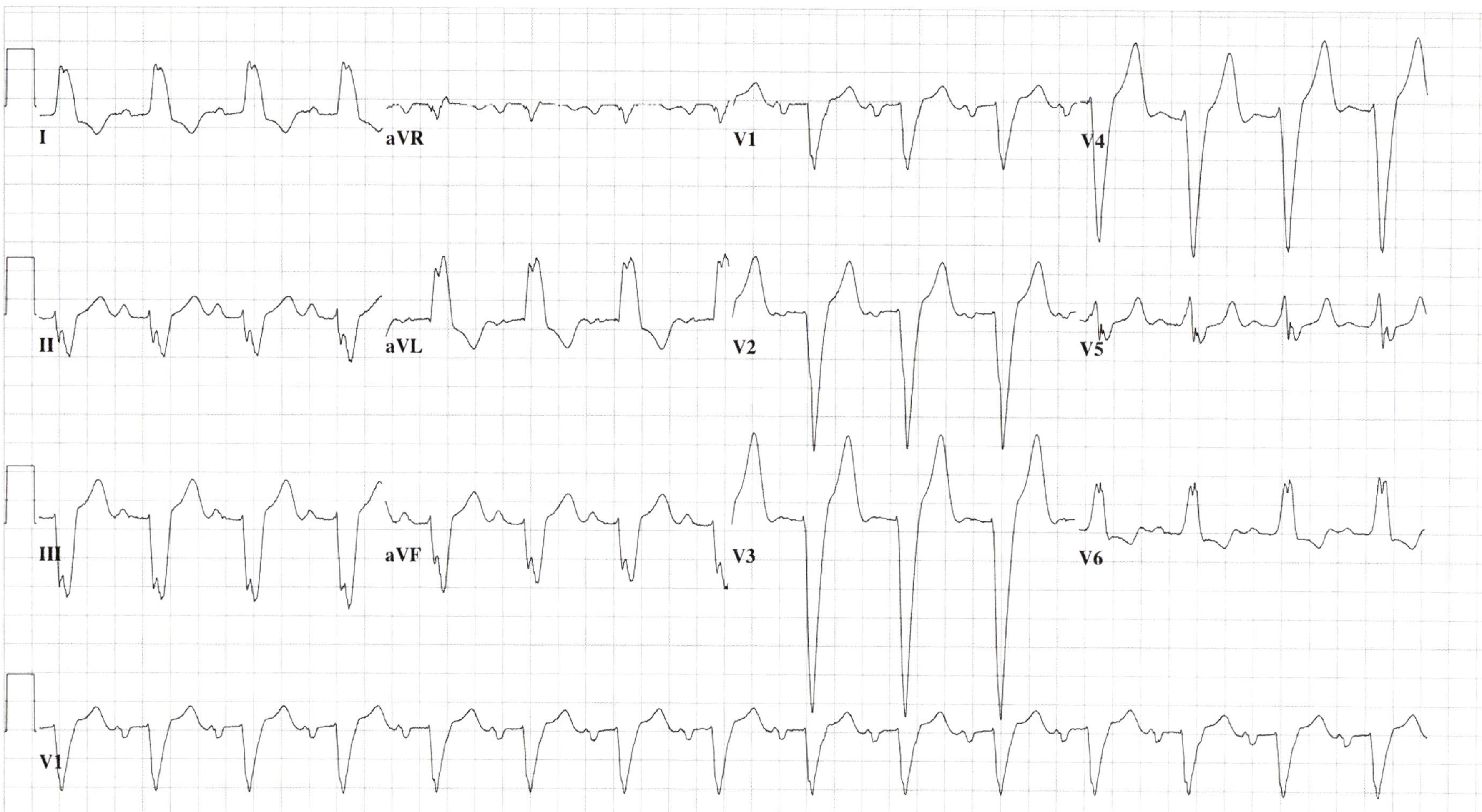

QUESTIONS

23-1. Interpret this ECG. What abnormalities are present?

23-2. Explain why the QRS complex has this particular morphology.

83
P2-4AC
15.0 cm MI 0.9
Gen TIs 1.1
[2d] G78/71 d
FA4/P90
HAR/FSI0
[C] G50/0.80 kHz
FA5/F1/8
TDI
S-T
interval
2.5
3
Time (s)
3.5

ANSWERS

23-1. Interpret this ECG. What abnormalities are present?

This tracing demonstrates normal sinus rhythm at a rate of 90 beats/min. There is left-axis deviation. There is AV conduction delay/first-degree AV block with a PR interval of 240 milliseconds. The QRS duration is prolonged at 200 milliseconds. The QRS has a left bundle branch block (LBBB) morphology with a broad QS complex in V1, and broad, notched R waves in leads I, aVL, and V6. The QT interval is normal. There are signs of left atrial abnormality, as the negative deflection of the P wave in lead V1 is longer than 40 milliseconds (1 small box), and deeper than 1 mV (1 small box) with hints of P wave notching in lead II. There are ST-segment and T-wave changes that are secondary to the LBBB.

23-2. Explain why the QRS complex has this particular morphology.

Similar to right bundle branch block (RBBB) resulting in slow and late *rightward*-directed forces, *LBBB* results in slow and late *leftward*-directed forces. In LBBB, unlike in RBBB, the initial part of the QRS complex *is* abnormal because the initial activation of the septum/ventricles normally proceeds via part of the left bundle branch. The normal initial r in V1 and q in V6 are therefore usually *absent* in LBBB (a small r wave in V1 can sometimes be seen as in the above example, but there should *not* be a small initial q wave in V6). The initial activation of the ventricles therefore occurs via the right bundle branch and then via ventricular myocardium. The right ventricle depolarizes first in a right to left direction. On the ECG this is manifest as an initial S or rS wave in V1 and initial R wave in I, aVL, and V6 (initial leftward-directed forces). Finally, there is *late* depolarization of the left ventricle, which causes the terminal part of the QRS complex to point toward the left side of the heart, and which corresponds to the wide terminal S wave in V1 and the wide terminal R wave in I, aVL, and V6. Putting this all together, LBBB is characterized by a wide and sometimes notched S wave in V1 (rightward leads), and a wide and sometimes notched R wave in I, aVL, and V6 (leftward leads).

Case #24. A 28-year-old cross-country runner has the following ECG obtained.

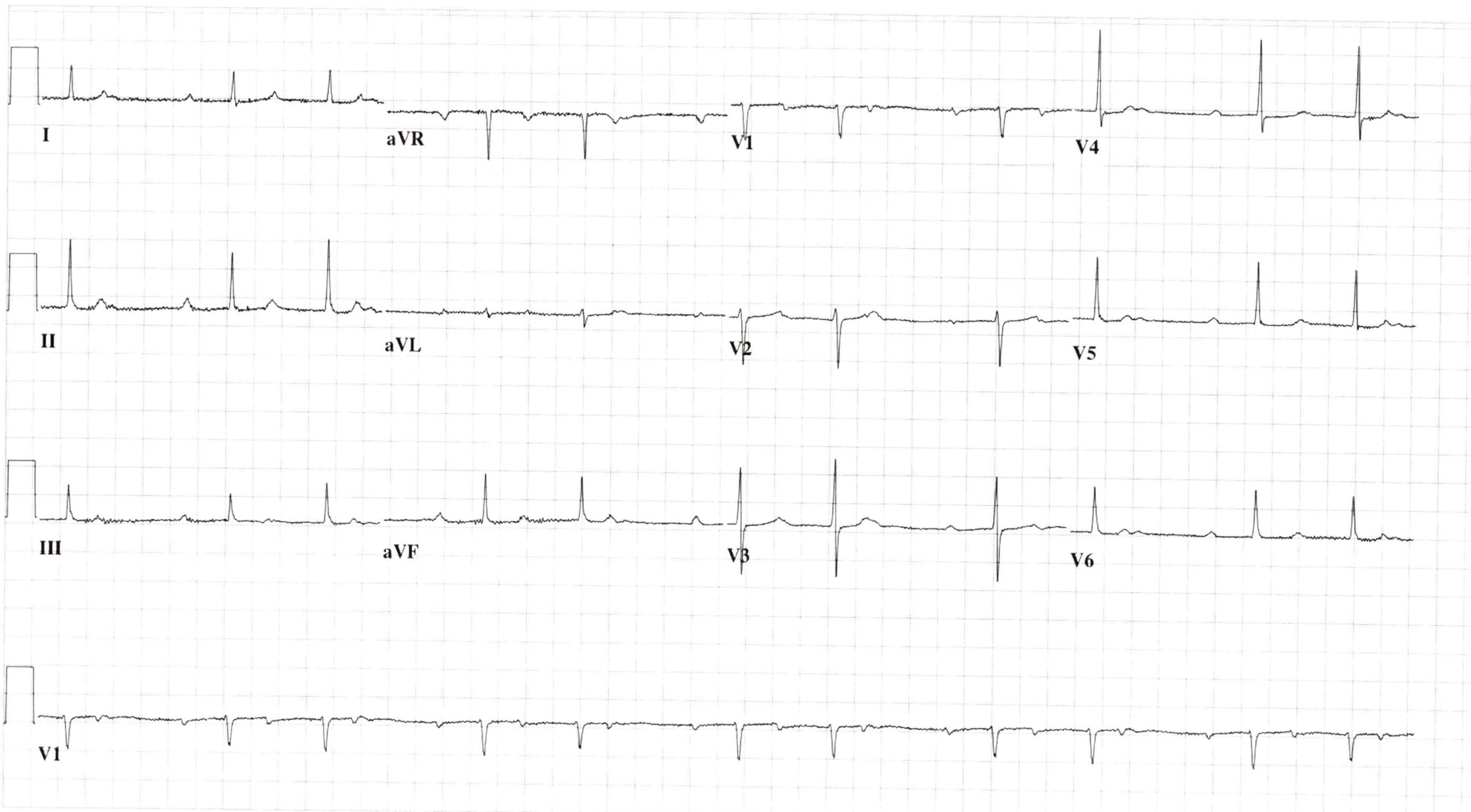

QUESTIONS

24-1. Interpret this ECG. What rhythm is present?

24-2. What intervention (if any) is needed for this patient?

83
P2-4AC
15.0 cm MI 0.9
Gen TIs 1.1
[2d] G78/71 d
FA4/P90
HAR/FSI0
[C] G50/0.80 kHz
FA5/F1/8
TDI
S-T
interval
2.5
3
3.5

ANSWERS

24-1. Interpret this ECG. What rhythm is present?

The ventricular rate is 66 beats/min. The rhythm is "regularly irregular" with grouped beating—one observes pairs of QRS complexes followed by a longer pause. Detailed rhythm analysis begins by first identifying the P waves and the QRS complexes, and then defining the relationship between the two. In the figure, P waves are marked with asterisks. If we start at the first QRS complex of each pair, we see a P wave conducted with a long PR interval. The next P wave conducts with an even longer PR interval (see the arrows in the figure). The third P wave in the cycle is nonconducted and the cycle then resets. The P-wave morphology is consistent with underlying sinus rhythm. The pattern of progressive lengthening of the PR interval followed by a nonconducted P wave and resetting of the PR interval after the nonconducted P wave is consistent with Mobitz Type I A-V block, or Wenckebach block. The remainder of the ECG reveals normal QRS axis, normal QT interval, and no evidence of chamber enlargement or ischemia.

P waves are noted with asterisks. The PR interval progressively lengthens, shown by arrows, prior to a nonconducted P wave. The cycle repeats.

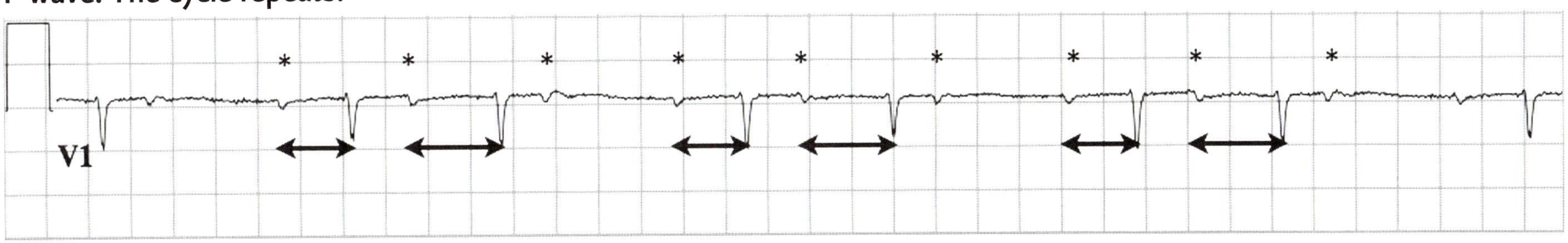

24-2. What intervention (if any) is needed for this patient?

This young athlete has Mobitz type I A-V block and is asymptomatic. In such scenarios, the anatomic location of the heart block is typically at the level of the A-V node rather than deeper in the cardiac conduction system. This ECG likely reflects high vagal tone, and the A-V block would be expected to dissipate with vagal withdrawal such as during exercise. Assuming heart rate increases as expected with an exercise challenge, no therapy is indicated.

Case #25. A 42-year-old woman presents with chest fluttering.

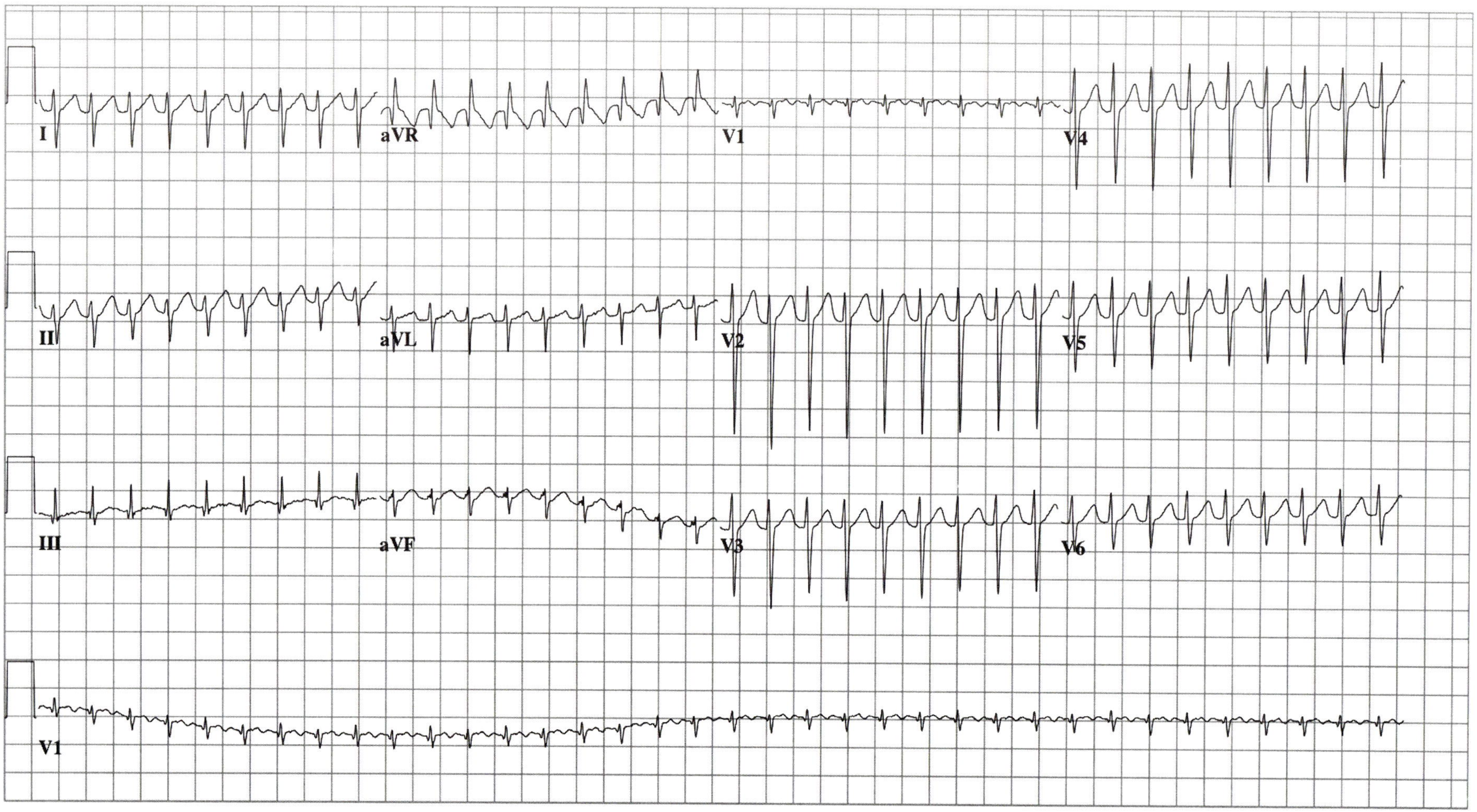

QUESTIONS

25-1. Interpret this ECG.

25-2. How could the diagnosis be clarified?

83
P2-4AC
15.0 cm MI 0.9
Gen TIs 1.1
[2d] G78/71 d
FA4/P90
HAR/FSI0
[C] G50/0.80 kHz
FA5/F1/8
TDI
Amplitude (V)
S-T
Interval
Time (s)
2.5
3
3.5

ANSWERS

25-1. Interpret this ECG.

This tracing reveals a very rapid narrow complex, regular tachycardia at 216 beats/min. The axis is rightward. Intervals are normal, and baseline motion artifact is present particularly in lead V1. The differential diagnosis of a narrow complex, regular tachycardia includes sinus tachycardia, ectopic atrial tachycardia, atrial flutter with constant block, junctional tachycardia, AV reentrant tachycardia (AVRT), and AV nodal reentrant tachycardia (AVNRT). To make this distinction, it is imperative to search and characterize any atrial activity on the ECG. Small negative deflections that may represent atrial activity can be seen in lead V1, approximately halfway between QRS complexes, shown with circles in the figure. From the surface ECG, it is not clear if these represent sinus beats, ectopic atrial beats, or retrograde conduction from a reentrant tachycardia. Thus, in the face of this uncertainty, this rhythm is best characterized as a supraventricular tachycardia.

Possible atrial activity is shown with circles, although it does not clearly discriminate between the diagnostic possibilities at this rapid heart rate. The rhythm is best categorized as supraventricular tachycardia.

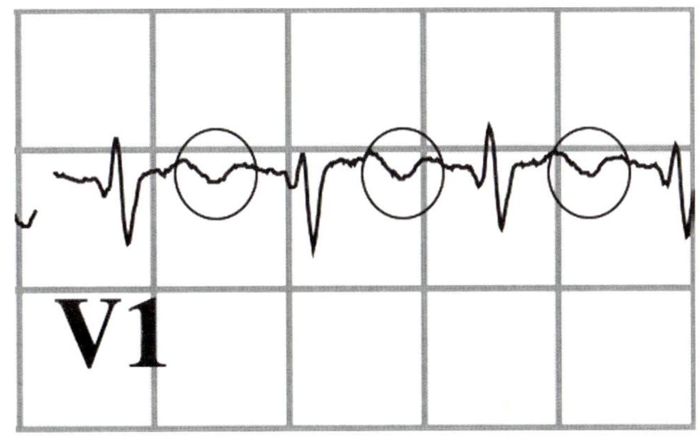

25-2. How could the diagnosis be clarified?

Vagal maneuvers, adenosine, or nodal blockade while continuously running a telemetry strip could help clarify the diagnosis. These maneuvers would cause transient AV block, which could terminate the tachycardia, suggesting a reentrant mechanism, or unmask underlying atrial activity consistent with sinus or ectopic atrial rhythm.

Case #26. A 65-year-old with a history of nonischemic cardiomyopathy presenting after a shock from his implantable defibrillator.

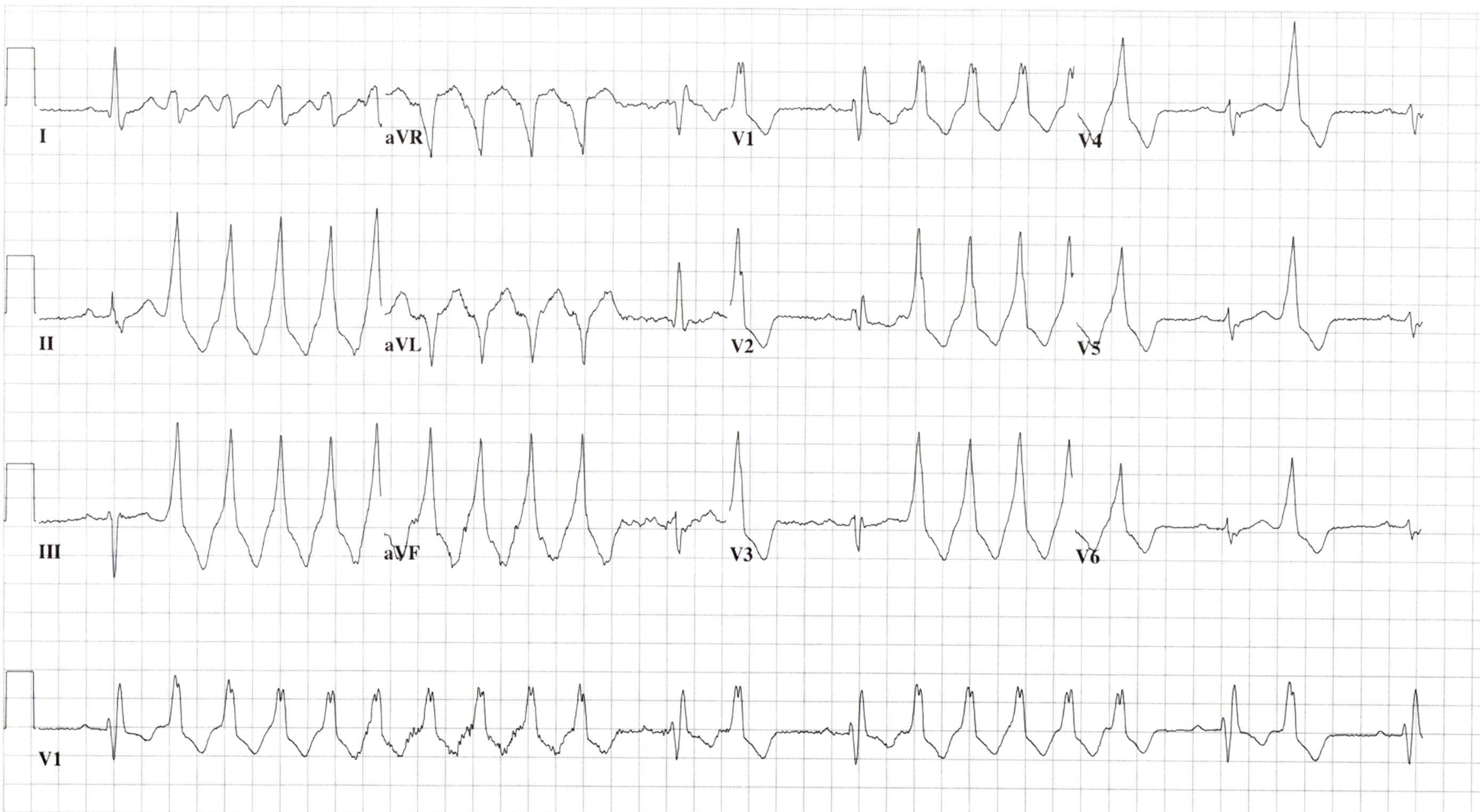

QUESTION

26-1. Please interpret this ECG. What arrhythmia is present?

83
P2-4AC
15.0 cm MI 0.9
Gen TIs 1.1
[2d] G78/71 d
FA4/P90
HAR/FS|0
[C] G50/0.80 kHz
FA5/F1/B
TDI
S-T
3
2.5

ANSWER

26-1. Please interpret this ECG. What arrhythmia is present?

There are two distinct rhythms and QRS morphologies. The first beat of the rhythm strip demonstrates normal sinus rhythm with normal frontal plane axis and right bundle branch block. There are several other sinus beats visualized throughout the rhythm strip interspersed with salvos of a monomorphic wide complex tachycardia. These beats demonstrate a completely positive polarity throughout leads V1 through V6. This finding is termed concordance and suggests nonsustained ventricular tachycardia as the diagnosis, particularly in this patient with underlying cardiomyopathy. Evaluating the sinus beats further reveals that, through leads V1 to V6, there is borderline low voltage and poor R-wave progression, which may suggest prior myocardial infarction.

In sum, this tracing reveals sinus rhythm with right bundle branch block and poor R-wave progression and nonsustained monomorphic ventricular tachycardia.

Case #27. An 18-year-old young man presents with nausea after cocaine use.

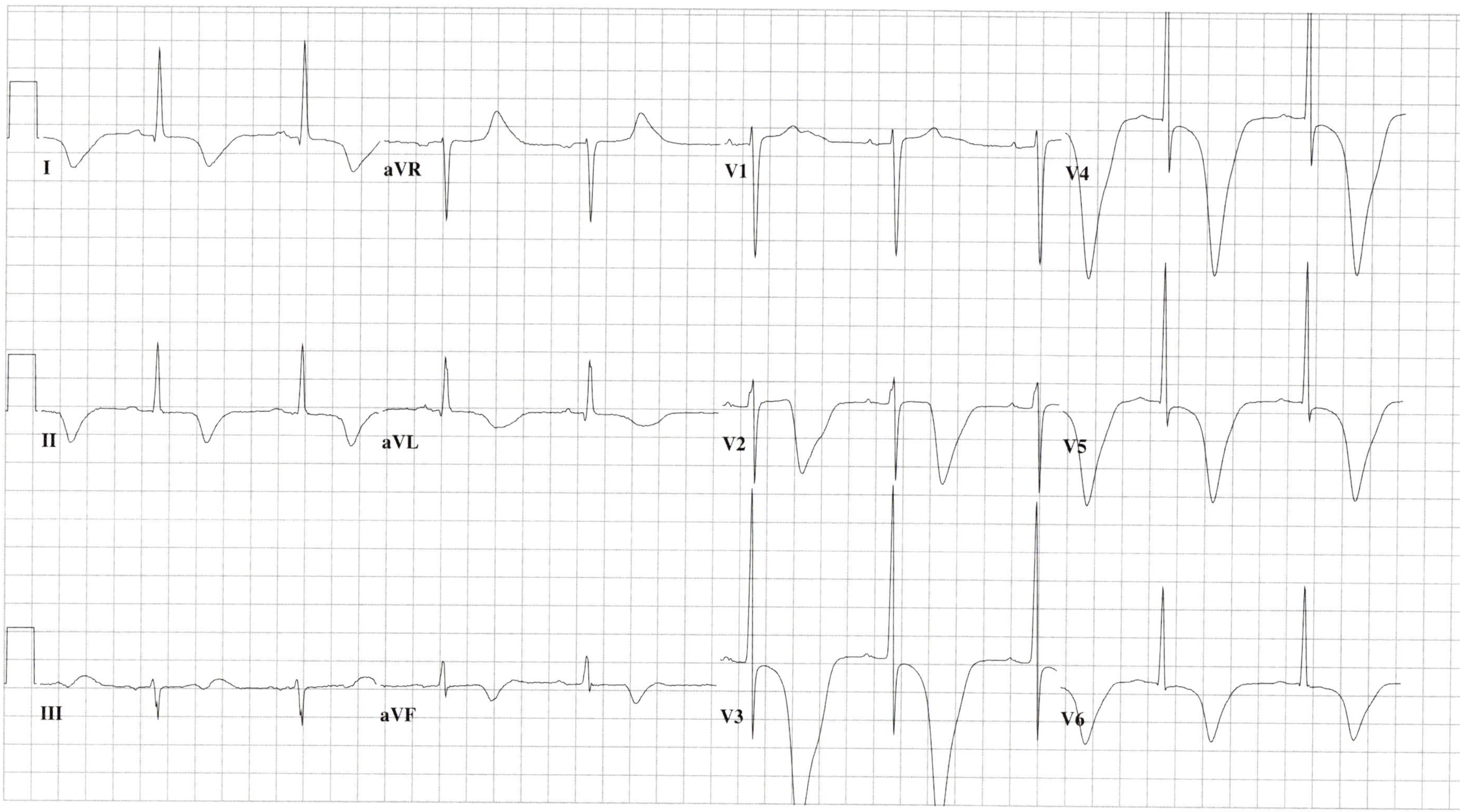

QUESTIONS

27-1. What abnormalities are present?

27-2. What is the differential diagnosis for the observed abnormalities?

27-3. What are the cardiovascular effects of cocaine?

83
P2-4AC
15.0 cm MI 0.9
Gen TIs 1.1
[2d] G78/71 d
FA4/P90
HAR/FS10
[C] G50/0.80 kHz
FA5/F1/8
TDI
Amplitude (V)
S-T
Interval
2.5
3
Time (s)

ANSWERS

27-1. What abnormalities are present?

There is sinus bradycardia at 53 beats/min with a normal QRS axis. The most striking finding is deep T-wave inversions throughout but most prominent in leads V2 through V6 with associated ST-segment depression. The QT interval is very prolonged to over 600 milliseconds.

27-2. What is the differential diagnosis for the observed abnormalities?

Causes of giant inverted T waves include myocardial ischemia, cerebrovascular accidents (in particular, hemorrhagic strokes), cardiomyopathies, medication toxicity (including class III antiarrhythmic medications), and toxins including cocaine, both in the acute and in the chronic settings.

27-3. What are the cardiovascular effects of cocaine?

Acutely, cocaine exerts sympathomimetic effect via inhibition of catecholamine reuptake. This high-catecholamine state causes increased vascular tone and increased inotropy leading in turn to increases in left ventricular afterload and wall stress. Heightened shear stresses may predispose to atherosclerotic plaque rupture and arterial dissection, with associated risk of acute coronary and acute aortic syndromes. Cocaine-induced vasospasm may produce ischemia in the coronary and other arterial beds. A hypercoagulable state is also induced.

Case #28. A 79-year-old female presents with dizziness and abdominal pain.

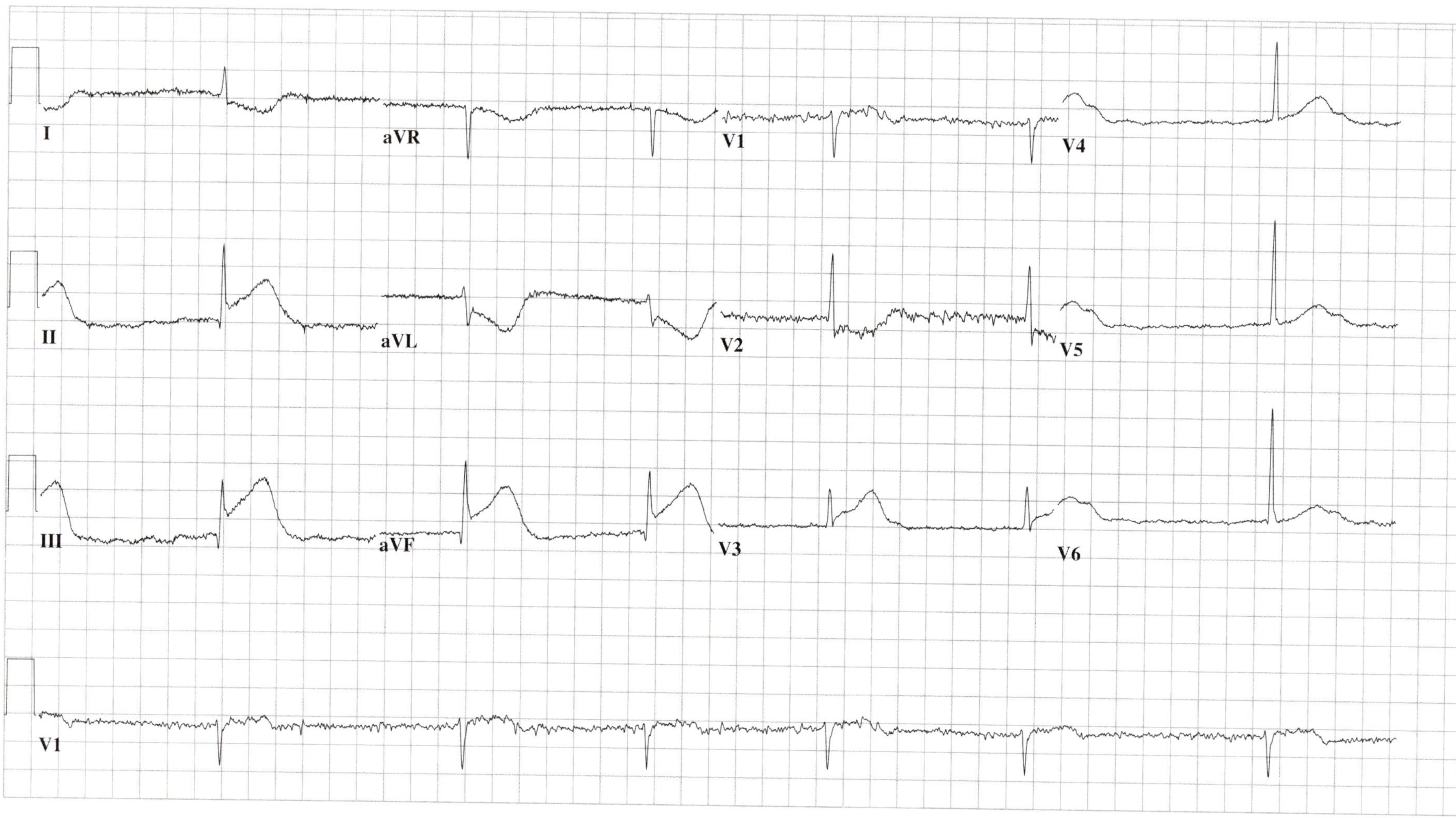

QUESTIONS

28-1. What is the diagnosis?

28-2. Explain the bradycardia.

83
P2-4AC
15.0 cm MI 0.9
Gen TIs 1.1
[2d] G78/71 d
FA4/P90
HAR/FS10
[C] G50/0.80 kHz
FA5/F1/8
TDI
S-T
S-T
interval
2.5
3
3.5
Time (s)
Amplitude (V)

ANSWERS

28-1. What is the diagnosis?

There is bradycardia with only 6 QRS complexes through the 10-second rhythm strip. Thus, the ventricular rate is 36 beats/min. The QRS complexes are narrow and the R–R interval is irregularly irregular with no atrial activity visible. Fine baseline artifact is present. Thus, the rhythm is atrial fibrillation with a bradycardic ventricular response. There are large ST-segment elevations in the inferior leads without pathologic Q waves and reciprocal ST-segment depressions in leads I and aVL. Assessing the R-wave progression across the precordium, normally, the S waves are more prominent than the R waves in leads V1 and V2; in this tracing, there is a dominant R wave present in V2 with ST-segment depression in this lead. This may represent posterior wall infarction. There is also ST-segment elevation in lead V3, which may represent apical ischemia. The distribution of ischemia, therefore, is infero-postero-apical and suggests occlusion of a large, dominant right coronary artery, which wraps around to supply the left ventricular apex.

28-2. Explain the bradycardia.

Inferior ST-segment elevation myocardial infarction can be caused by occlusion of the right coronary or the left circumflex coronary artery. In this case, the ST elevations of greater magnitude in lead III compared to lead II coupled with ST depressions in leads I and aVL make the RCA a more likely culprit vessel. The blood supply to the AV node is via the AV nodal artery, a branch off of the posterior descending coronary artery (PDA). In a significant majority of patients, the PDA is a branch off of the right coronary artery (so called "right dominant" patients); in a minority of patients, the PDA is a branch off of the left circumflex (so-called "left dominant" patients). In this case, the patient has likely occluded her right coronary artery leading to inferior and posterior ischemia and attendant ischemia of the AV node leading to slowed conduction and the bradycardia.

Case #29. A 24-year-old presents with pleuritic chest pain.

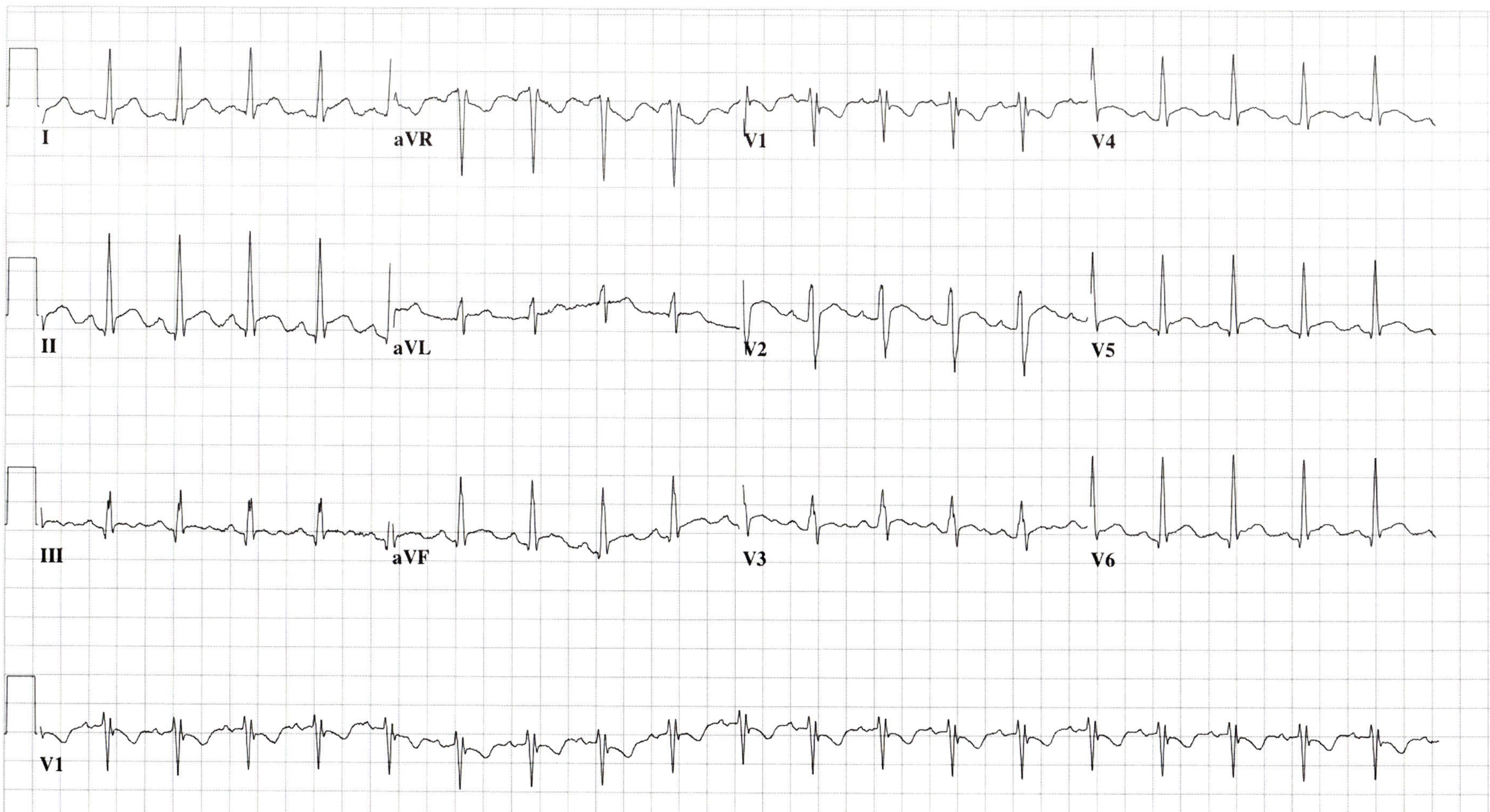

QUESTIONS

29-1. Interpret this ECG.

29-2. What is the differential diagnosis for these ECG findings?

83
P2-4AC
15.0 cm MI 0.9
Gen TIs 1.1
[2d] G78/71 d
FA4/P90
HAR/FSI0
[C] G50/0.80 kHz
FA5/F1/8
TDI
Amplitude (V)
S-T
S-T
interval
Time (s)
2.5
3
3.5

ANSWERS

29-1. Interpret this ECG.

Sinus rhythm is present at a rate of approximately 100 beats/min. The axis is normal. There is no chamber enlargement. An incomplete right bundle branch block is present, diagnosed on the basis of the RSR′ ("rabbit ears") appearance of the QRS complex in lead V1 with a normal QRS duration. There are ST-segment elevations of 1 to 3 mm present in all leads: the inferior (II, III, and aVF), lateral (V5, V6, I, and aVL), and anterior (V2-V4) leads. In addition, there is depression of the PR segment best visualized in lead II. In lead aVR, there is PR-segment elevation.

29-2. What is the differential diagnosis for these ECG findings?

The differential diagnosis for ST-segment elevation in general includes transmural ischemia, left ventricular aneurysm, hyperkalemia, repolarization abnormalities as in left ventricular hypertrophy, and the early-repolarization pattern, as well as pericarditis. This tracing demonstrating diffuse, concave upward ST-segment elevation coupled with PR-segment depression in lead II and PR-segment elevation in lead aVR is most consistent with pericarditis.

Case #30. A 65-year-old woman with hypertension presents for routine primary care follow-up.

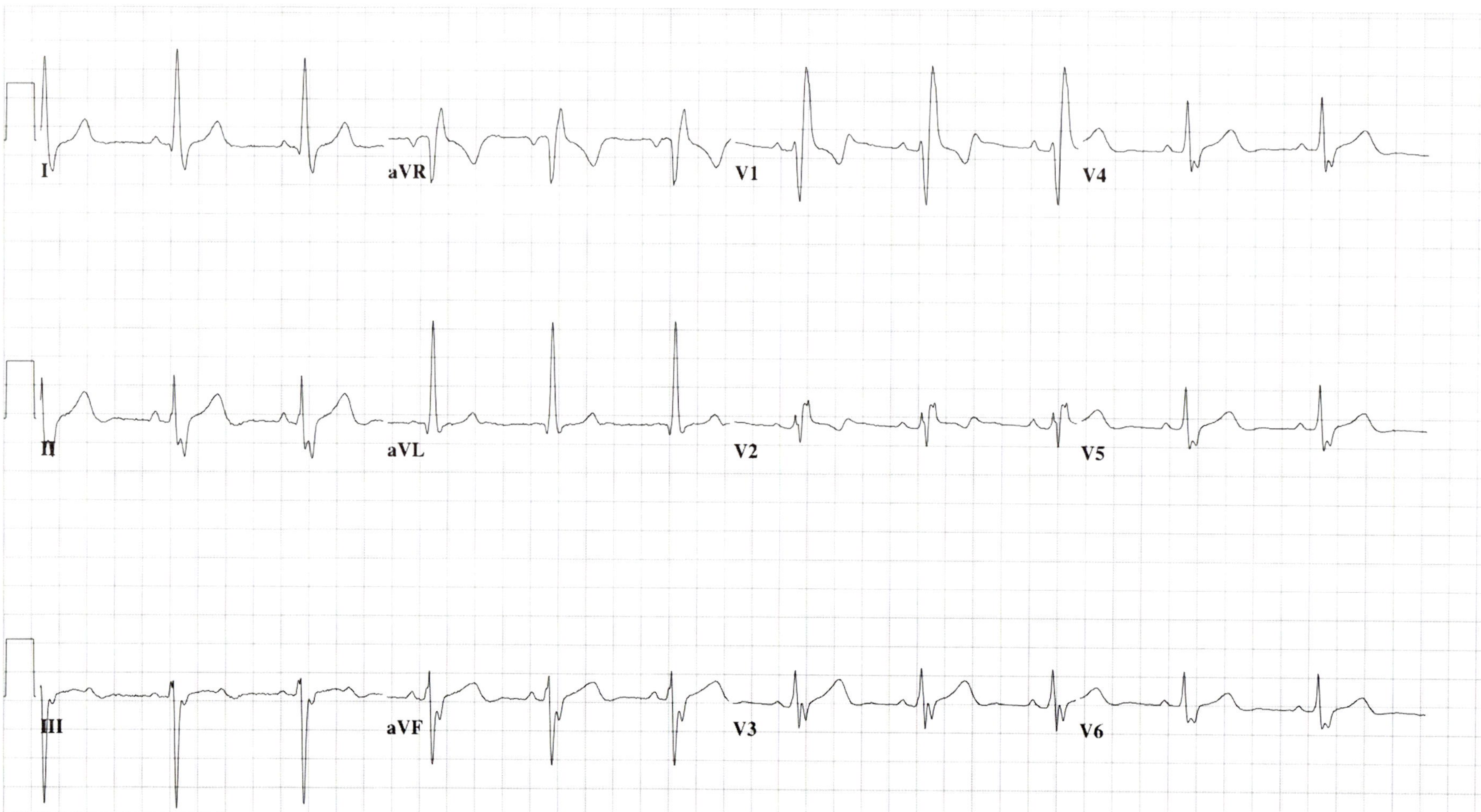

QUESTIONS

30-1. Interpret this ECG. What abnormalities are present on this tracing?

30-2. How is the electrocardiographic diagnosis of left ventricular hypertrophy affected by the presence of right bundle branch block?

83
P2-4AC
15.0 cm MI 0.9
Gen TIs 1.1
[2d] G78/71 d
FA4/P90
HAR/FS|0
[C] G50/0.80 kHz
FA5/F1/8
TDI
Amplitude (V)
3
2.5

ANSWERS

30-1. Interpret this ECG. What abnormalities are present on this tracing?

This tracing demonstrates normal sinus rhythm at a rate of 65 beats/min. The QRS axis is normal. The QRS duration is prolonged to 140 milliseconds with a right bundle branch block pattern. The QT interval is normal. There is probable left ventricular hypertrophy on the basis of the R-wave amplitude in lead aVL of 17 mV. There are T-wave inversions in leads V1 and V2, which are normal in the setting of right bundle branch block.

30-2. How is the electrocardiographic diagnosis of left ventricular hypertrophy affected by the presence of right bundle branch block?

The standard electrocardiographic methods for determining left ventricular hypertrophy can be used in the setting of a right bundle branch block.

Case #31. A 62-year-old male presents with palpitations and breathlessness.

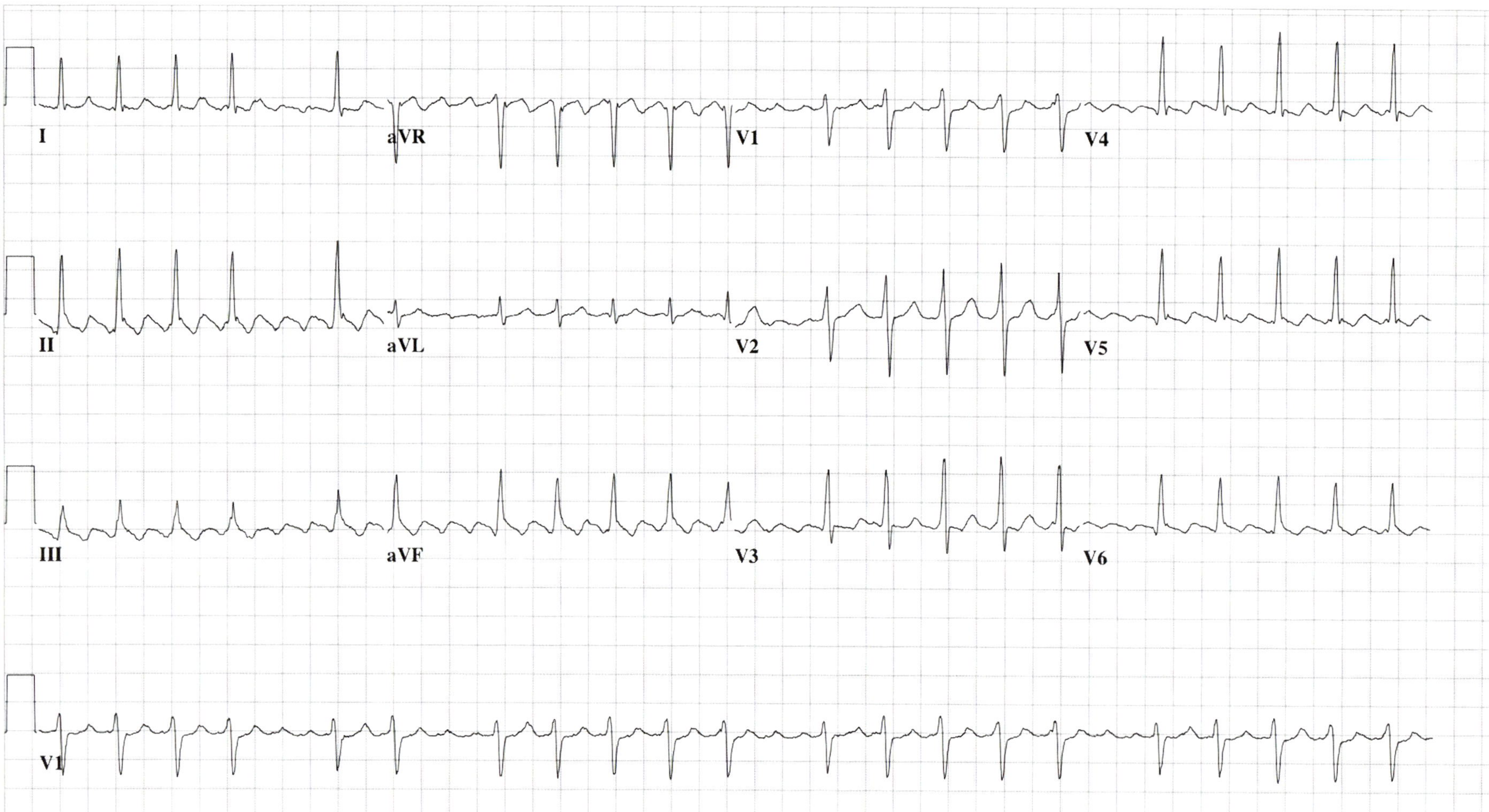

QUESTION

31-1. What abnormalities are present on this tracing?

83
P2-4AC
15.0 cm MI 0.9
Gen TIs 1.1
[2d] G78/71 d
FA4/P90
HAR/FS10
[C] G50/0.80 kHz
FA5/F1/8
TDI
Amplitude (V)
Interval
2.5
3
Time (s)
3.5

ANSWER

31-1. What abnormalities are present on this tracing?

There is a rapid, irregular, narrow complex rhythm. There are 21 QRS complexes throughout the 10-second rhythm strip yielding an approximate average ventricular rate of 126 beats/min. Most pairs of QRS complexes on this tracing are separated by an RR interval of 420 milliseconds. All of the wider RR intervals are also identical (720 milliseconds). This is not a chaotic irregularly irregular rhythm as is seen with atrial fibrillation. A search for atrial waveforms reveals the characteristic sawtooth waves of atrial flutter in the inferior leads II, III, and aVF. The flutter waves have a rate of 300 beats/min, which is typical for this arrhythmia. The short RR intervals are the result of 2 to 1 conduction of flutter waves to the ventricles, whereas the long RR intervals are the result of 4 to 1 conduction. The figure demonstrates the flutter waves with 2 to 1 and 4 to 1 conduction. Axis and intervals are normal, and there is no evidence of hypertrophy or ischemia.

Flutter waves at a rate of 300 beats/min with both 2 to 1 and 4 to 1 conduction patterns.

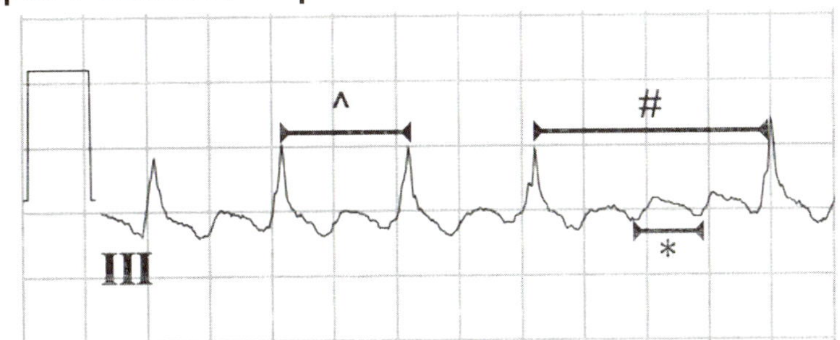

*Flutter waves at 300 beats per minute
#Four to one A-V conduction
^Two to one A-V conduction

Case #32. A 68-year-old gentleman presents with chest pain.

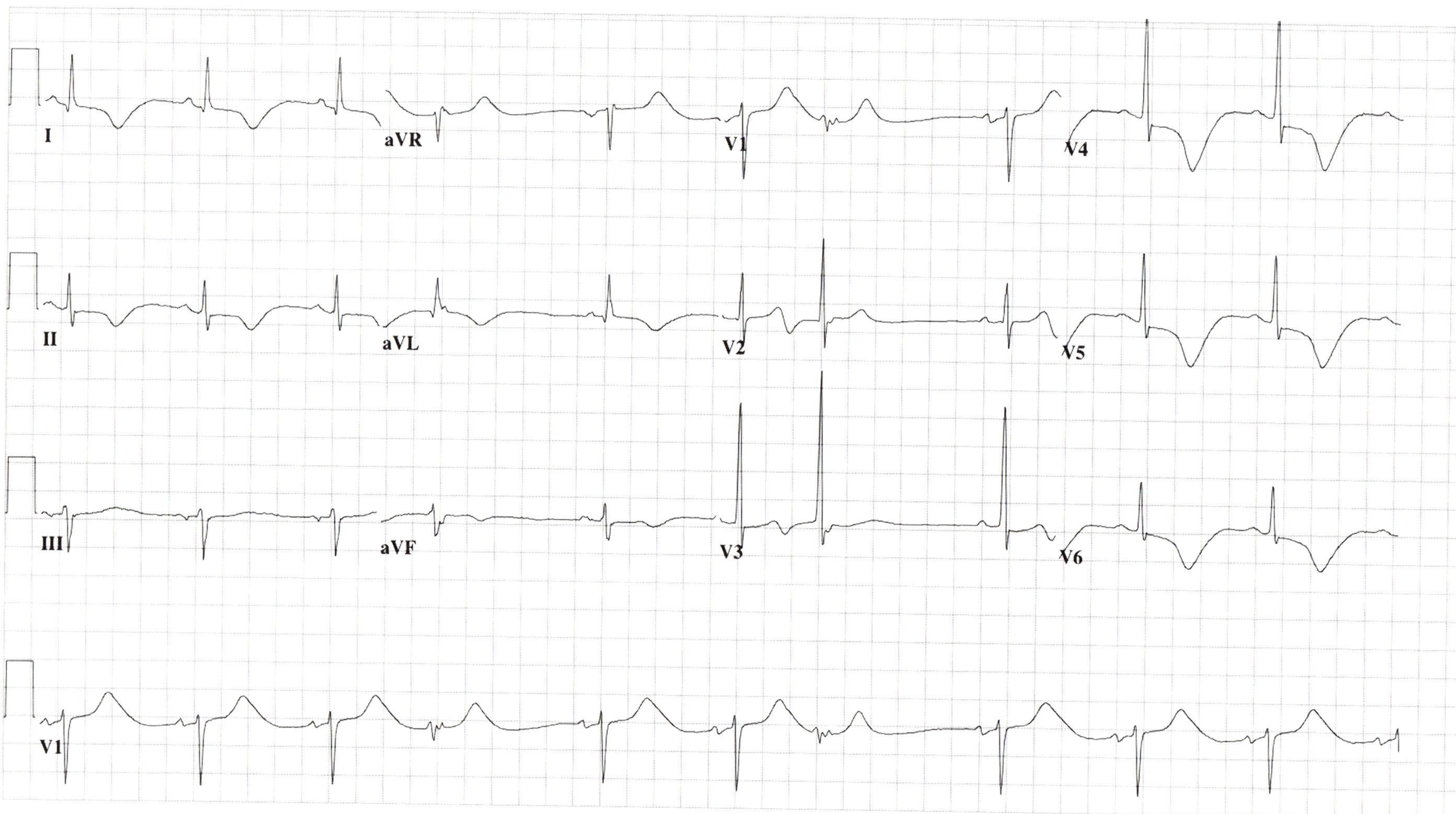

QUESTIONS

32-1. What abnormalities are present?

32-2. What is the differential diagnosis of the T-wave abnormalities?

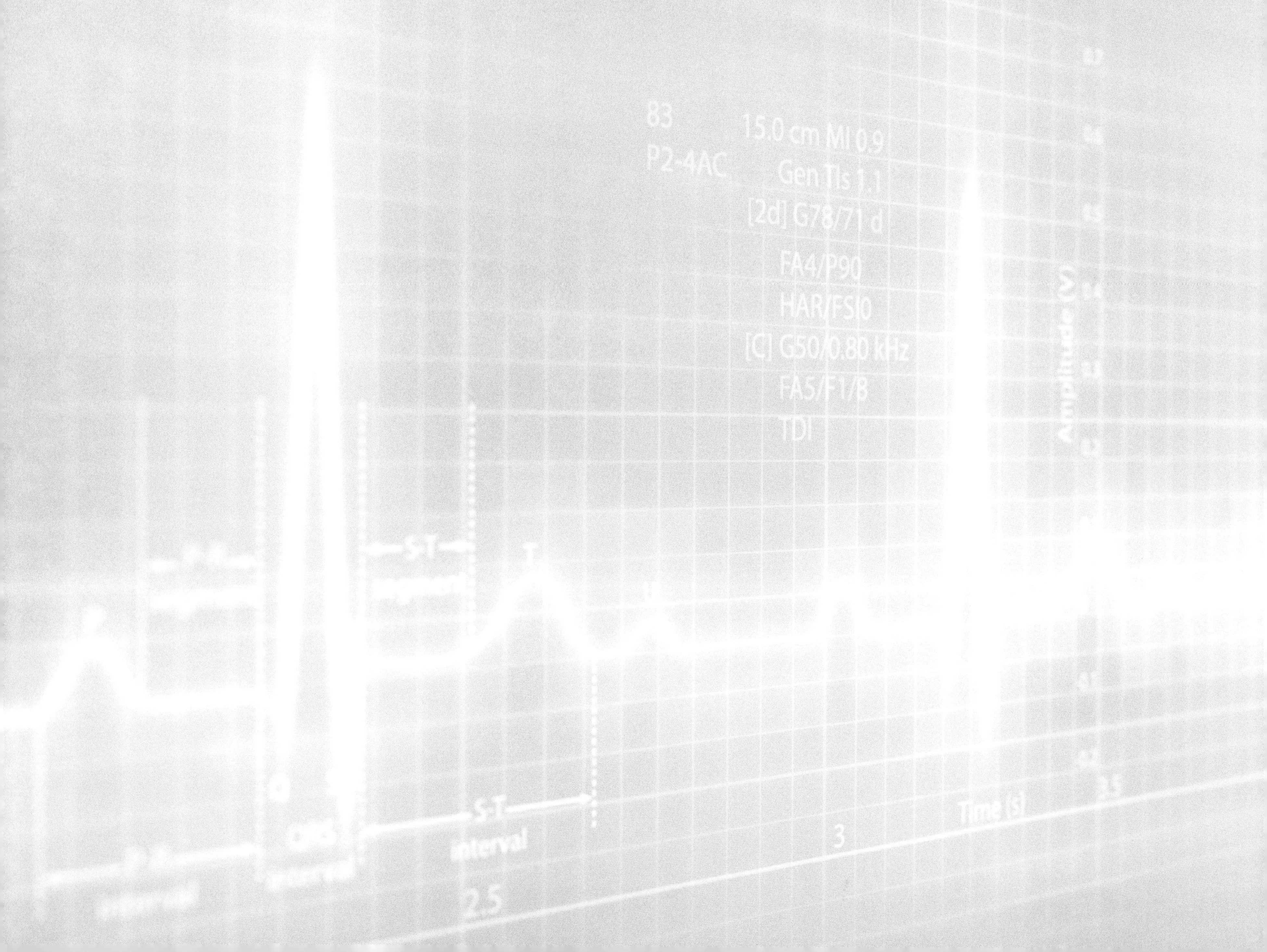
83
P2-4AC
15.0 cm MI 0.9
Gen TIs 1.1
[2d] G78/71 d
FA4/P90
HAR/FSI0
[C] G50/0.80 kHz
FA5/F1/8
TDI
Amplitude (V)
S-T
T
S-T
interval
3
Time (s)
2.5

ANSWERS

32-1. What abnormalities are present?

This ECG demonstrates sinus rhythm at a rate of approximately 60 beats/min. The fourth and seventh QRS complexes represent junctional premature beats with retrograde P waves visible just after the QRS complexes. The axis is normal, whereas the QT interval is markedly prolonged. Downsloping ST-segment depression and deep T-wave inversions are present and most prominent in the anterior and lateral leads.

32-2. What is the differential diagnosis of the T-wave abnormalities?

Deep T-wave inversions and QT-interval prolongation can be caused by myocardial ischemia, electrolyte abnormalities, cardiomyopathies, central nervous system insults, and toxins or medications such as cocaine or antiarrhythmic drugs. In this case, the clinical scenario suggested ischemia as the most likely cause, and the patient underwent coronary angiography and stenting of a severe left circumflex stenosis.

Case #33. A 42-year-old woman with 2 months of palpitations and exertional dyspnea. She has a distant history of rheumatic fever.

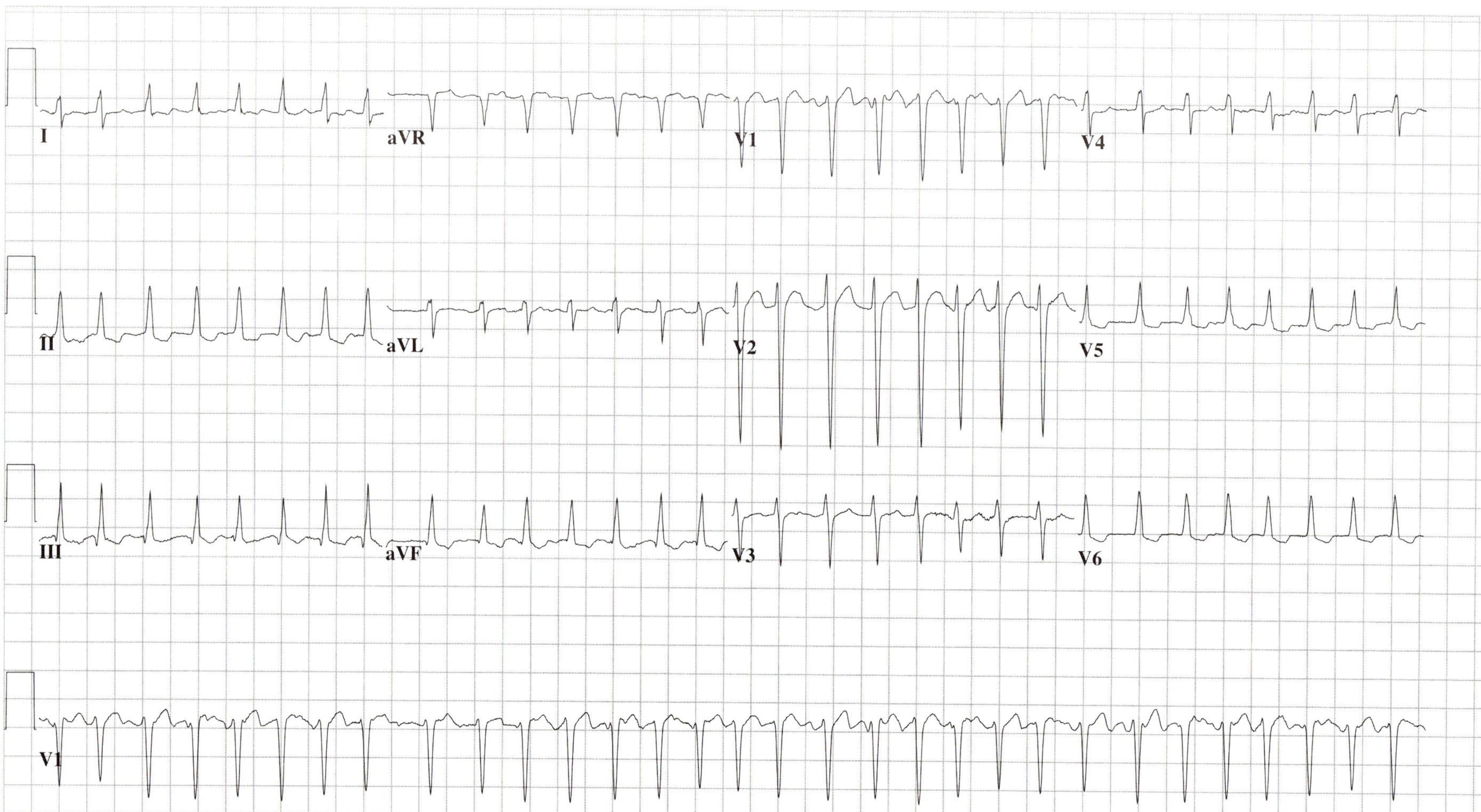

QUESTIONS

33-1. What abnormalities are present on this ECG?

33-2. What is the suspected underlying diagnosis, and what diagnostic test should be ordered next for this patient?

33-3. What medical management is indicated while the patient awaits definitive repair of the underlying problem?

83
P2-4AC
15.0 cm MI 0.9
Gen TIs 1.1
[2d] G78/71 d
FA4/P90
HAR/FSI0
[C] G50/0.80 kHz
FA5/F1/8
TDI
S-T
S-T
interval
2.5
3
Time (s)
3.5
Amplitude (V)

ANSWERS

33-1. What abnormalities are present on this ECG?

This is a rapid, irregular, narrow-complex tachycardia. There are 31 QRS complexes in the 10-second rhythm strip—a ventricular rate of 186 beats/min. The irregularly irregular rhythm narrows the differential diagnosis to either atrial fibrillation or multifocal atrial tachycardia. There are no obvious P waves before every QRS complex; hence, the rhythm is atrial fibrillation. The QRS axis is normal, and there are no pathologic Q waves. There are ST-segment depressions with T-wave inversions in the inferolateral leads which are nonspecific.

33-2. What is the suspected underlying diagnosis, and what diagnostic test should be ordered next for this patient?

New-onset atrial fibrillation in a patient with a history of rheumatic fever may suggest mitral stenosis. Mitral stenosis is classically secondary to rheumatic heart disease and leads to left atrial enlargement and atrial fibrillation. The classic findings of an opening snap and low-pitched, diastolic rumbling murmur can be notoriously soft and difficult to hear, particularly at high heart rates. This patient should undergo transthoracic echocardiography to estimate the transmitral gradient, define mitral valve anatomy, and estimate pulmonary artery systolic pressure. Depending on the valvular anatomy and whether concomitant mitral regurgitation is present, this patient may be a candidate for either percutaneous mitral balloon valvotomy or surgical repair.

33-3. What medical management is indicated while the patient awaits definitive repair of the underlying problem?

β-Blockers appear to be well tolerated in mitral stenosis and can be used for rate control while the patient awaits balloon valvulotomy or surgical intervention. Compared to patients with nonvalvular AF, patients with AF and mitral stenosis have a higher risk of thromboembolic stroke. Anticoagulation is indicated.

Case #34. A 61-year-old man presents for follow-up.

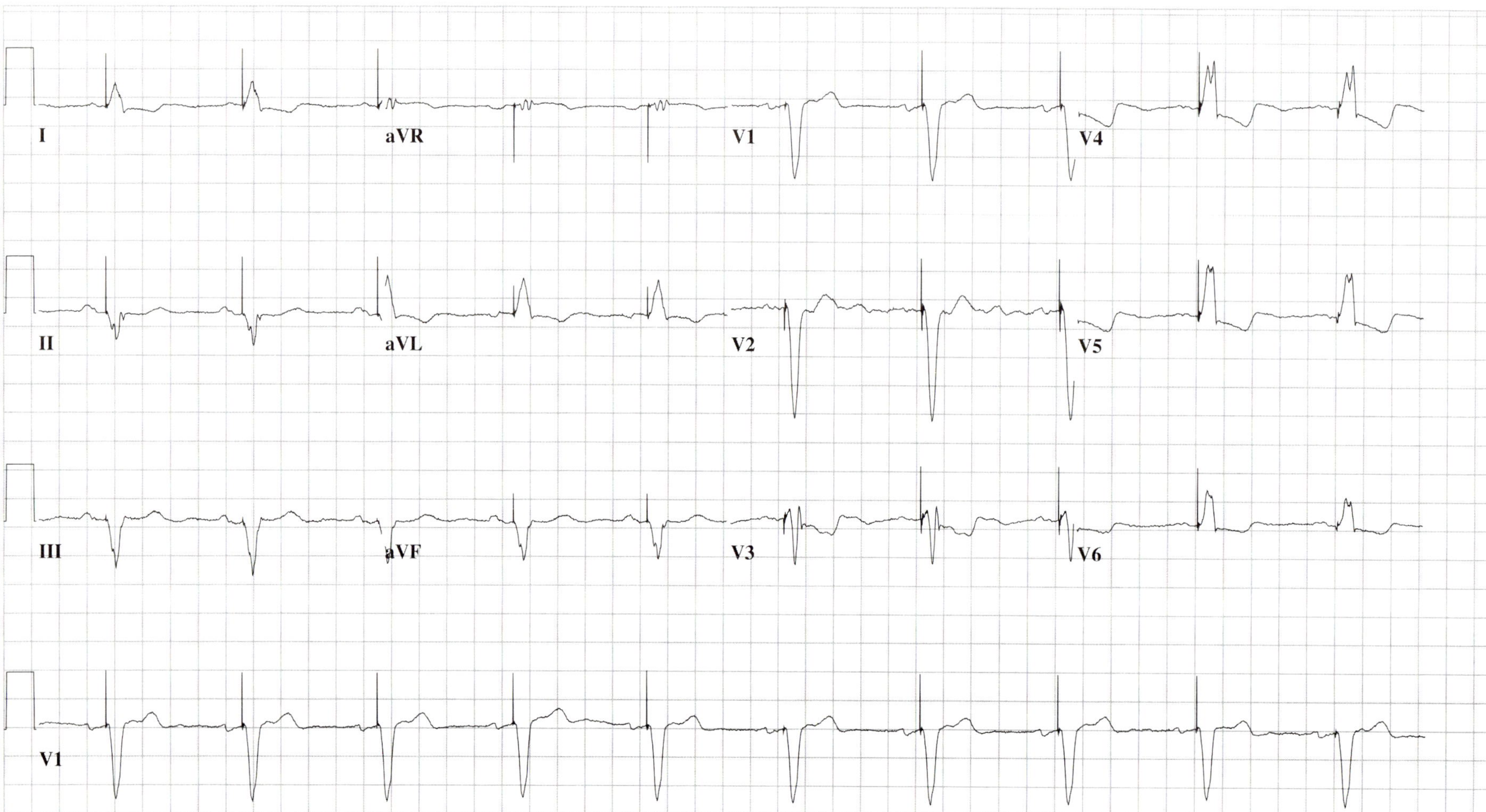

QUESTIONS

34-1. What is the rhythm?

34-2. Where are the pacemaker leads located?

83
P2-4AC
15.0 cm MI 0.9
Gen TIs 1.1
[2d] G78/71 d
FA4/P90
HAR/FS0
[C] G50/0.80 kHz
FA5/F1/B
TDI
S-T
Amplitude (V)
2.5
3

ANSWERS

34-1. What is the rhythm?

P waves are present at 60 beats/min. The P waves are upright in the inferior leads and lead I consistent with normal sinus rhythm. Each P wave is followed by a paced ventricular beat with a left bundle branch configuration and a leftward axis consistent with a ventricular pacemaker located in the right ventricular apex. The PR interval is constant. Thus, the patient has a dual-chamber pacemaker with atrial sensing and ventricular pacing. Other findings include a notched and broad P wave in lead II indicative of left atrial abnormality. There are ST-segment deviations with T-wave inversions in I, aVL, and V3 through V6 that are normal in the setting of ventricular pacing. In summary, this tracing demonstrates sinus rhythm with a dual-chamber pacemaker with atrial sensing and ventricular pacing in addition to left atrial abnormality.

34-2. Where are the pacemaker leads located?

The presence of ventricular pacing implies the obvious presence of a ventricular pacemaker. The left bundle branch configuration and the negative QRS polarity in the inferior leads imply that the pacemaker is in the right ventricular apex, with current flowing opposite the orientation of the inferior leads. The fact that there are native P waves and a constant PR interval followed by paced beats implies that there is atrial sensing and hence a right atrial lead is also present.

Case #35. A 65-year-old woman with poorly controlled hypertension presenting for routine office follow-up.

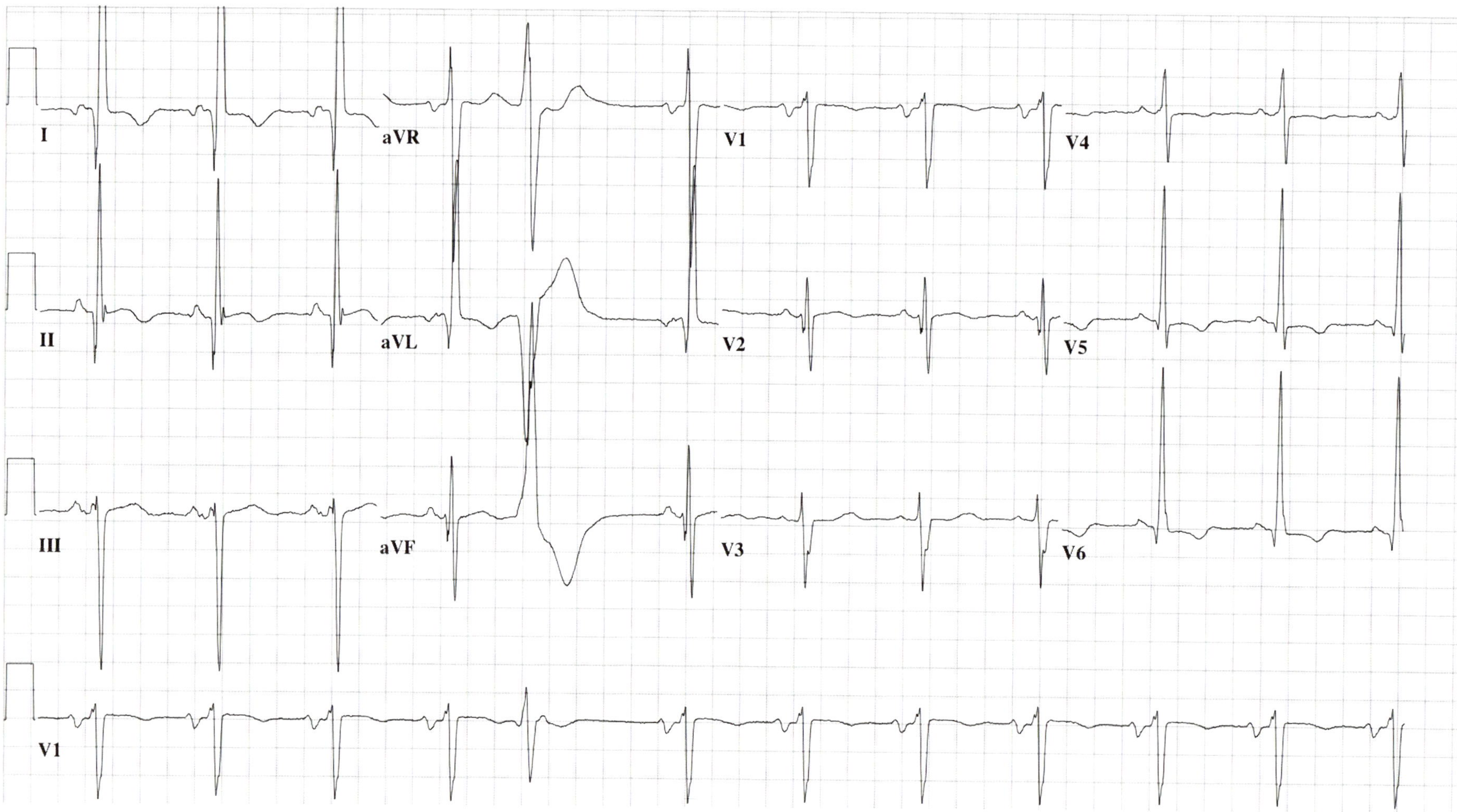

QUESTIONS

35-1. What abnormalities are present?

35-2. What is the differential diagnosis?

83
P2-4AC
15.0 cm MI 0.9
Gen TIs 1.1
[2d] G78/71 d
FA4/P90
HAR/FSI0
[C] G50/0.80 kHz
FA5/F1/8
TDI
S-T
Interval
2.5
3
Time (s)

ANSWERS

35-1. What abnormalities are present?

The heart rate is 70 beats per minute. The P waves have abnormal biphasic morphology in lead I consistent with an ectopic atrial rhythm rather than sinus rhythm." The fifth beat is a premature ventricular contraction. Axis is normal. The QRS complex is widened to greater than 100 milliseconds and is best classified as an intraventricular conduction delay because the QRS morphology is neither that of a left bundle branch block nor of a right bundle branch block. There is left ventricular hypertrophy on the basis of the R-wave magnitude greater than 11 mV in lead aVL and the magnitude of the S wave in lead V1 plus magnitude of the S wave in lead V6 greater than 35 mV. There are T-wave inversions and ST-segment abnormalities in leads with the most prominent R-wave voltage, which are secondary to the left ventricular hypertrophy. Finally, Q waves are present in leads I, II, and aVL consistent with lateral myocardial infarction of indeterminate age versus hypertrophy of the interventricular septum.

35-2. What is the differential diagnosis?

Left ventricular hypertrophy is associated with hypertensive heart disease, cardiomyopathy, aortic stenosis or insufficiency, and mitral regurgitation. In general, diseases that cause pressure and volume overload of the left ventricle can result in left ventricular hypertrophy.

Case #36. A 59-year-old gentleman presents with 20 minutes of substernal chest pain that abated spontaneously.

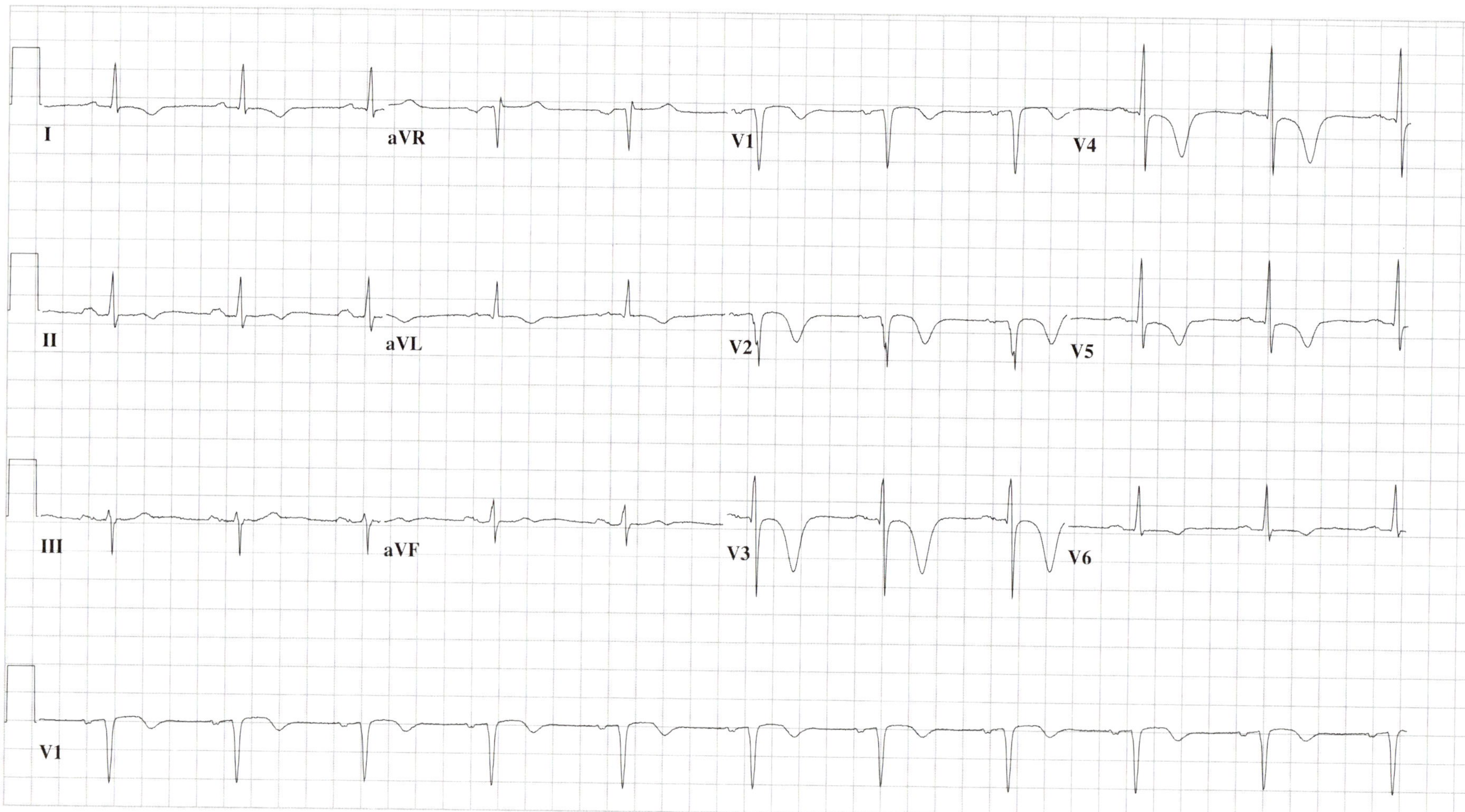

QUESTIONS

36-1. What is the diagnosis?

36-2. What would you do next?

83
P2-4AC
15.0 cm MI 0.9
Gen TIs 1.1
[2d] G78/71 d
FA4/P90
HAR/FSI0
[C] G50/0.80 kHz
FA5/F1/B
TDI
S-T
interval
2.5
3
Time (s)
3.5

ANSWERS

36-1. What is the diagnosis?

This ECG demonstrates normal sinus rhythm with normal axis and intervals. There are broad Q waves in V1 and V2 consistent with a myocardial infarction of indeterminate age in the septal distribution. Deep, symmetric T-wave inversions are present in the septal leads V1 and V2 and the anterior leads V3, V4, and V5. The presence of T-wave inversions with this deep, narrow, symmetric morphology in an anterior distribution and a chest pain history is called Wellens syndrome. This syndrome suggests a severe stenosis of the proximal left anterior descending coronary artery.[1]

36-2. What would you do next?

This patient presents with self-limited chest pain and a Wellens ECG. The natural history of Wellens syndrome is to progress to anterior ST-segment elevation myocardial infarction; therefore, this patient should be treated with aggressive medical therapy for unstable angina and referred for expeditious coronary angiography with PCI if the anticipated finding of proximal LAD stenosis is confirmed.

[1] Rhinehardt J, Brady WJ, Perron AD, et al. Electrocardiographic manifestations of Wellens' syndrome. *Am J Emerg Med* 2002; 20: 638-643.

Case #37. A 62-year-old gentleman transferred for further management of ST elevation MI.

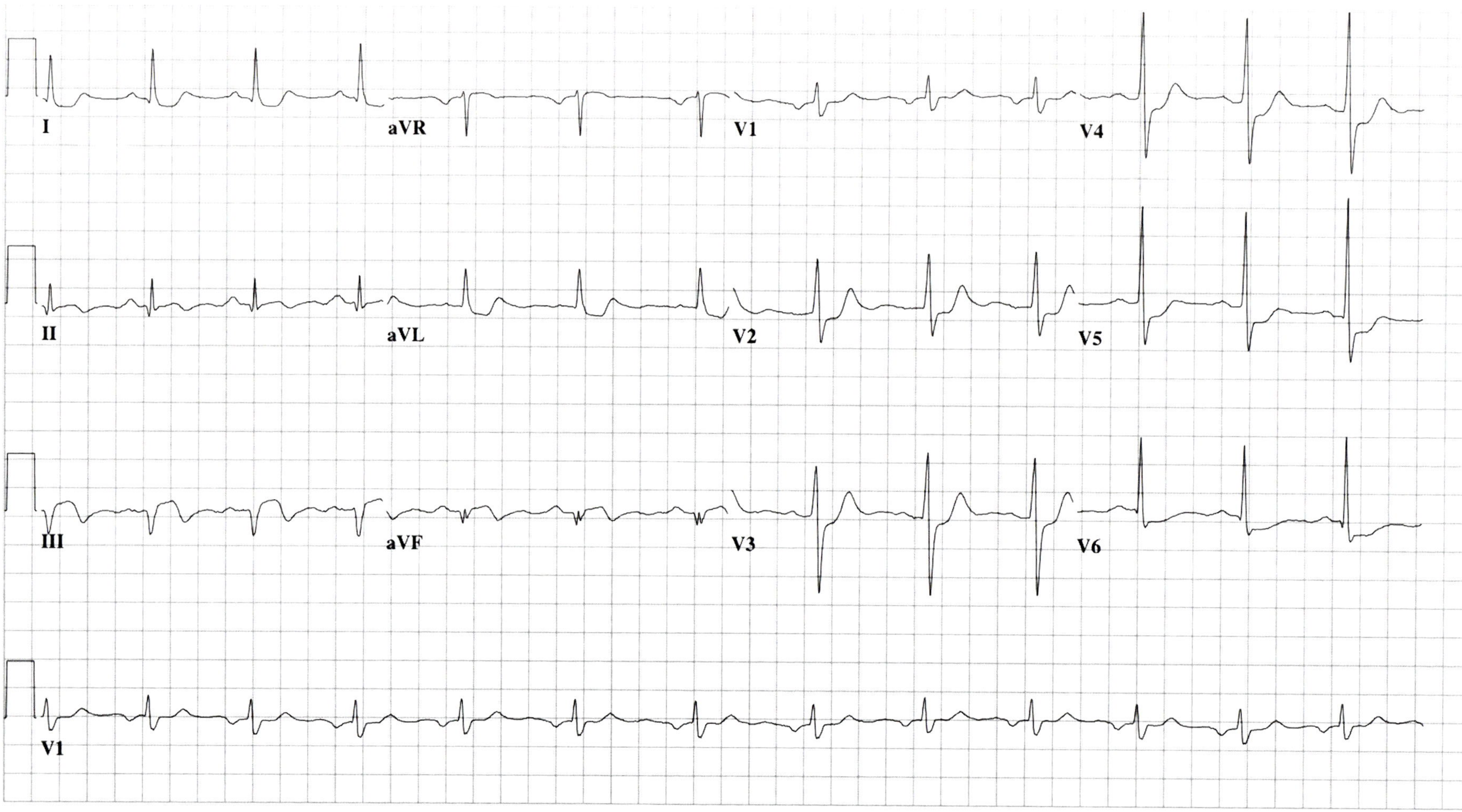

QUESTIONS

37-1. What abnormalities are present?

37-2. What is the differential diagnosis of the tall R wave in lead V1?

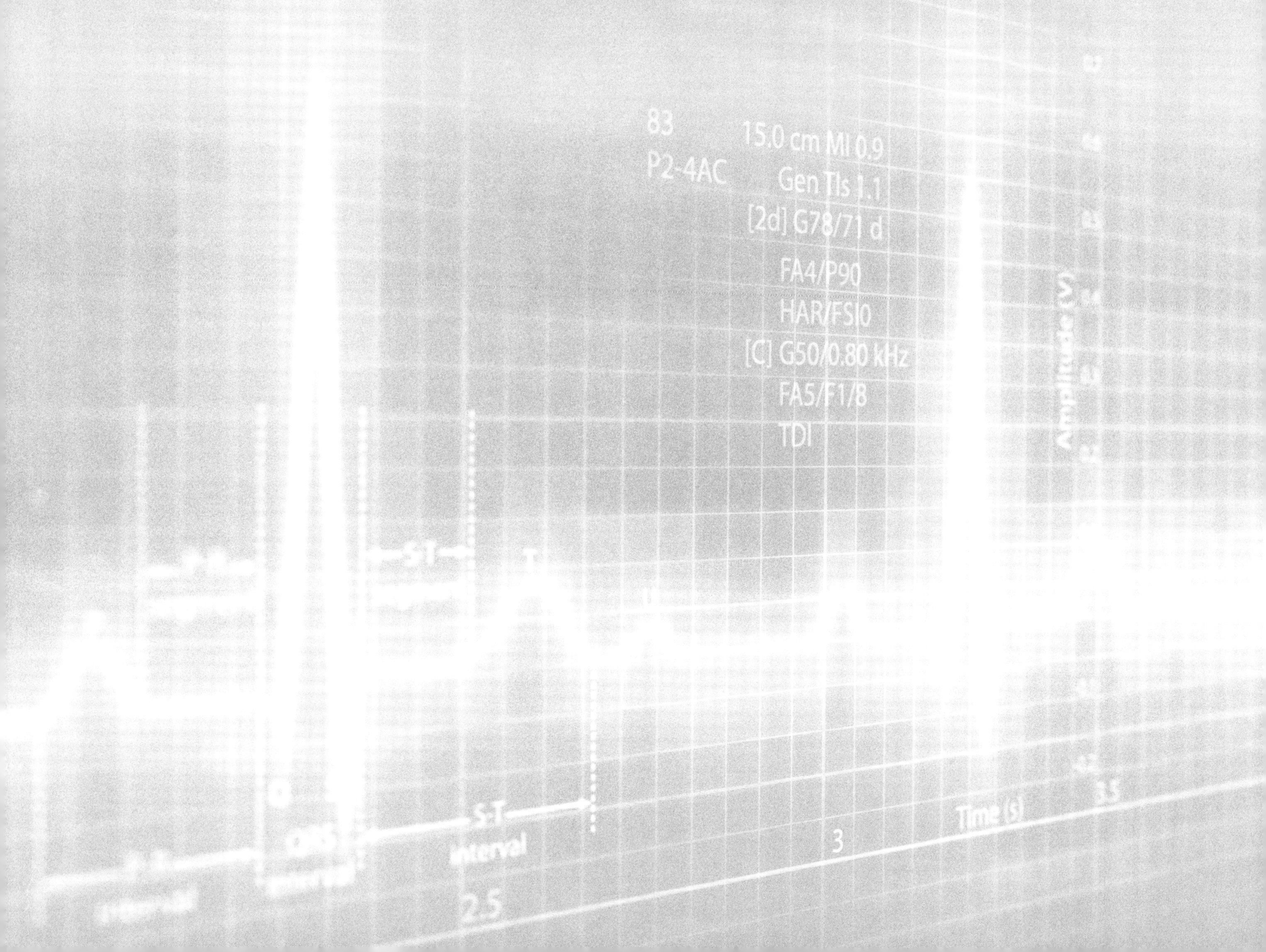
83
P2-4AC
15.0 cm MI 0.9
Gen TIs 1.1
[2d] G78/71 d
FA4/P90
HAR/FSI0
[C] G50/0.80 kHz
FA5/F1/8
TDI
Amplitude (V)
S-T
T
S-T
interval
2.5
3
Time (s)
3.5

ANSWERS

37-1. What abnormalities are present?

This tracing demonstrates sinus rhythm at a rate of 75 beats/min. The axis and intervals are normal. Q waves and ST-segment elevation are seen in leads III and aVF, suggesting an inferior ST-segment elevation myocardial infarction. ST-segment depressions are seen in I, aVL, and V2 through V6 along with an R wave taller than the S wave in V1.

37-2. What is the differential diagnosis of the tall R wave in lead V1?

The differential diagnosis of a tall R wave in V1 includes posterior transmural infarction (posterior STEMI), right ventricular hypertrophy, certain muscular dystrophies, misplacement of the precordial leads, and the Wolff-Parkinson-White pattern. In the setting of inferior STEMI, a tall R wave in V1 coupled with anterior ST depressions is most likely to represent posterior ischemia and infarction (the R wave in V1 is really a posterior Q wave; similarly anterior ST depression is really posterior ST elevation). When patients present with an inferior infarct, closely inspect the right precordial and anterior leads for evidence of posterior involvement.

Case #38. A 74-year-old woman with paroxysmal atrial fibrillation maintained on digoxin.

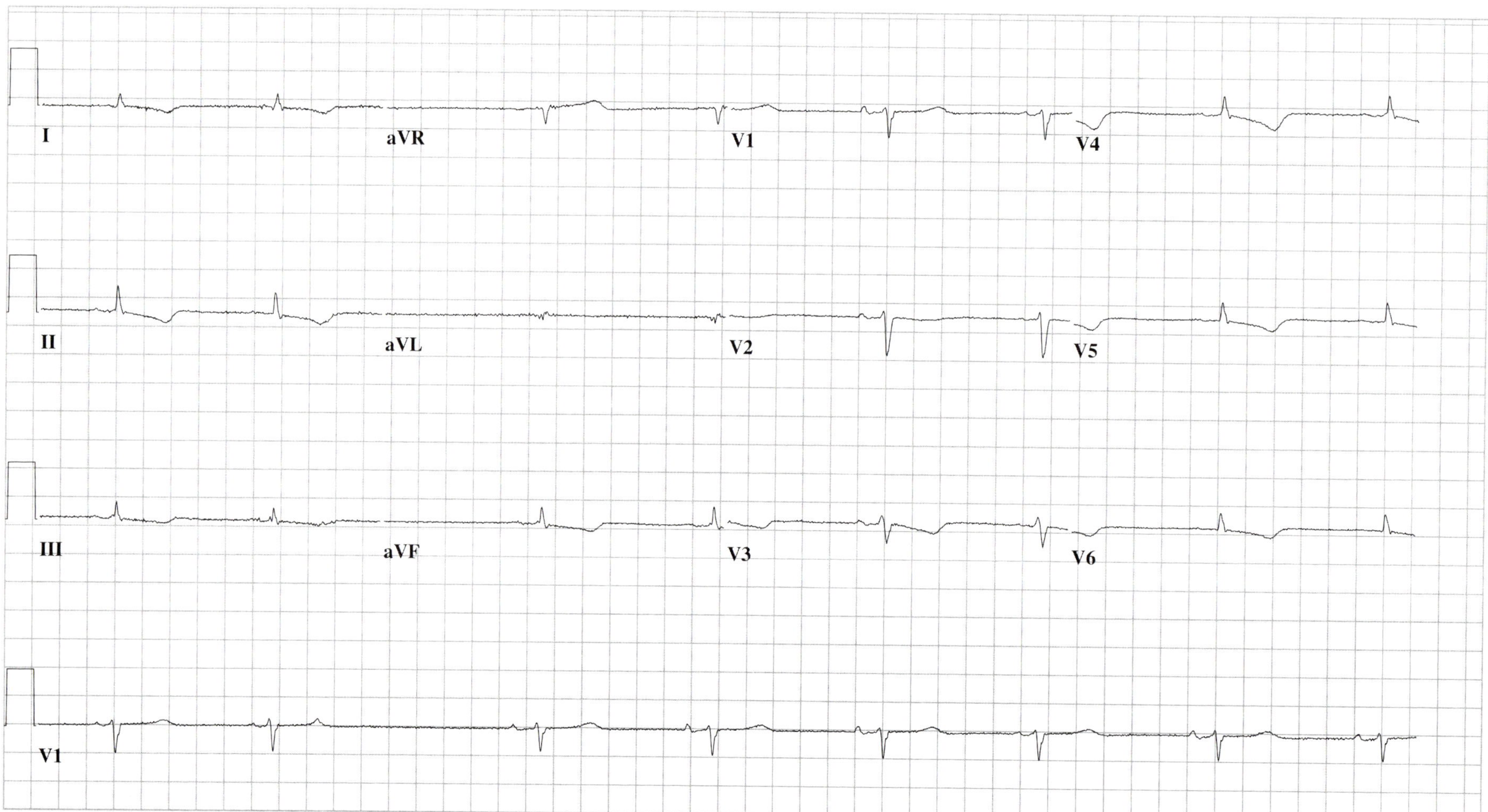

QUESTIONS

38-1. Interpret this tracing.

38-2. How does digitalis affect the heart, and how do serum electrolyte levels impact its action?

38-3. Describe the potential electrocardiographic manifestations of digitalis toxicity.

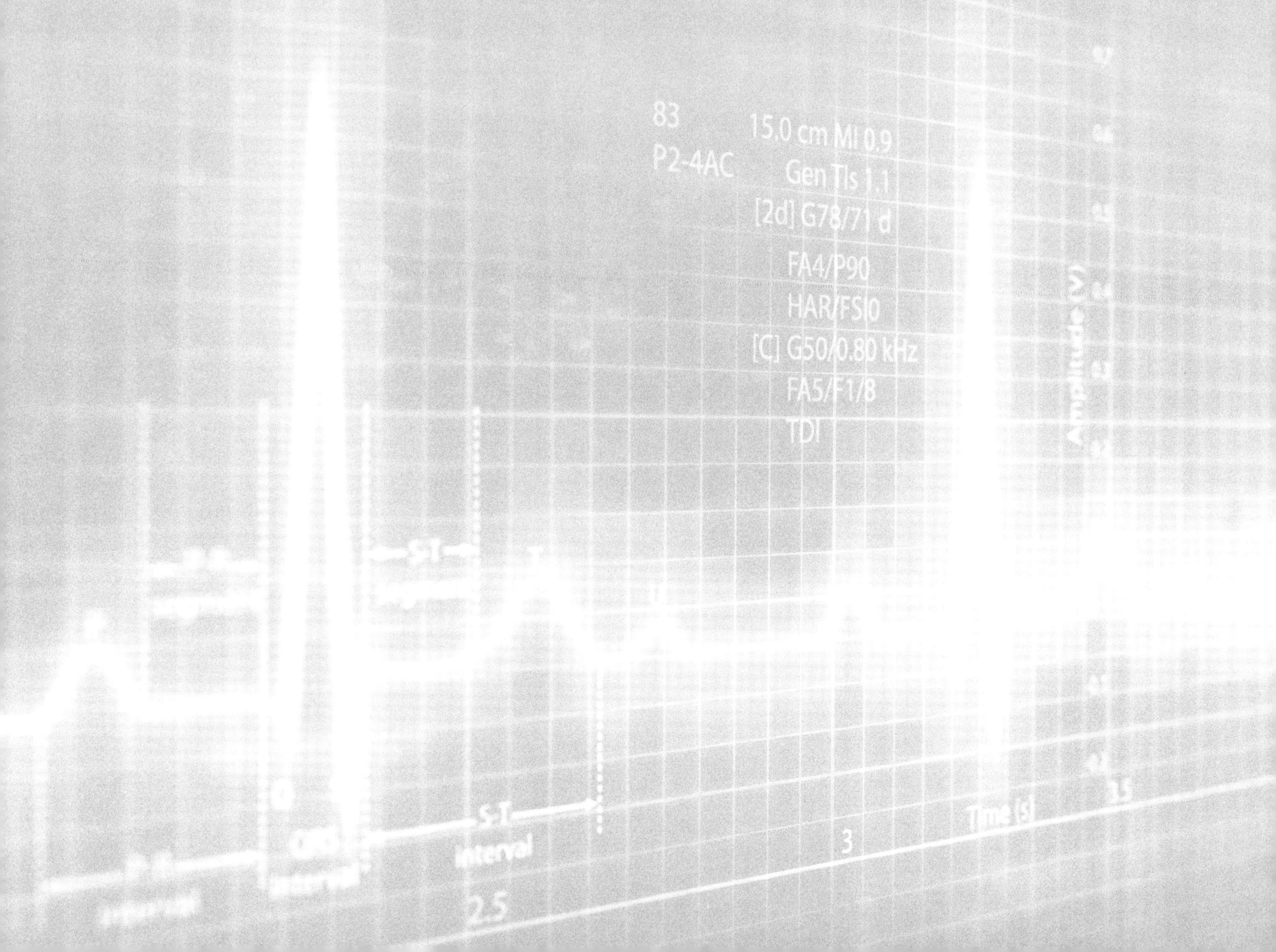
83
P2-4AC
15.0 cm MI 0.9
Gen TIs 1.1
[2d] G78/71 d
FA4/P90
HAR/FS|0
[C] G50/0.80 kHz
FA5/F1/8
TDI
Amplitude (V)
S-T
interval
Time (s)
3
2.5

ANSWERS

38-1. Interpret this tracing.

This ECG reveals a bradycardic rhythm at 46 beats/min. The P waves have multiple morphologies with subtly varying PR and P–P intervals most consistent with a wandering atrial pacemaker. After the second P wave, there is a nearly 2-second pause. Close inspection of the preceding T wave reveals a nonconducted P wave that occurs during the ventricular refractory period as shown in the figure. The QRS axis is normal and the PR, QRS, and corrected QT intervals are normal. QRS voltages are low, as indicated by amplitude of the QRS complex less than 5 mV in all limb leads and less than 10 mV in all precordial leads. There are diffuse abnormalities of the ST segments with inverted T waves—the ST segments slope downward with a "scooped" morphology. This ST-segment appearance is typical of digoxin effect.

38-2. How does digitalis affect the heart, and how do serum electrolyte levels impact its action?

Digitalis directly inhibits sodium/potassium adenosine triphosphatase (Na/K ATPase) at the myocardial cell membrane. In an energy-dependent manner, this enzyme transports sodium and potassium against concentration gradients to maintain the myocardial resting membrane potential and high potassium and low sodium concentrations within cardiac myocytes. Inhibition of Na/K ATPase by digitalis results in an increase in intracellular sodium concentration. This increase in intracellular sodium inhibits activity of a second transporter, a sodium/calcium (Na/Ca) exchanger, which moves calcium out of cells in exchange for inward flux of sodium down its concentration gradient. In this manner, digitalis results in an increase in intracellular calcium concentration. Effects of digitalis include increased inotropy, slowed conduction velocity and increased refractoriness in conducting tissue, and enhanced automaticity. Digitalis effect may be potentiated by hypokalemia, as reduced extracellular potassium concentrations further decrease the activity of Na/K ATPase; hypomagnesemia, which also inhibits Na/K ATPase; and hypercalcemia, as higher extracellular calcium concentrations further decrease Na/Ca exchange.

ANSWERS (Cont.)

38-3. Describe the potential electrocardiographic manifestations of digitalis toxicity.

Early digitalis toxicity is mediated by increased vagal tone and manifests as depression of SA and AV nodal conduction. Enhanced automaticity can precipitate ectopic rhythms, including atrial premature beats and tachyarrhythmias, junctional tachycardia, ventricular premature beats, ventricular tachycardia (including bidirectional ventricular tachycardia), and ventricular fibrillation. Advanced depression of SA and AV nodal conduction may lead to high-grade second-degree and third-degree SA and AV block.

A P wave that occurs during the ventricular refractory period is shown with an arrow, slightly deforming the preceding T wave.

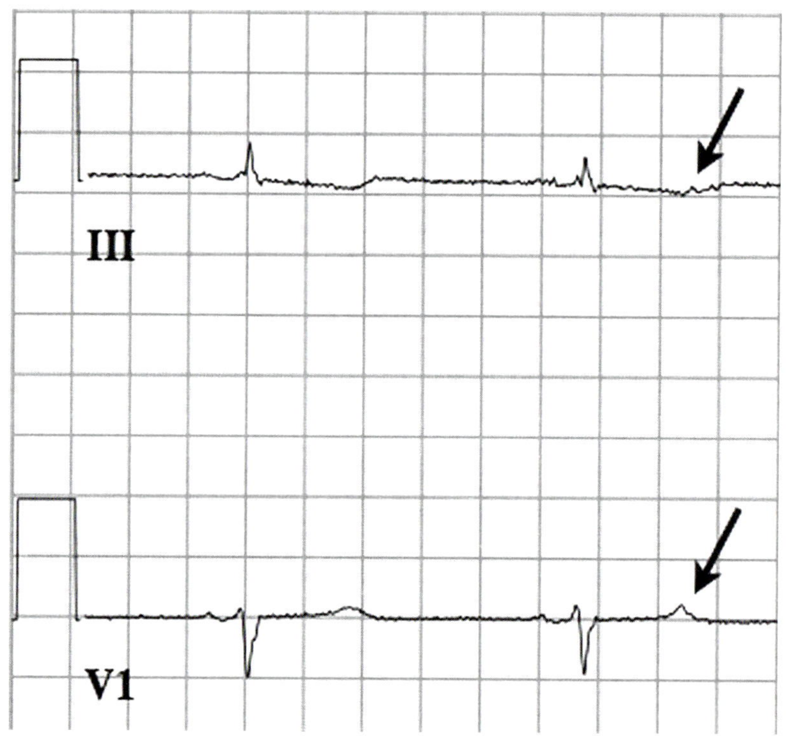

Case #39. An 81-year-old woman with COPD presents for follow-up.

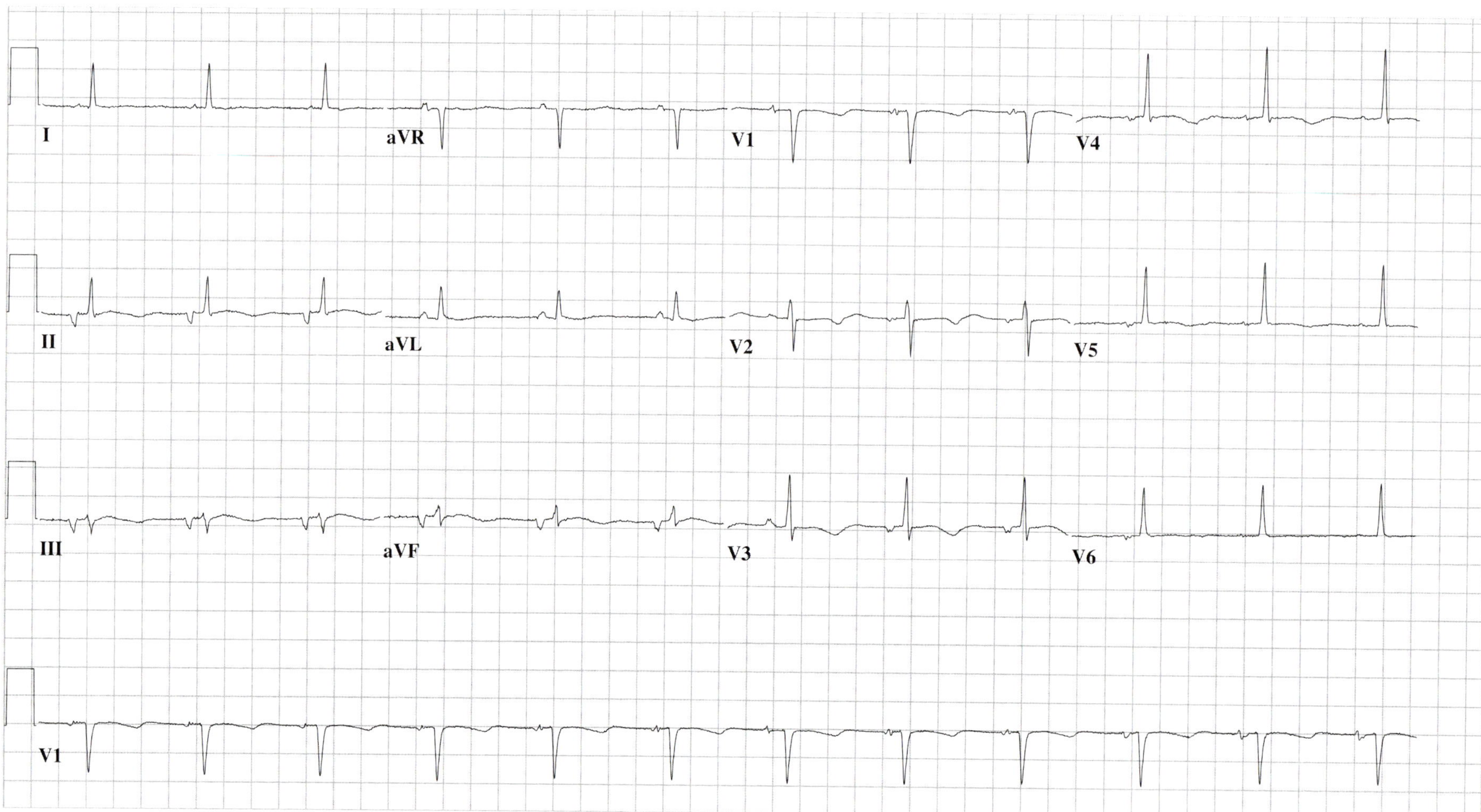

QUESTION

39-1. What does the ECG show? What is the rhythm?

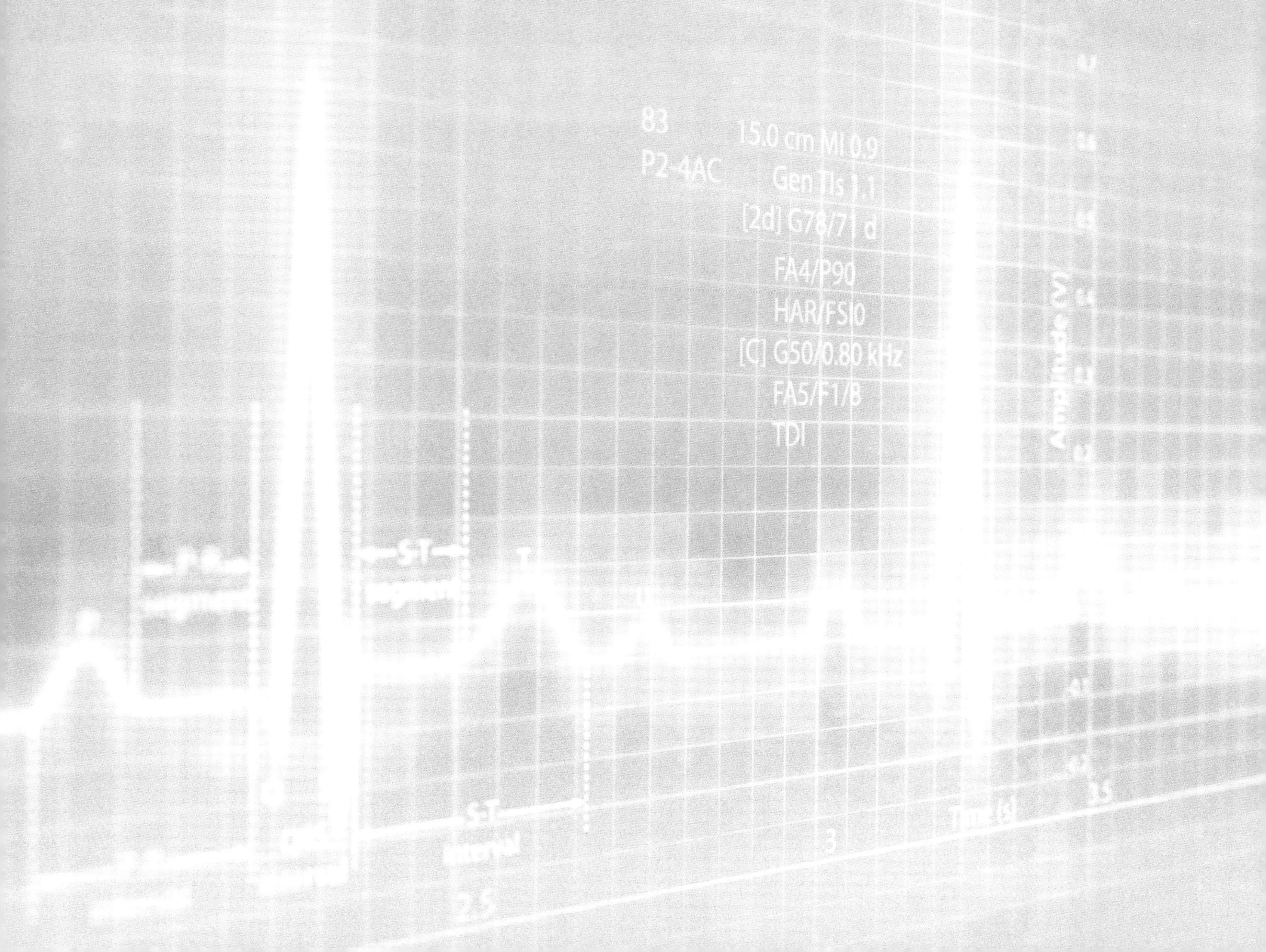
83
P2-4AC
15.0 cm MI 0.9
Gen TIs 1.1
[2d] G78/71 d
FA4/P90
HAR/FSI0
[C] G50/0.80 kHz
FA5/F1/8
TDI
Amplitude (V)
S-T
Time (s)
2.5
3
3.5

ANSWER

39-1. What does the ECG show? What is the rhythm?

The heart rate is 72 beats/min. There is atrial activity preceding each QRS complex, but the P waves are not normal in morphology. Normal sinus P waves should be upright in leads I and II and inverted or biphasic in lead V1. This polarity reflects the anatomic fact that the sinus node is located in the upper right atrium, with impulses depolarizing the atria by moving inferiorly and laterally generating positive P waves in those leads. In contrast, the P waves seen in this tracing have a sharp negative contour in the inferior leads, are isoelectric in lead I, and triphasic in lead V1. These are nonsinus P waves, and the rhythm is categorized as an ectopic atrial rhythm. Otherwise, the axis is normal, the T waves are diffusely flat-to-inverted, and the QT interval is prolonged. There is a U wave seen in lead V2.

Atrial arrhythmias are common in patients with severe COPD and likely reflect right heart strain and right atrial enlargement. If this rhythm is well tolerated, there is no indication for specific treatment aside from optimizing management of the underlying lung disease.

Case #40. A 63-year-old man with hypertension appreciates "skipped beats" when measuring his radial pulse.

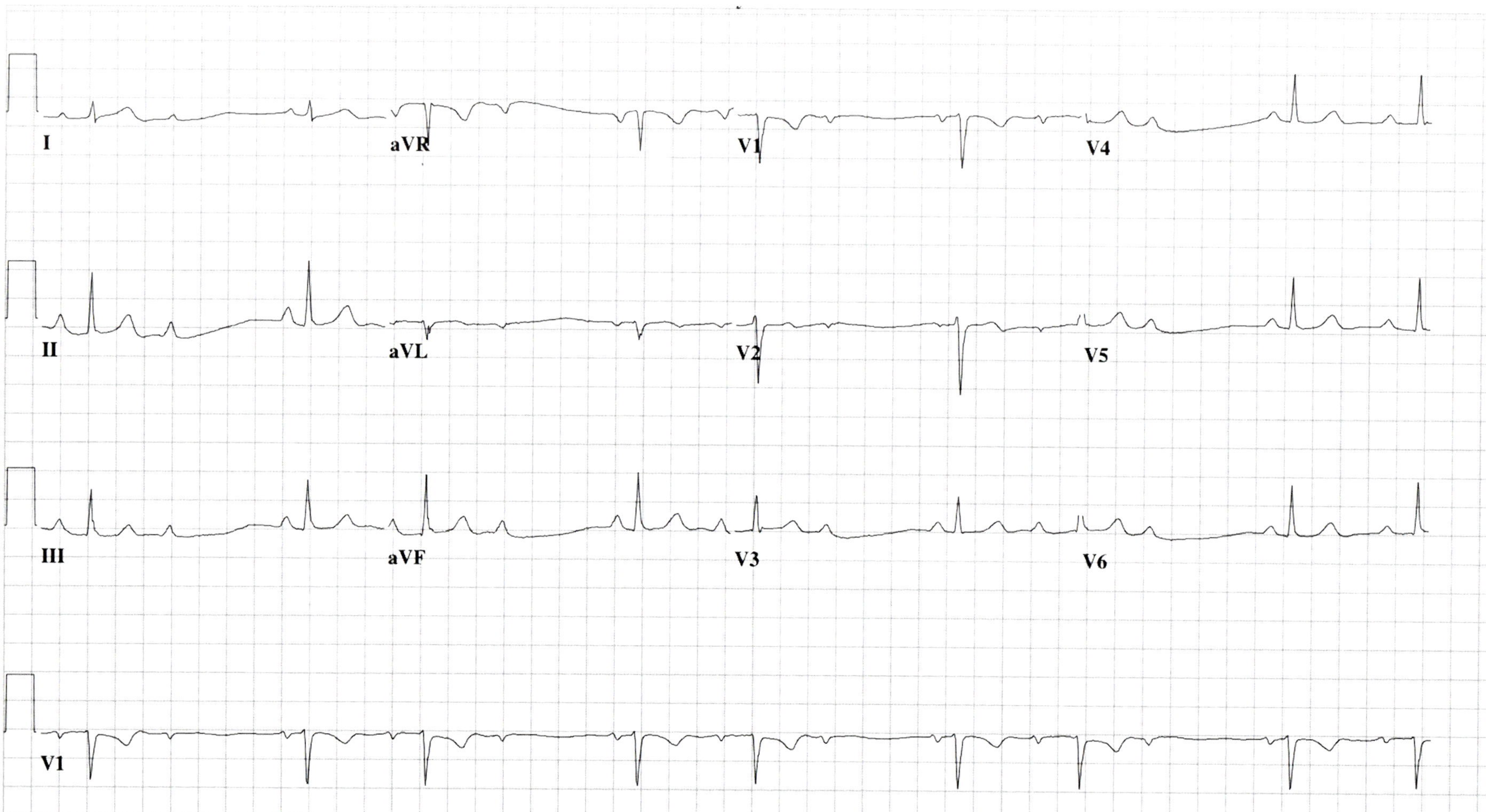

QUESTION

40-1. Interpret this ECG. What rhythm is present?

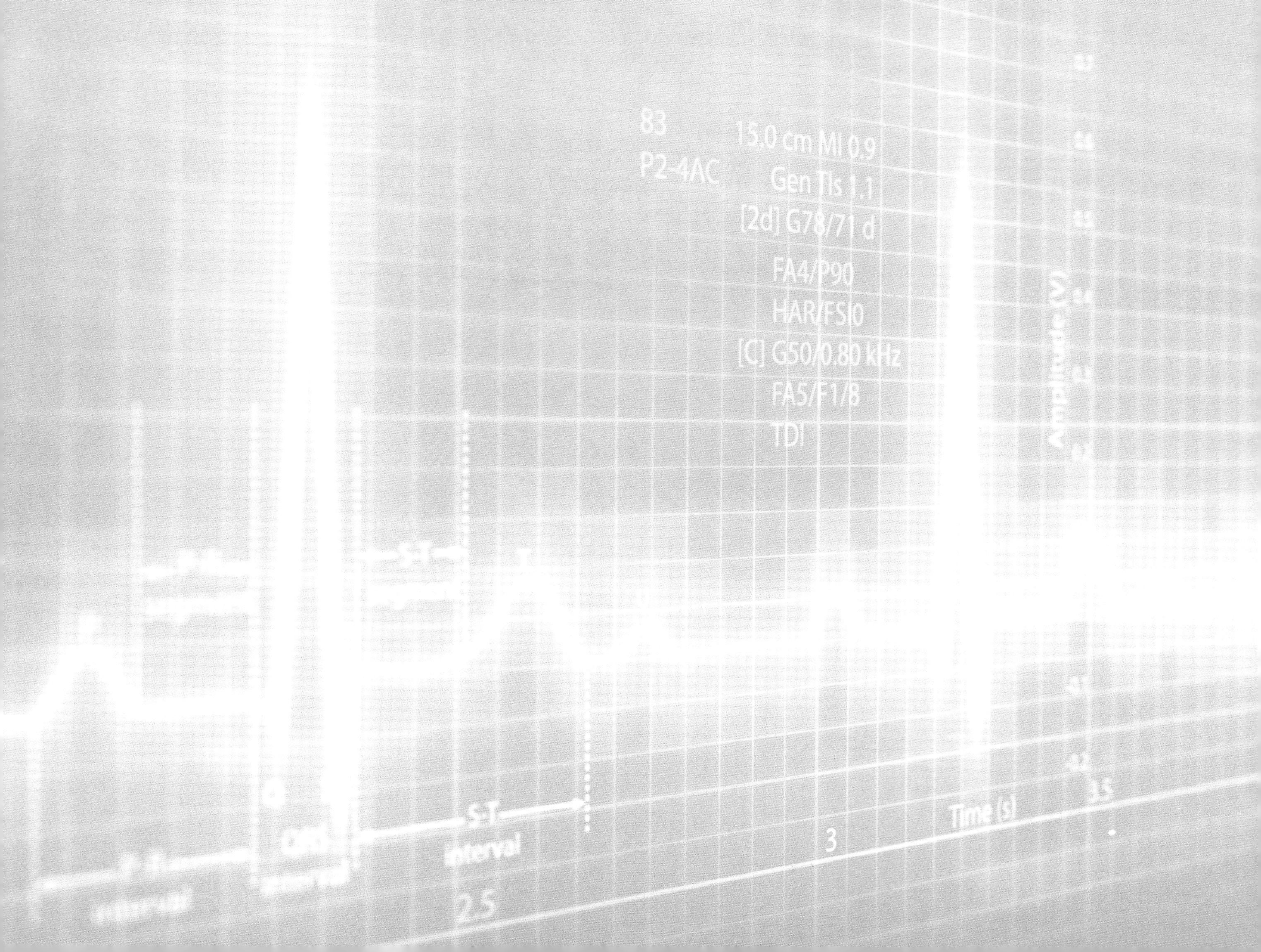
83
15.0 cm MI 0.9
P2-4AC
Gen TIs 1.1
[2d] G78/71 d
FA4/P90
HAR/FSI0
[C] G50/0.80 kHz
FA5/F1/8
TDI
Amplitude (V)
S-T
interval
2.5
3
Time (s)
3.5

ANSWER

40-1. Interpret this ECG. What rhythm is present?

Normal sinus rhythm is present—there are regular P waves at a rate of 75 beats/min. The P waves are upright in the inferior leads and biphasic in lead V1 confirming sinus origin. Each QRS is preceded by a P wave, yet not each P wave is followed by a QRS, suggesting that A-V block is present. The rhythm strip demonstrates cycles of two conducted QRS complexes with progressive lengthening of the PR interval followed by a nonconducted P wave. This confirms a diagnosis of Mobitz I second-degree heart block, or Wenckebach-type heart block. The frontal plane QRS axis is normal, the QRS is narrow, and QT interval is normal, and there are no ST-segment or T-wave abnormalities.

Case #41. A 48-year-old gentleman presents with dyspnea. A diastolic rumbling murmur is heard over the cardiac apex.

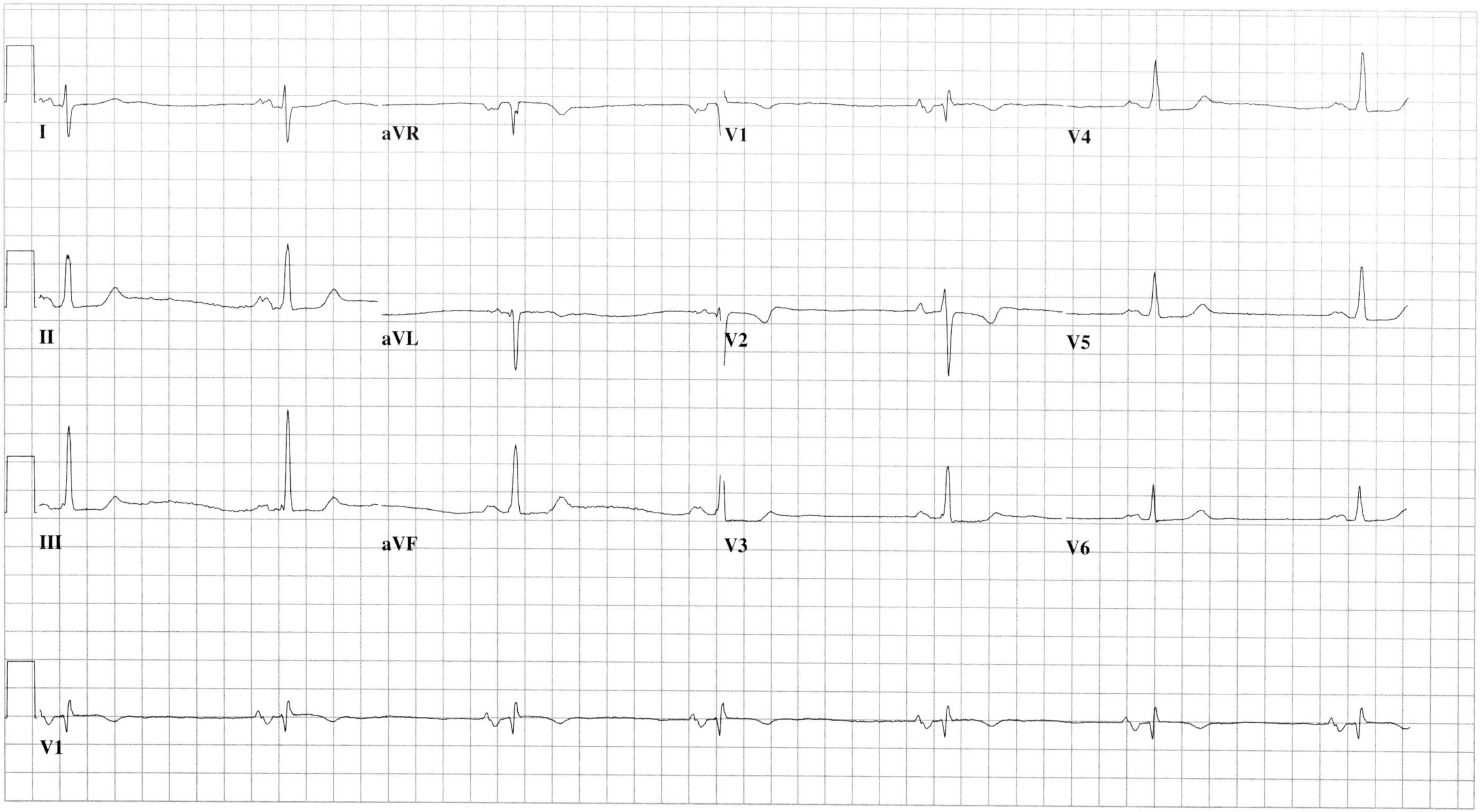

QUESTIONS

41-1. What are the ECG findings?

41-2. What might you visualize on an echocardiogram?

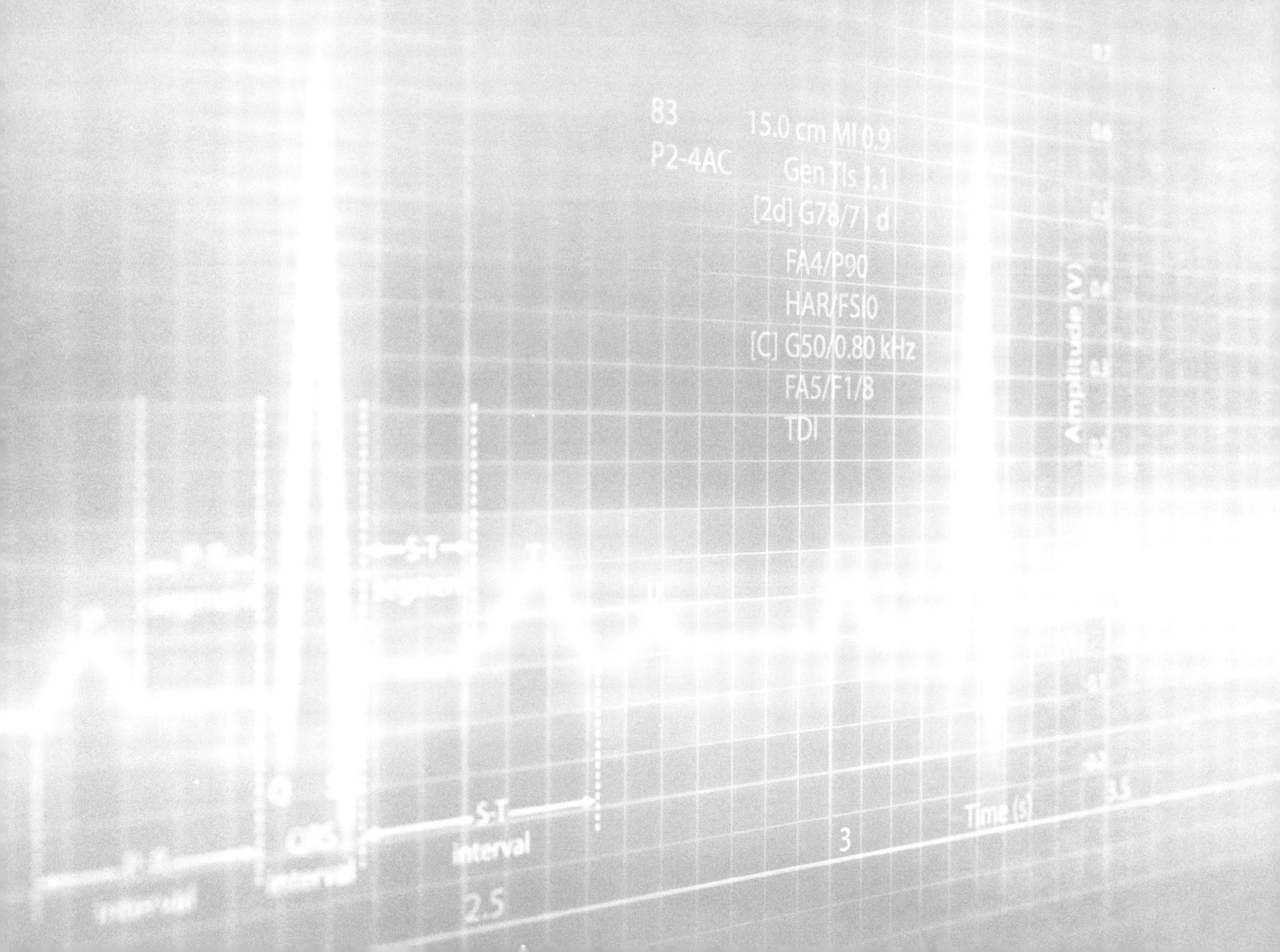
83
P2-4AC
15.0 cm MI 0.9
Gen TIs 1.1
[2d] G78/71 d
FA4/P90
HAR/FSI0
[C] G50/0.80 kHz
FA5/F1/8
TDI
Amplitude (V)
S-T
interval
2.5
3
Time (s)
3.5

ANSWERS

41-1. What are the ECG findings?

There is sinus bradycardia at a rate of 42 beats/min. The QRS axis is rightward (negative polarity in lead I and positive polarity in leads II and aVF). The QRS complex is narrow, and QT and PR intervals are normal. There is a qR complex in lead V1 with the R-wave amplitude equal to the q-wave amplitude. This finding in combination with the rightward axis suggests right ventricular hypertrophy. Furthermore, there is a notched P wave broader than 120 milliseconds in lead II consistent with left atrial abnormality. There are T-wave inversions in leads V1 and V2 with nonspecific ST-segment abnormalities in V1 through V3, aVL, and the inferior limb leads.

41-2. What might you visualize on an echocardiogram?

The ECG combination of right ventricular hypertrophy and left atrial abnormality suggests mitral stenosis. The stenotic and obstructed mitral valve leads to increased left atrial pressure and, over time, that pressure is transmitted back across the pulmonary circuit leading to pulmonary hypertension and right ventricular hypertrophy. The diastolic murmur described is also consistent with mitral stenosis. On echocardiogram, features of rheumatic mitral stenosis include fusion of the mitral valve commissures, a characteristic "fish-mouth" appearance of the mitral valve, and variable amounts of calcification of the valvular apparatus.

Case #42. A 56-year-old gentleman with end-stage renal disease presents with nausea after missing a dialysis treatment.

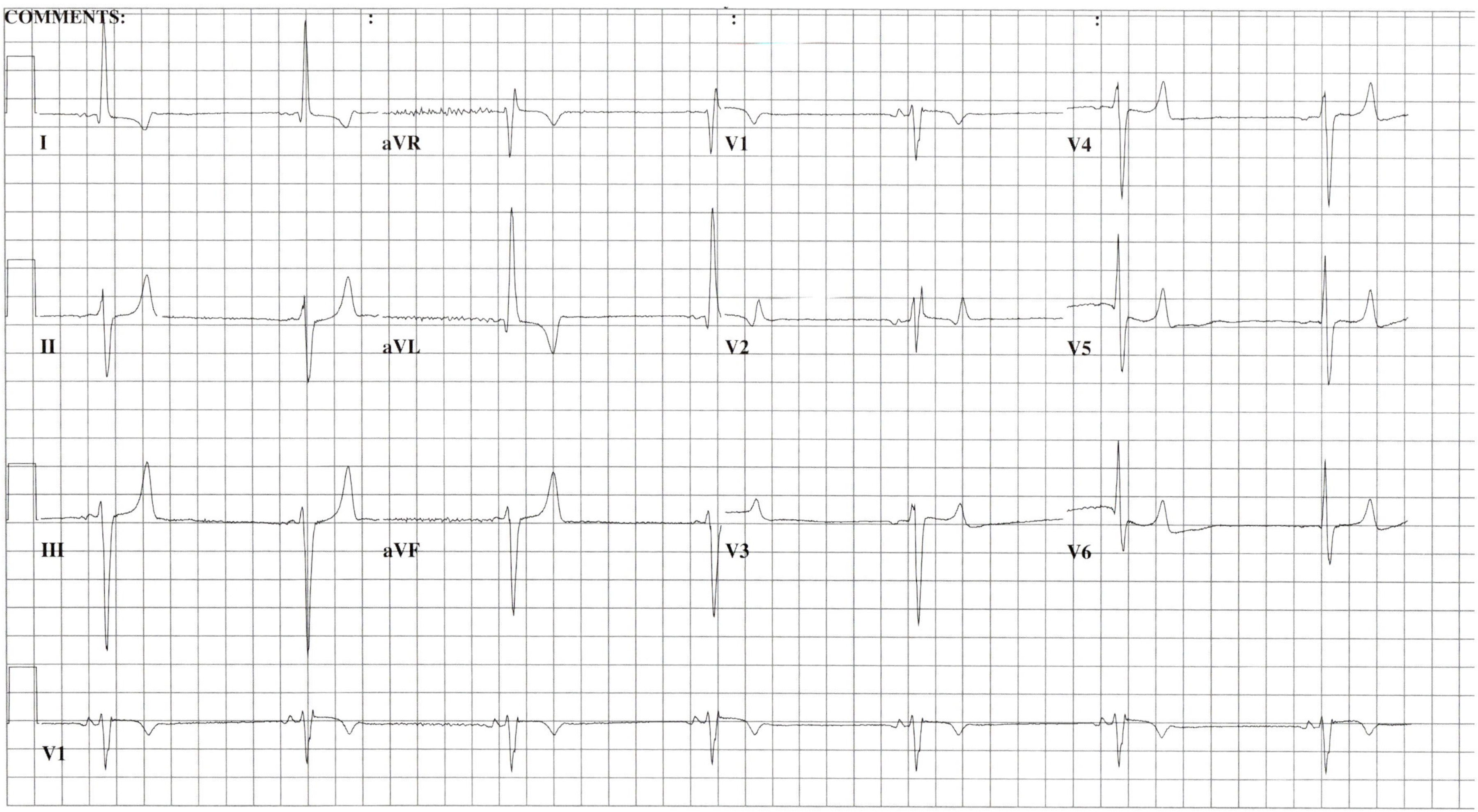

QUESTION

42-1. **What findings are present on this tracing?**

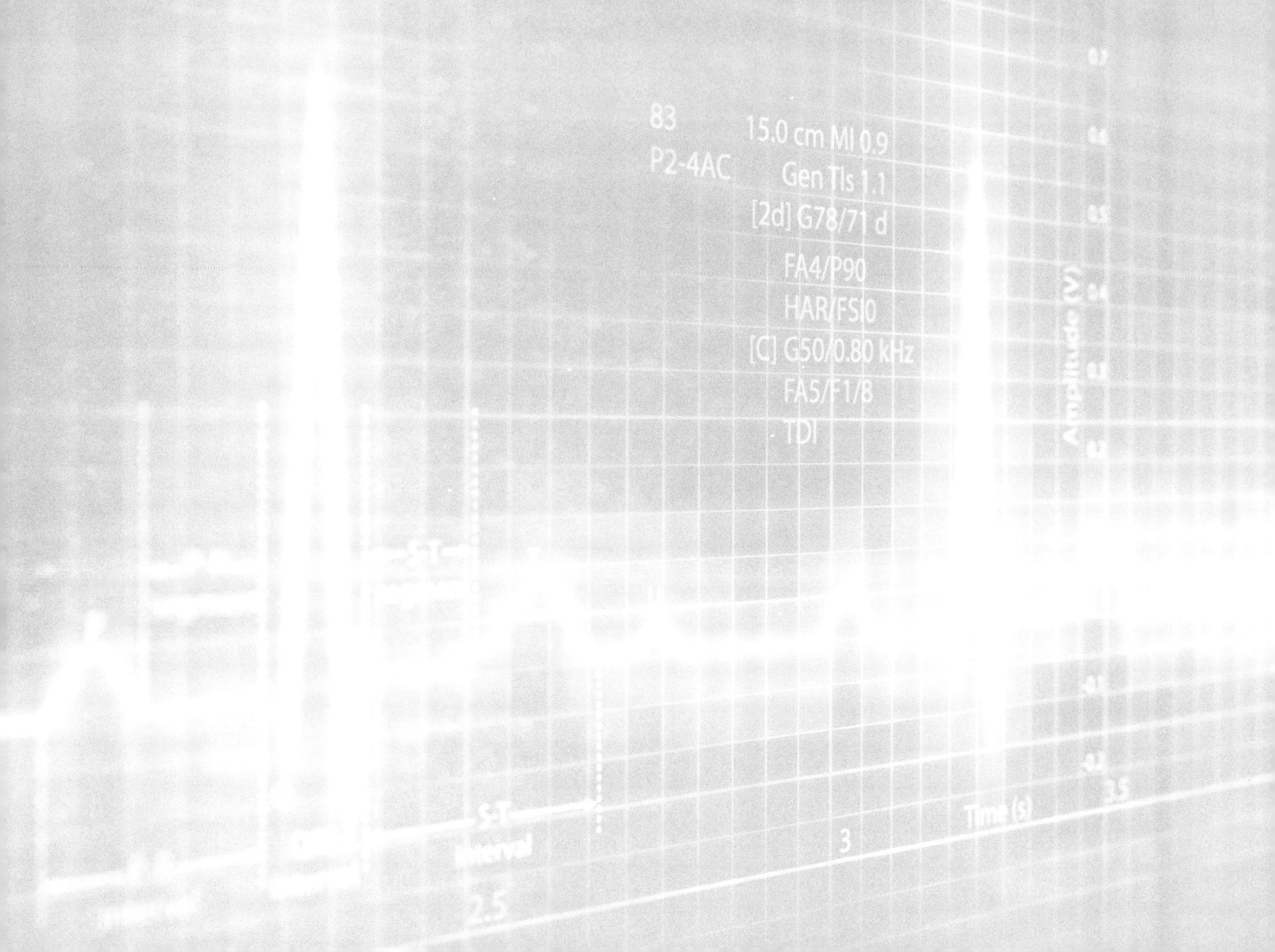
83
P2-4AC
15.0 cm MI 0.9
Gen TIs 1.1
[2d] G78/71 d
FA4/P90
HAR/FS|0
[C] G50/0.80 kHz
FA5/F1/8
TDI
Amplitude (V)
S-T
Interval
Time (s)
2.5
3
3.5

ANSWER

42-1. What findings are present on this tracing?

The rate is bradycardic at 42 beats/min. There are P waves seen before each QRS, but the P waves have an abnormal morphology—biphasic in lead I and isoelectric in lead II consistent with an ectopic atrial rhythm. Given the heart rate, the rhythm is best classified as an ectopic atrial bradycardia. The axis is leftward with small R waves and large S waves inferiorly and small Q waves with large R waves in leads I and aVL consistent with left anterior fascicular block. When left anterior fascicular block is present, the diagnosis of left ventricular hypertrophy becomes more complicated and necessitates both the presence of voltage abnormalities and the presence of ST-segment abnormalities. Both are present in this tracing diagnostic of left ventricular hypertrophy. In addition, there are narrow-based, sharply pointed T waves consistent with hyperkalemia. The abnormal T waves are best visualized in leads II, III, and aVF as well as the anterior precordial leads. It is important to evaluate not only T-wave height but also T-wave morphology when assessing hyperkalemia—the T waves become narrow based and pointed.

Case #43. A 62-year-old gentleman with chest pain.

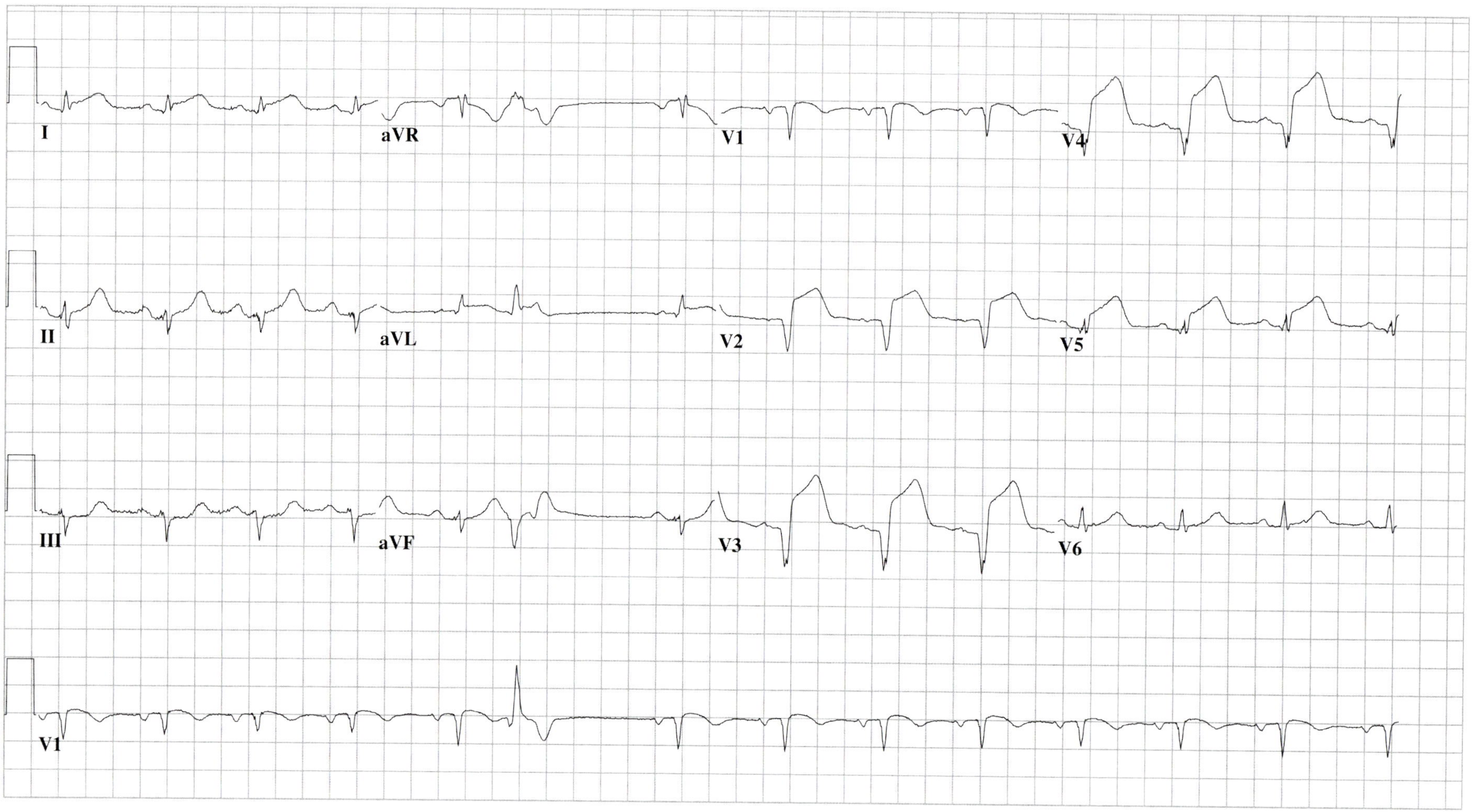

QUESTIONS

43-1. Interpret this ECG: which coronary artery is diseased?

43-2. Which drugs would you prescribe while arranging reperfusion?

83
P2-4AC
15.0 cm MI 0.9
Gen Tls 1.1
[2d] G78/71 d
FA4/P90
HAR/FSI0
[C] G50/0.80 kHz
FA5/F1/B
TDI
Amplitude (V)
S-T
Segment
S-T
interval
T
2.5
3
Time (s)

ANSWERS

43-1. Interpret this ECG: which coronary artery is diseased?

This ECG demonstrates sinus rhythm at a rate of approximately 90 beats/min. The sixth beat is a premature ventricular contraction with a retrograde P wave seen hidden in the ST segment. The axis is leftward. The most striking finding is pathologic Q waves with ST-segment elevation in leads V1 and V2 (septal leads) and V3 through V5 (anterior leads). In leads I and aVL (the "high-lateral" leads), there is ST-segment elevation with very subtle, small Q waves that do not yet meet criteria to be called pathologic. Q waves can be considered pathologic if they are broader than 20 milliseconds in leads V2 and V3 or broader than 40 milliseconds and deeper than 1 mV in all other leads.[1] Thus, this tracing provides evidence for ST-segment elevation myocardial infarction in the anteroseptal and lateral leads. This most likely represents occlusion of the left anterior descending coronary artery.

43-2. Which drugs would you prescribe while arranging reperfusion?

Immediate medical therapy of myocardial infarction should include aspirin to inhibit platelet activity, typically 4 baby aspirin chewed to speed absorption and avoid first-pass metabolism in the liver. Supplemental oxygen should be utilized, and nitroglycerine and morphine can be given to control pain and decrease myocardial oxygen consumption, assuming the patient is not hypotensive. Finally, urgent reperfusion via percutaneous coronary intervention or thrombolytic therapy should be arranged.

[1]Thygesen K, Alpert JS, Simoons ML, et al. Third universal definition of myocardial infarction. *J Am Coll Cardiol* 2012; 60: 1581-1598.

Case #44. A 62-year-old male complains of a racing heart.

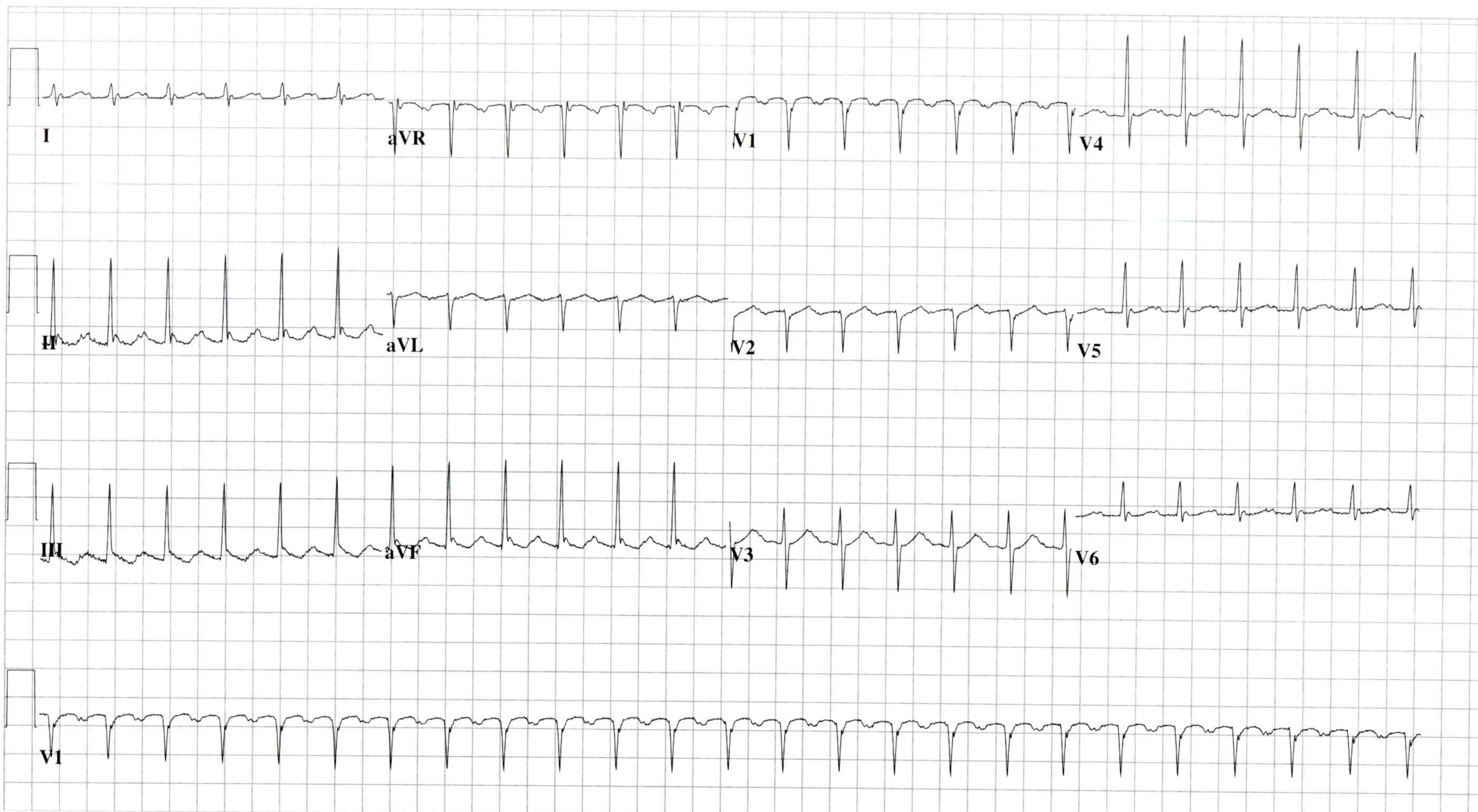

QUESTIONS

44-1. What is the rhythm disturbance?

44-2. What is the recommended management strategy?

83
P2-4AC
15.0 cm MI 0.9
Gen TIs 1.1
[2d] G78/71 d
FA4/P90
HAR/FS|0
[C] G50/0.80 kHz
FA5/F1/B
TDI
Amplitude (V)
S-T
S-T
interval
QRS
interval
P-R
interval
2.5
3
3.5
Time (s)

ANSWERS

44-1. What is the rhythm disturbance?

This is a regular narrow complex tachycardia with ventricular rate of almost exactly 150 beats/min. Atrial activity with a "sawtooth" morphology is seen best in the inferior leads illustrated in the figure. This represents atrial flutter with 2:1 AV block—meaning only every other flutter wave is conducted. The underlying atrial rate is 300 beats/min leading to a ventricular rate of 150 beats/min. Atrial flutter should be strongly considered in any patient presenting with a regular supraventricular tachycardia at a rate of 150 beats/min. Additional findings include normal axis, normal intervals, no evidence of enlargement or hypertrophy, and Q waves in leads V1 and V2.

44-2. What is the recommended management strategy?

Similar to atrial fibrillation, the ventricular rate of atrial flutter can be managed using AV nodal blockers such as calcium channel blockers, β-blockers, and digoxin. Ventricular rate is often more challenging to control as compared to patients with atrial fibrillation. Hemodynamically unstable patients with atrial flutter should undergo urgent DC cardioversion. Typical atrial flutter is caused by a reentrant circuit involving the cavo-tricuspid isthmus. Radiofrequency ablation in this anatomic area can be curative and is the preferred long-term management.

Sawtooth waves are marked with bold line. These sawtooth waves are classic for atrial flutter.

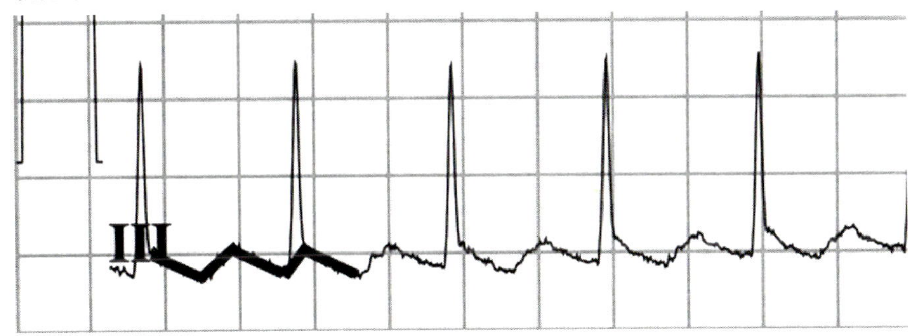

Case #45. A 45-year-old woman undergoing chemotherapy for lymphoma presents with chest pain, cough, and hypoxemia.

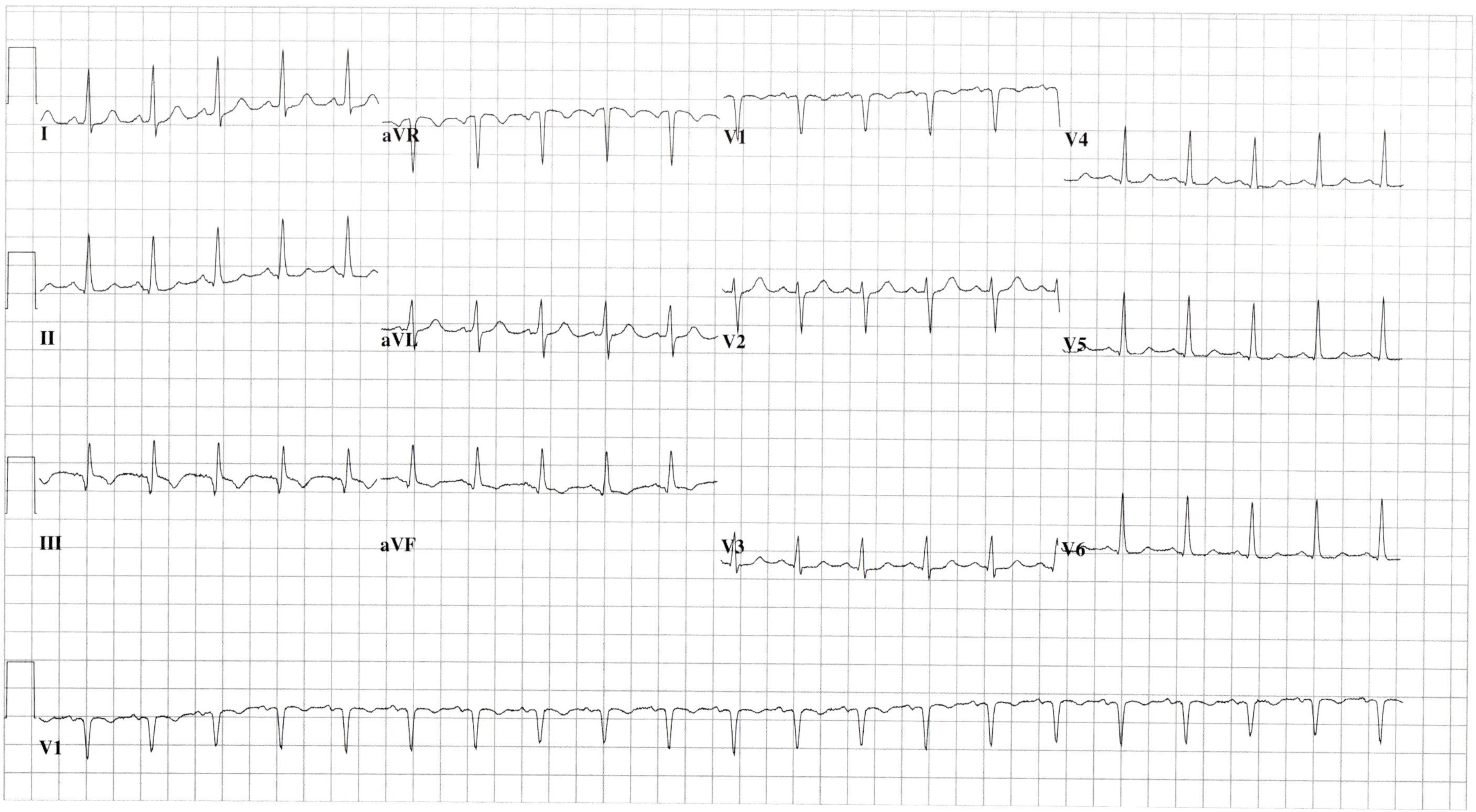

QUESTIONS

45-1. What are the findings?

45-2. What study would you order next?

83
P2-4AC
15.0 cm MI 0.9
Gen Tls 1.1
[2d] G78/71 d
FA4/P90
HAR/FS10
[C] G50/0.80 kHz
FA5/F1/8
TDI
Amplitude (V)
S-T
interval
2.5
3
Time (s)
3.5

ANSWERS

45-1. What are the findings?

The rhythm is sinus tachycardia at a rate of 126 beats/min. The QRS axis is normal. There is a Q wave in lead III with an inverted T wave in this lead coupled with an S wave in lead I. The "S1-QIII-TIII" pattern is associated with pulmonary embolism as well as any syndrome that causes acute right heart strain. The $S_1Q_3T_3$ pattern is uncommon, however, and often only sinus rhythm or sinus tachycardia is present.

45-2. What study would you order next?

The clinical history and ECG suggest pulmonary embolism; the patient's active malignancy also places her at risk. Anticoagulation should be initiated empirically, while CT pulmonary angiogram or ventilation-perfusion scanning is performed to confirm the diagnosis.

Case #46. A 33-year-old gentleman with familial hypercholesterolemia presenting with 28 hours of ongoing severe jaw pain and vomiting.

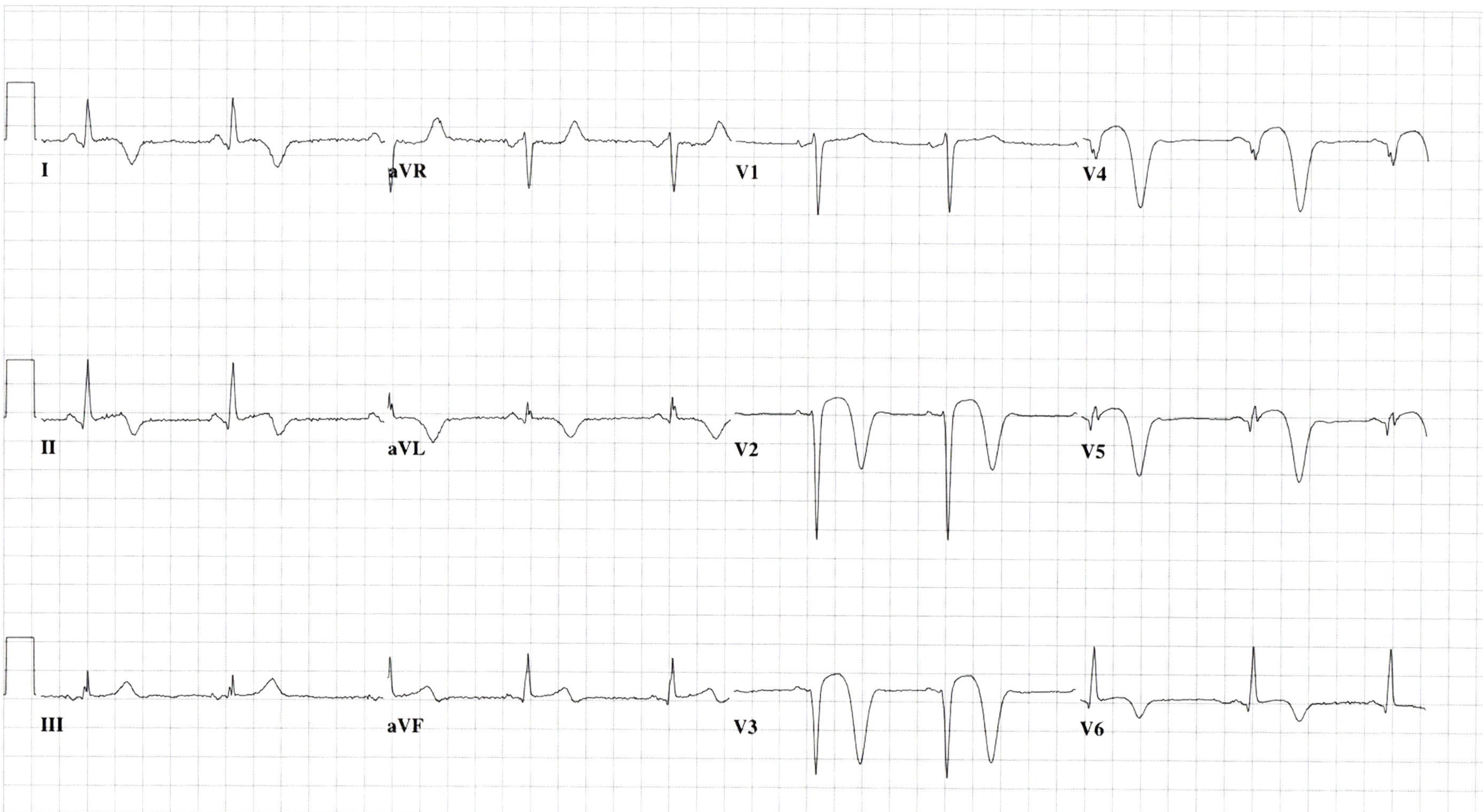

QUESTIONS

46-1. What is the ECG diagnosis?

46-2. What would you do next?

83
P2-4AC
15.0 cm MI 0.9
Gen TIs 1.1
[2d] G78/71 d
FA4/P90
HAR/FSI0
[C] G50/0.80 kHz
FA5/F1/8
TDI
Amplitude (V)
S-T
interval
2.5
3
Time (s)
3.5

ANSWERS

46-1. What is the ECG diagnosis?

There is sinus bradycardia at 60 beats/min. The axis is normal. There are Q waves, ST-segment elevation, and deep symmetric T-wave inversions best seen in leads V2 through V5. T-wave inversion alone is present in leads I, aVL, V6, and II. The pathologic Q waves and deep T-wave inversions suggest myocardial injury with infarction that has been evolving over time, as the deep T-wave inversions with Q waves often appear late in the course of acute infarction. This ECG demonstrates classic findings and the typical appearance of an acute infarction presenting late in the course of illness.

46-2. What would you do next?

Despite the late presentation, this patient has ongoing ST-segment elevation and ongoing ischemic symptoms. For patients who present with symptom onset greater than 12 hours prior and have ongoing ischemic symptoms, hemodynamic instability, or malignant arrhythmia, it is recommended to pursue revascularization. Angioplasty and stenting of the infarct-related artery is preferable to administration of fibrinolysis for patients presenting late as in this case.

Case #47. A 46-year-old man with chest pain and rhinorrhea.

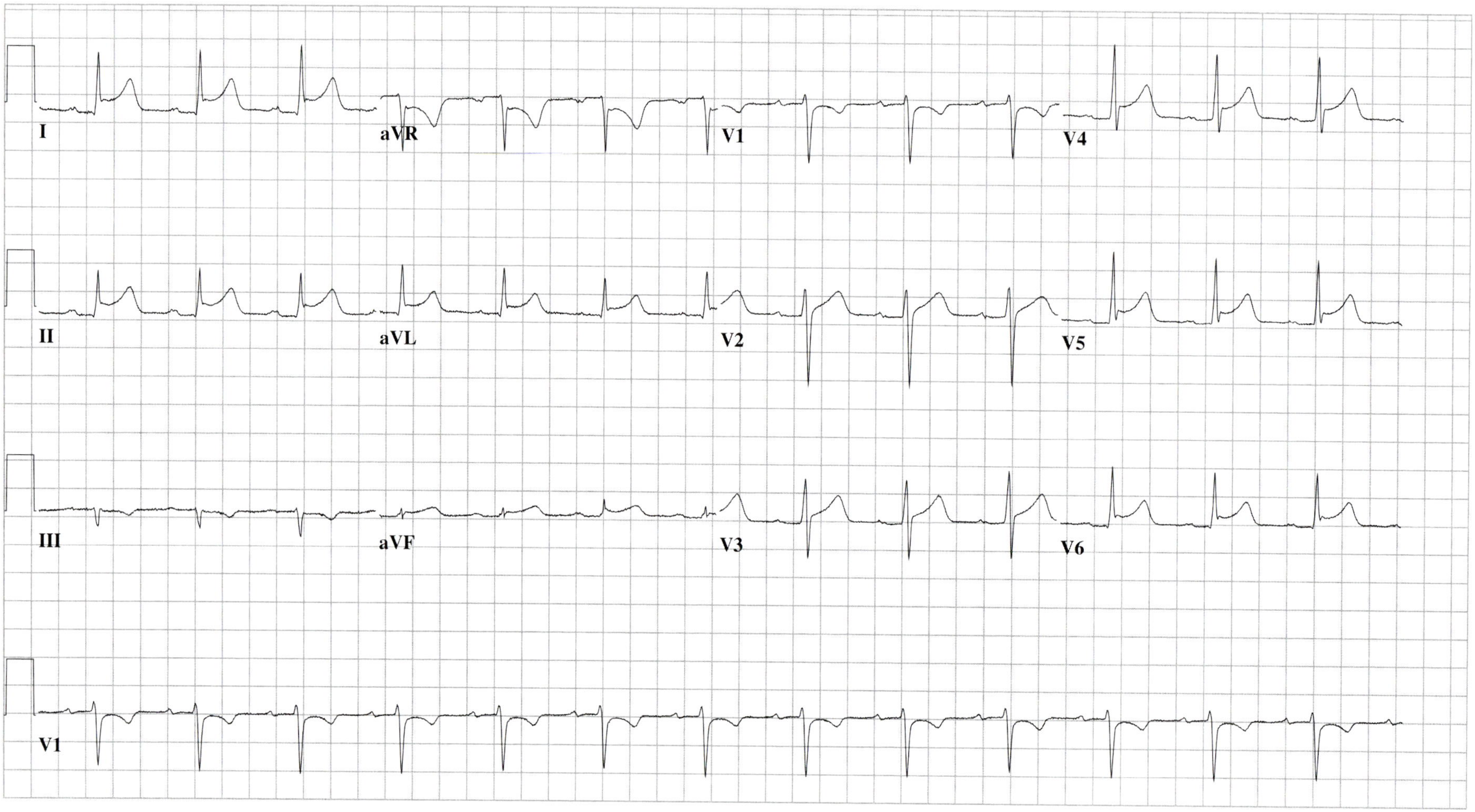

QUESTIONS

47-1. Interpret this ECG.

47-2. What other history is the patient likely to describe?

83
P2-4AC
15.0 cm MI 0.9
Gen TIs 1.1
[2d] G78/71 d
FA4/P90
HAR/FSI0
[C] G50/0.80 kHz
FA5/F1/8
TDI
Amplitude (V)
S-T
Time (s)
3
2.5

ANSWERS

47-1. Interpret this ECG.

This tracing reveals sinus rhythm at approximately 75 beats/min. The PR interval is prolonged to 200 milliseconds consistent with borderline first-degree AV block. The QRS axis and intervals are normal. ST elevations with concave upward morphology are seen in I and aVL, II and aVF, and V2 through V6. No Q waves are present. Furthermore, subtle PR-segment depression is seen in leads I and II. The differential diagnosis for ST-segment elevation includes, among other things, acute myocardial infarction, pericarditis, and left ventricular aneurysm. In this case, the upward concavity of the ST segment, the PR-segment depression, the lack of Q waves, and the diffuse nature of the ST-segment elevation in more than one coronary artery distribution make pericarditis the likely etiology.

47-2. What other history is the patient likely to describe?

Patients with pericarditis will complain of chest pain, typically described as sharp and pleuritic. Radiation is to the trapezius ridge. The pain is improved with sitting up and leaning forward and worsened by leaning backward.

Case #48. A 78-year-old man presents with substernal chest pain at rest.

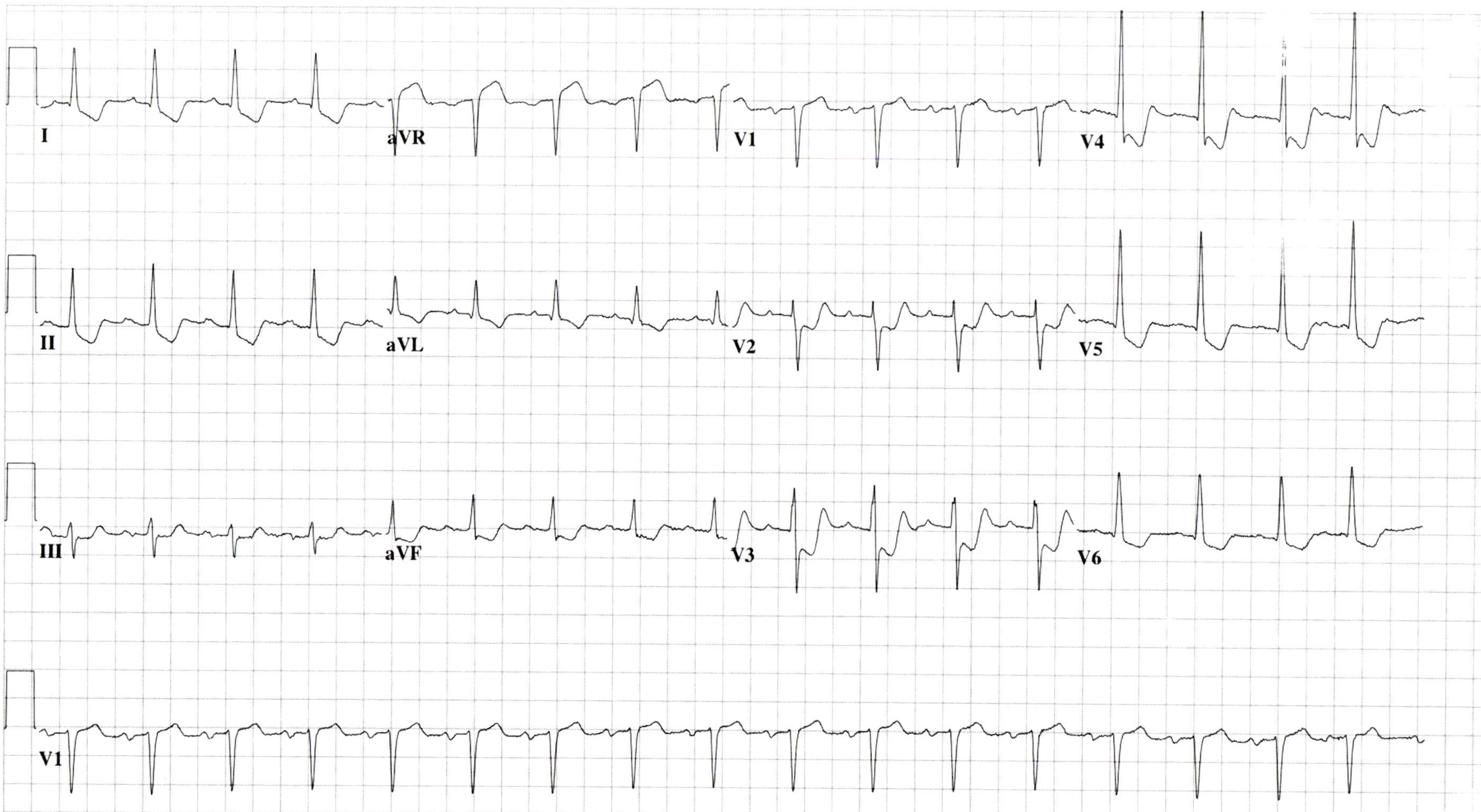

QUESTION

48-1. What abnormality is present?

83
P2-4AC
15.0 cm MI 0.9
Gen TIs 1.1
[2d] G78/71 d
FA4/P90
HAR/FS10
[C] G50/0.80 kHz
FA5/F1/8
TDI
Amplitude (V)
S-T
interval
2.5
3
Time (s)
3.5

ANSWER

48-1. What abnormality is present?

There is sinus tachycardia at a rate slightly higher than 100 beats/min. Examining the rhythm strip, the final (17th) QRS complex and its associated P wave represent a premature atrial contraction. The axis and intervals are normal. Prominent ST-segment depressions are present in the anterior leads of V2 through V4, with ST-segment abnormalities present to a lesser degree in the lateral leads I, V5, and V6 as well as the inferior leads II and aVF. There are no pathologic Q waves. The ST-segment depressions are consistent with subendocardial ischemia. Causes of subendocardial ischemia include primary acute coronary syndromes as well as clinical syndromes that globally decrease myocardial oxygen supply such as aortic stenosis or severe anemia, or conditions that increase myocardial oxygen demand such as severe sepsis or high-output heart failure. This patient underwent coronary angiography that revealed severe 3-vessel coronary disease with greater than 90% stenoses in the left anterior descending, left circumflex, and right coronary arteries. He was referred for coronary artery bypass grafting. When considering the ECG findings in a patient with myocardial infarction, it is important to note that, unlike the distribution of ST-segment elevations that can suggest the specific coronary artery involved, the distribution of ST-segment depressions cannot be used to localize the ischemia to a particular coronary territory.

Case #49. An 83-year-old woman with severe chronic obstructive pulmonary disease is admitted to the hospital with community-acquired pneumonia.

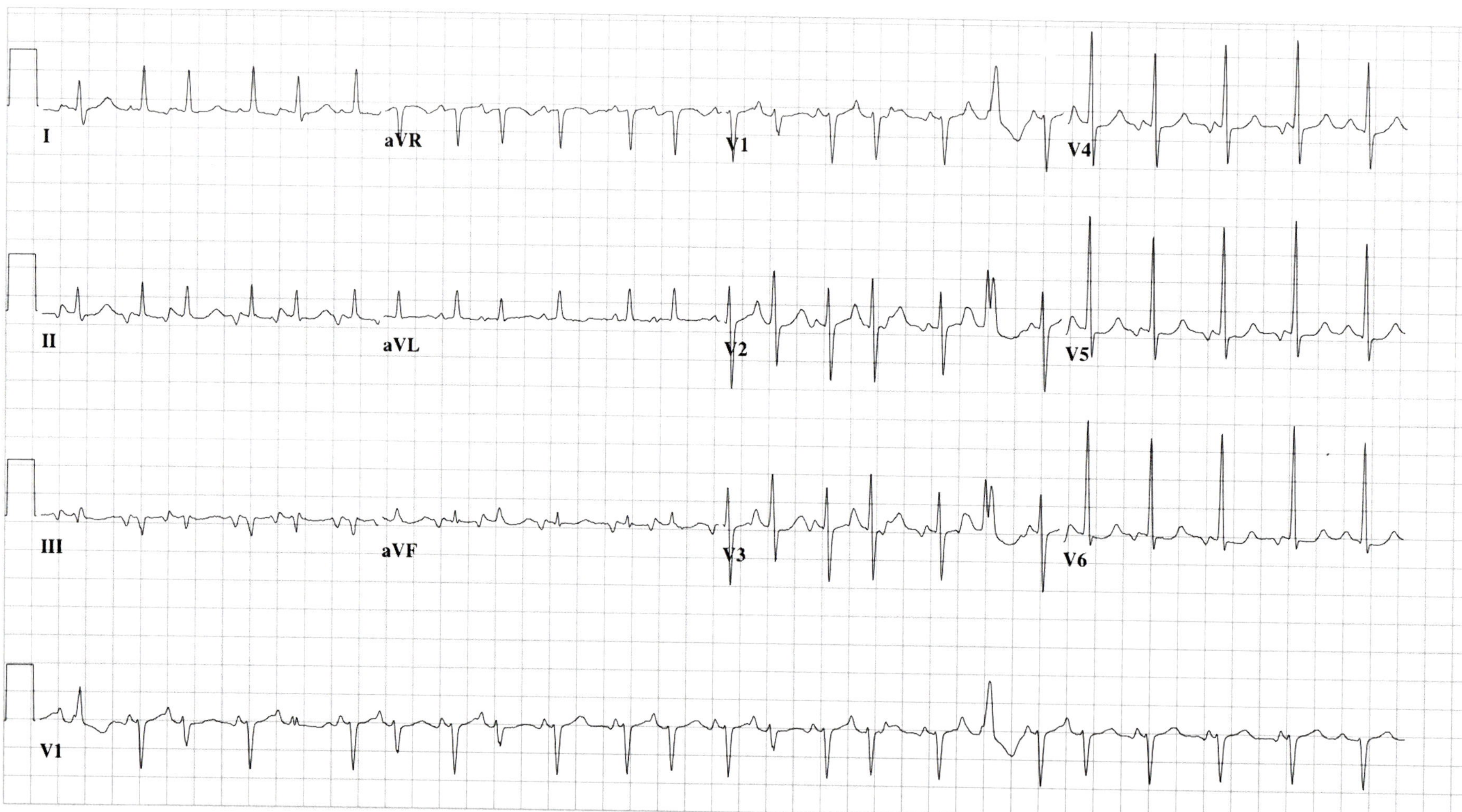

QUESTIONS

49-1. Interpret this ECG: what is the rhythm?

49-2. Why is QRS complex 18 wider than the others?

49-3. What are risk factors for development of this arrhythmia, and how is it managed?

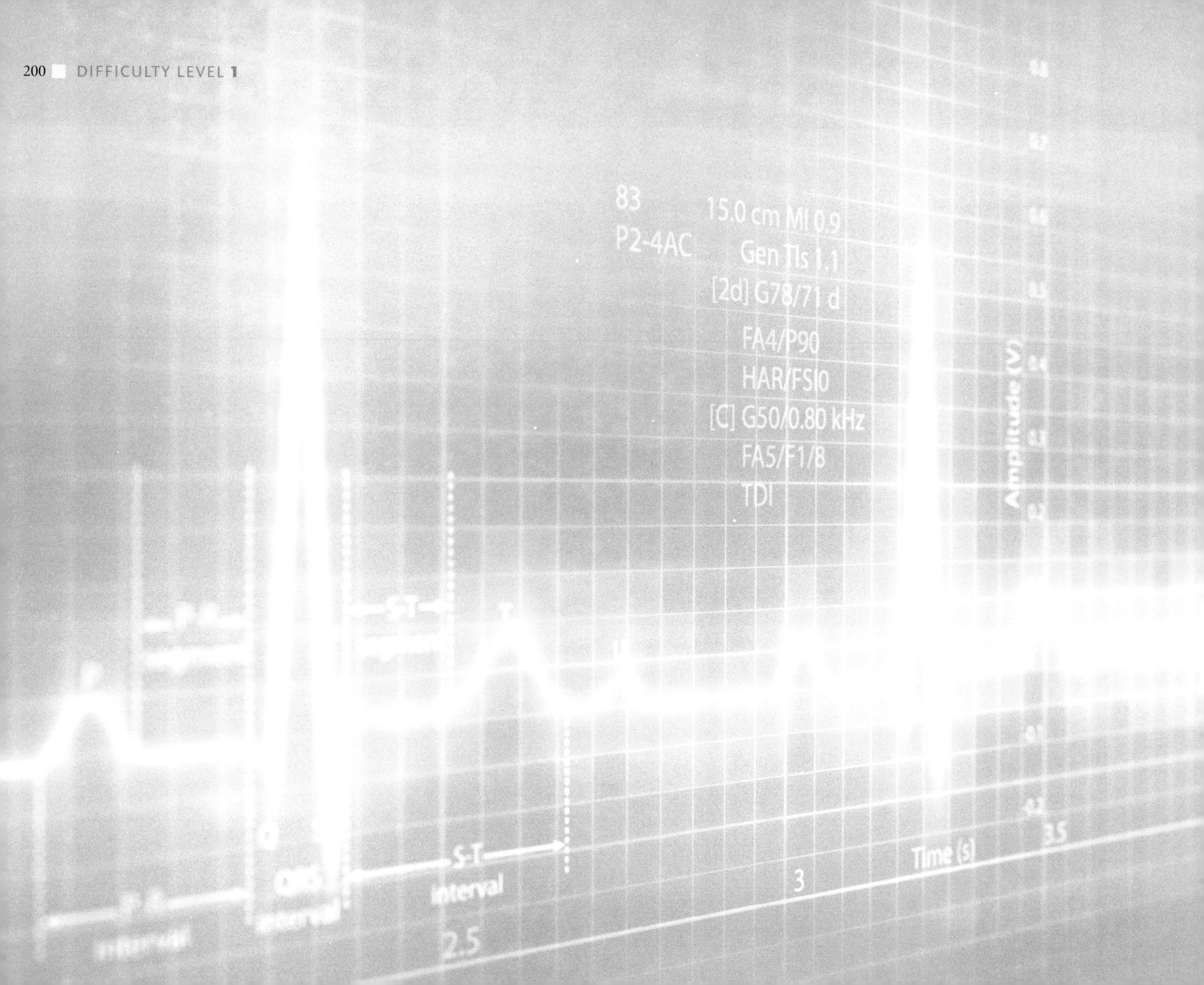
83
P2-4AC
15.0 cm MI 0.9
Gen TIs 1.1
[2d] G78/71 d
FA4/P90
HAR/FSI0
[C] G50/0.80 kHz
FA5/F1/8
TDI
Amplitude (V)
S-T
interval
QRS
interval
2.5
3
3.5
Time (s)

ANSWERS

49-1. Interpret this ECG: what is the rhythm?

The heart rate is rapid and the QRS complexes are narrow with the exception of the 18th QRS complex. The average ventricular rate can be estimated by counting the 24 QRS complexes across the 10-second rhythm strip, then multiplying by 6 to arrive at 144 beats/min. The RR intervals are irregular, and the irregularity lacks a pattern. Thus, this is an "irregularly irregular" narrow-complex tachycardia, which implies that the rhythm is either atrial fibrillation or multifocal atrial tachycardia. In this case, there are visible P waves present before each QRS; however, the P waves have varying morphology. In the V1 rhythm strip, there are at least three different morphologies of P wave: the first, "P1," is tall and peaked, is associated with a slightly longer PR interval (approximately 120 milliseconds), and can be found preceding the first, third, fifth, seventh, ninth, twelfth, and fourteenth QRS complexes. The second P wave "P2," has a tiny initial negative deflection and then a smaller positive peak and a shorter PR interval (approximately 100 milliseconds), and can be found preceding the second, fourth, sixth, eighth, tenth, eleventh, and thirteenth QRS complexes. The third P-wave morphology can be seen prior to the final QRS complex on the strip, with a smooth positive deflection and an even longer PR interval of approximately 160 milliseconds. This makes the diagnosis of multifocal atrial tachycardia (MAT) most likely. Within the ST segment of the 16th QRS complex is a nonconducted, or blocked, P wave. Otherwise, the axis is normal, and there is no evidence of ischemia or hypertrophy.

ANSWERS (Cont.)

49-2. Why is QRS complex 18 wider than the others?

This finding is secondary to Ashman's phenomenon, which is sometimes associated with irregular narrow-complex tachycardias. Ashman's phenomenon occurs when a long RR interval is followed by a short RR interval, as is the case with the RR interval between QRS complexes 16 and 17 (500 milliseconds), and the interval between QRS complexes 17 and 18 (340 milliseconds). The longer the RR interval, the longer the refractory period. When a short RR interval abruptly follows a long RR interval, the supraventricular impulse is conducted with aberrancy—right bundle branch block aberrancy in this case. The first and fifth QRS complexes demonstrate incomplete right bundle branch block also consistent with Ashman's phenomenon.

49-3. What are risk factors for development of this arrhythmia, and how is it managed?

MAT is an arrhythmia that is often seen in patients with intrinsic lung disease. It is associated with COPD, asthma, pneumonia, pulmonary embolism, hypokalemia, and hypomagnesemia. The mainstay of treatment for MAT is to treat the underlying cause. AV nodal agents including calcium channel blockers and β-blockers can be used. Electrolytes including calcium, potassium, and magnesium should be aggressively repleted.

Case #50. A 48-year-old woman with diabetes and smoking history presents with nausea, diaphoresis, and upper epigastric discomfort.

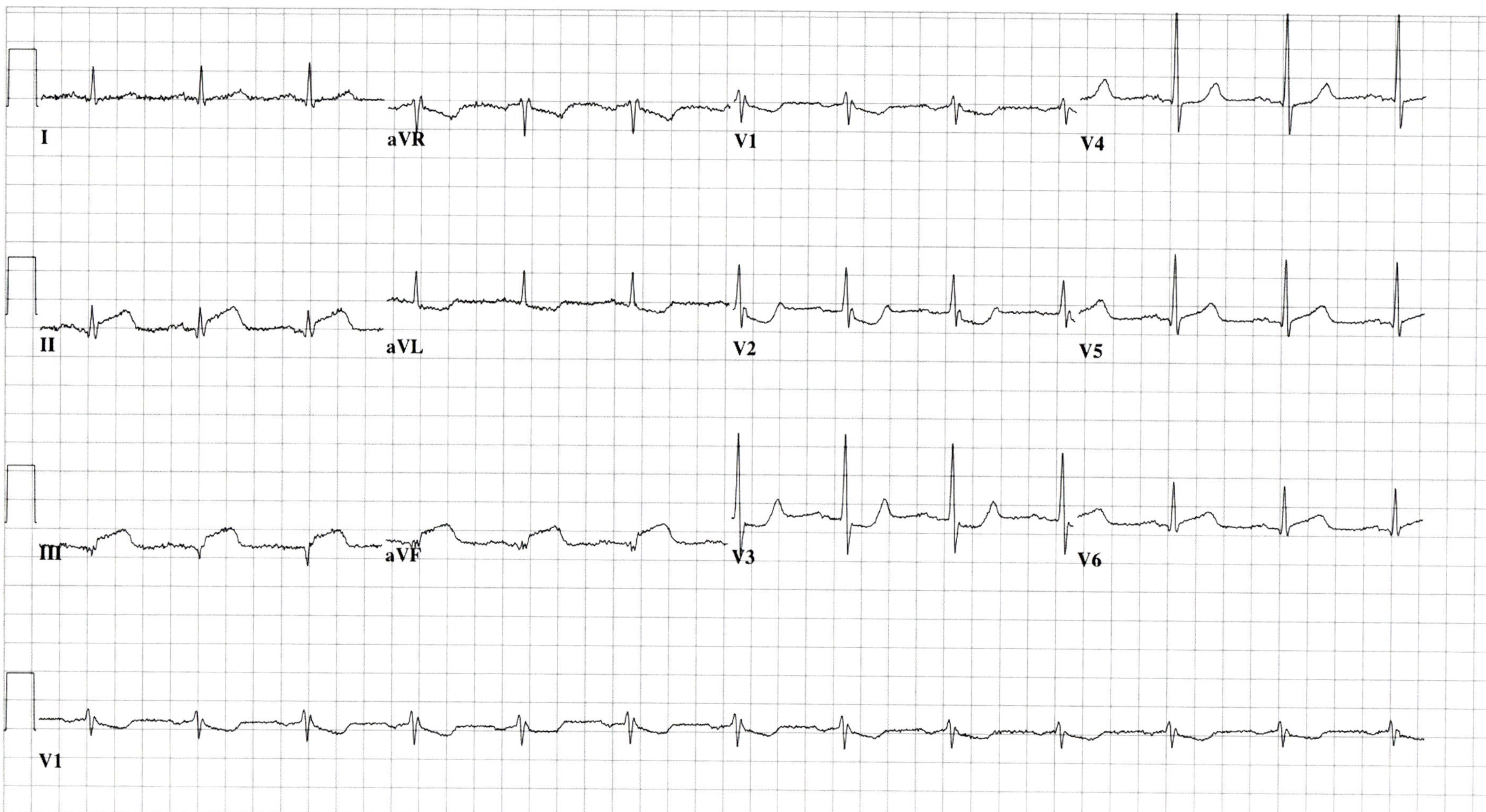

QUESTIONS

50-1. What is the diagnosis?

50-2. Which coronary artery might be causing the symptoms?

83
P2-4AC
15.0 cm MI 0.9
Gen TIs 1.1
[2d] G78/71 d
FA4/P90
HAR/FS10
[C] G50/0.80 kHz
FA5/F1/8
TDI
Amplitude (V)
Time (s)
2.5
3
3.5

ANSWERS

50-1. What is the diagnosis?

Sinus rhythm is present at a rate of 75 beats/min. Axis is normal. The QRS complex is narrow but has an RSR′ configuration in lead V1 consistent with incomplete right bundle branch block, sometimes called right ventricular conduction delay. There are ST-segment elevations with small Q waves in the inferior leads II, III, and aVF with slight and subtle ST-segment elevation in leads V5 and V6. There is 0.5 mm of ST-segment depression in lead aVL with ST-segment depression also seen in leads V2 and V3. In the setting of inferior infarction, ST-segment depression anteriorly often connotes posterior infarction; that is, posterior ST-segment elevation typically manifests as ST-segment depression in the anterior leads. The overall diagnosis, therefore, is inferoposterolateral myocardial ischemia with inferior infarction.

50-2. Which coronary artery might be causing the symptoms?

Inferior infarction is usually due to occlusion of the right coronary artery and less commonly due to occlusion of a dominant left circumflex artery. In this patient, the fact that the magnitude of ST-segment elevation is greater in lead II (which is oriented leftward) than lead III (which is oriented rightward), and the presence of ST-segment elevations in the lateral precordial leads suggests the possibility that the left circumflex is the infarct-related artery. At coronary angiography, a large, dominant left circumflex coronary was occluded in the mid portion and was successfully stented.

Section II

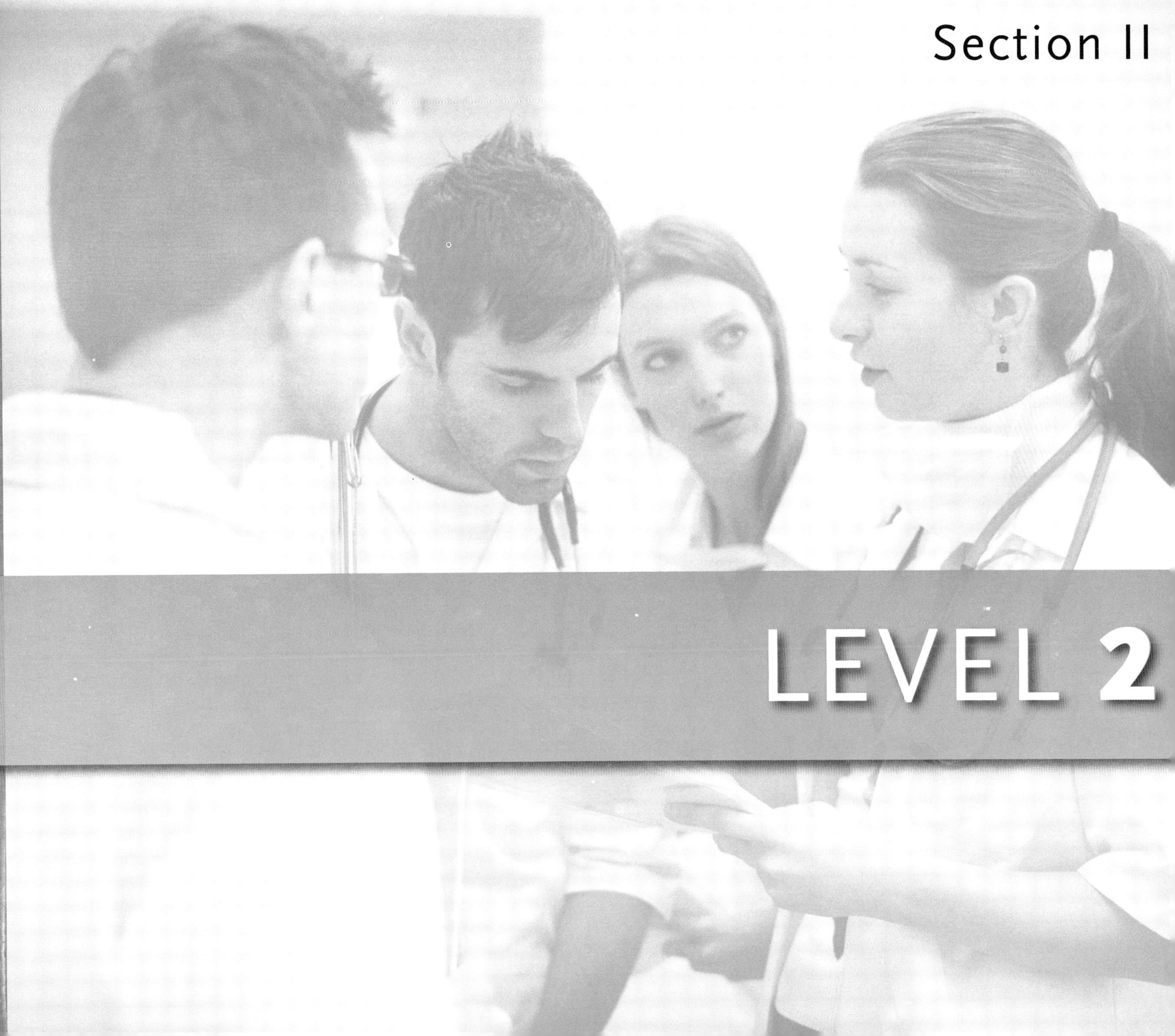

LEVEL 2

Case #51. An asymptomatic 30-year-old woman.

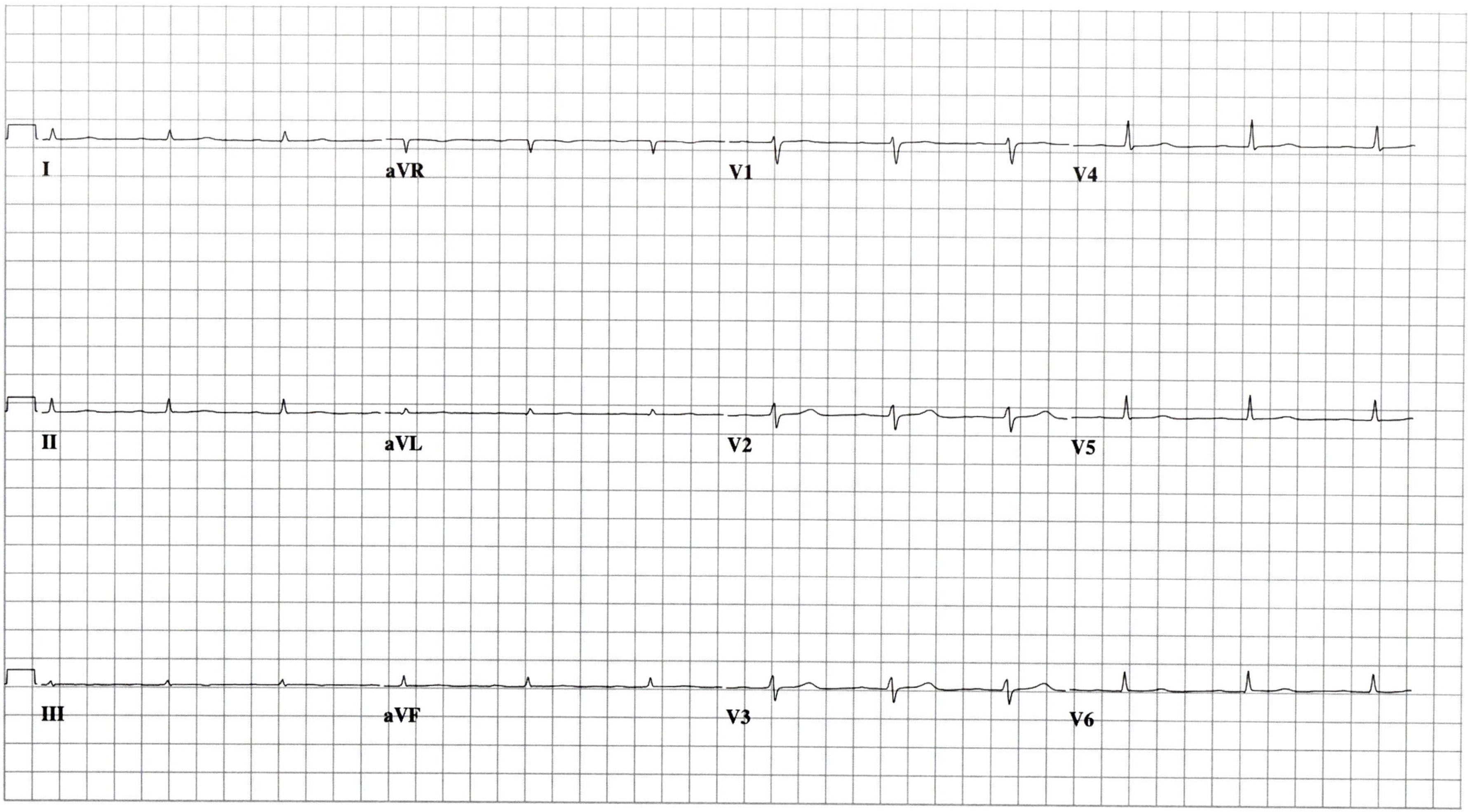

QUESTION

51-1. What does the ECG reveal?

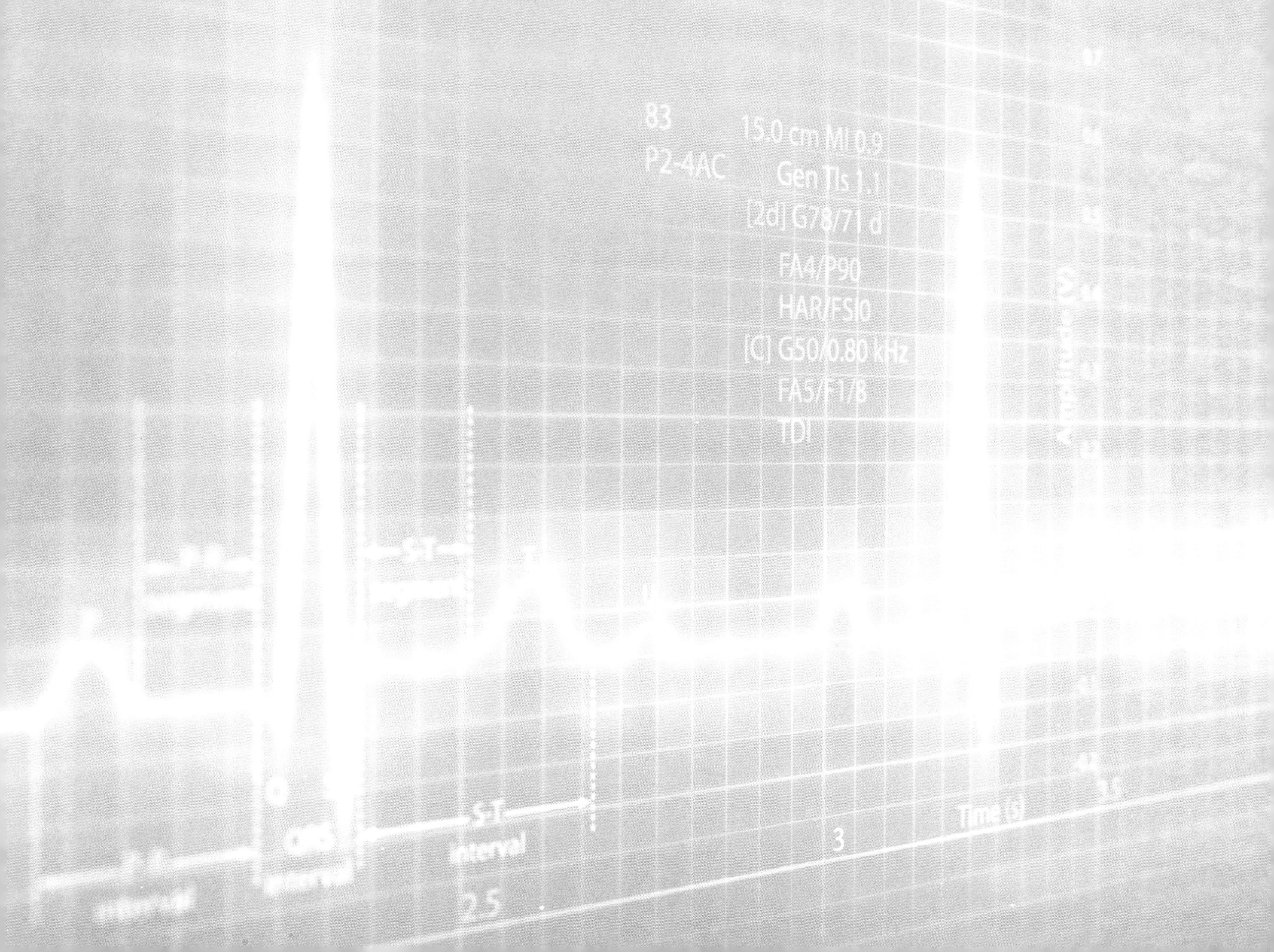
83
P2-4AC
15.0 cm MI 0.9
Gen Tls 1.1
[2d] G78/71 d
FA4/P90
HAR/FSI0
[C] G50/0.80 kHz
FA5/F1/8
TDI
S-T
interval
2.5
3
Time (s)

ANSWER

51-1. What does the ECG reveal?

The rate is slightly slower than 75 beats/min. P waves are difficult to visualize but can be seen in leads V3, I, and II. The PR interval is slightly prolonged at just greater than 200 milliseconds. Hence, the rhythm is sinus rhythm with first-degree AV block. The intervals are otherwise normal, as is the QRS frontal plane axis. At a glance, there may appear to be low voltage. Before settling on this diagnosis, however, look closely at the voltage standardization of recording, represented by the rectangle at the far left of the tracing and noted in the figure. This rectangle corresponds to 10 mV. The standard 12-lead ECG is recorded such that 1 little box of vertical amplitude is equivalent to 1 mV. Thus, the standardization rectangle would be 10 little boxes tall, as shown in the figure. When an ECG is recorded at "half-standard" voltage, 1 little box is equivalent to 2 mV, and the standardization rectangle would be 5 little boxes tall, as shown in the figure. Thus, this ECG does not represent low voltage, but rather is a normal tracing recorded at half standardization. This case illustrates the importance of a systematic approach to ECG interpretation including an evaluation of recording quality and standardization.

Normal standardization

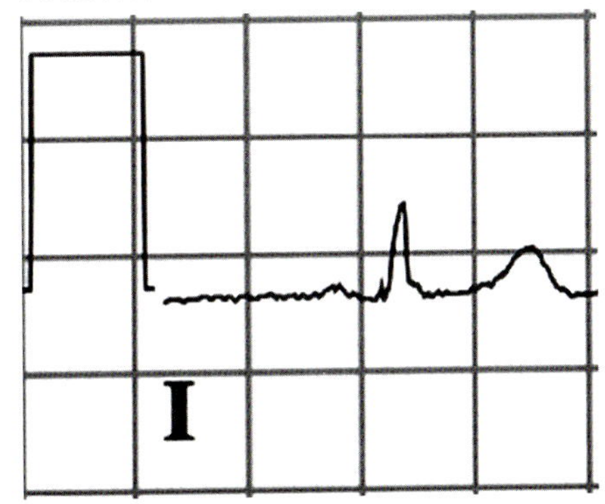

Half standardization

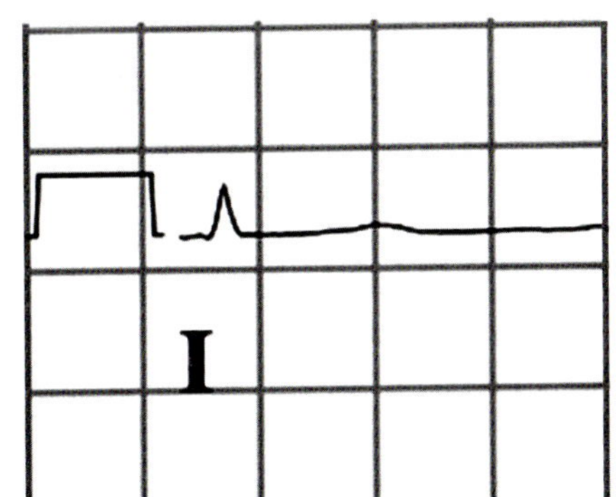

Case #52. A 53-year-old woman with long-standing mitral valve prolapse.

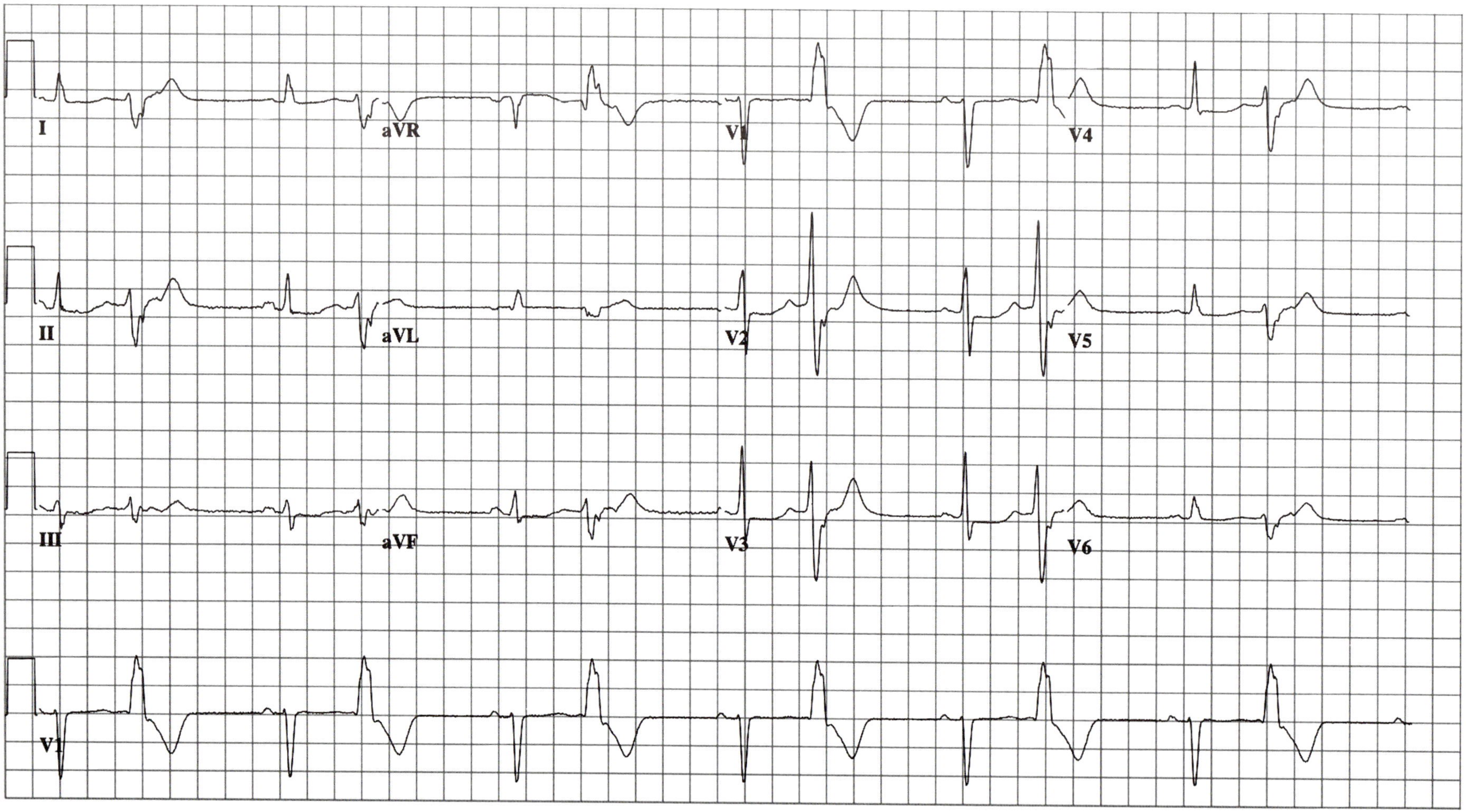

QUESTIONS

52-1. What abnormalities are present on this ECG?

52-2. How would these abnormalities affect the qualities of the murmur of mitral valve prolapse?

83
15.0 cm MI 0.9
P2-4AC
Gen TIs 1.1
[2d] G78/71 d
FA4/P90
HAR/FSI0
[C] G50/0.80 kHz
FA5/F1/8
TDI
S-T
interval
2.5
3
Time (s)
3.5

ANSWERS

52-1. What abnormalities are present on this ECG?

Sinus rhythm is present with frequent premature ventricular contractions in a bigeminal pattern—a premature ventricular contraction alternating with a sinus beat. The axis is normal. There is an early R-wave transition in the precordial leads with an R wave greater than an S wave in lead V2; normally, the transition from dominant S wave to dominant R wave occurs at lead V4 in the precordium. There are nonspecific ST-segment and T-wave abnormalities in leads V3 to V6.

52-2. How would these abnormalities affect the qualities of the murmur of mitral valve prolapse?

The classic auscultatory findings of mitral valve prolapse include a midsystolic click and late systolic murmur that continues with constant intensity through S2. These findings are caused by redundant, billowing tissue of the myxomatous mitral valve, much like a parachute in the wind. Maneuvers that increase left ventricular (LV) cavity diameter stretch the mitral valve annulus, leading to a decrease in the amount of redundant tissue (like a parachute being pulled taut), while decreasing LV cavity diameter has the opposite effect, increasing the amount of redundant tissue. A smaller LV cavity will cause the prolapse to occur earlier in systole, moving the click closer to S1 and increasing the intensity of the murmur, while a large LV cavity has the opposite effect. Given the tracing above, a shorter R–R interval, such as that between a native beat and a premature ventricular contraction, will lead to decreased LV filling and the click–murmur complex of mitral valve prolapse will occur earlier in systole. Conversely, the longer R–R interval following a PVC will increase LV filling and move the click–murmur complex later in systole.

Case #53. An 89-year-old gentleman with hypertension, presenting for routine follow-up.

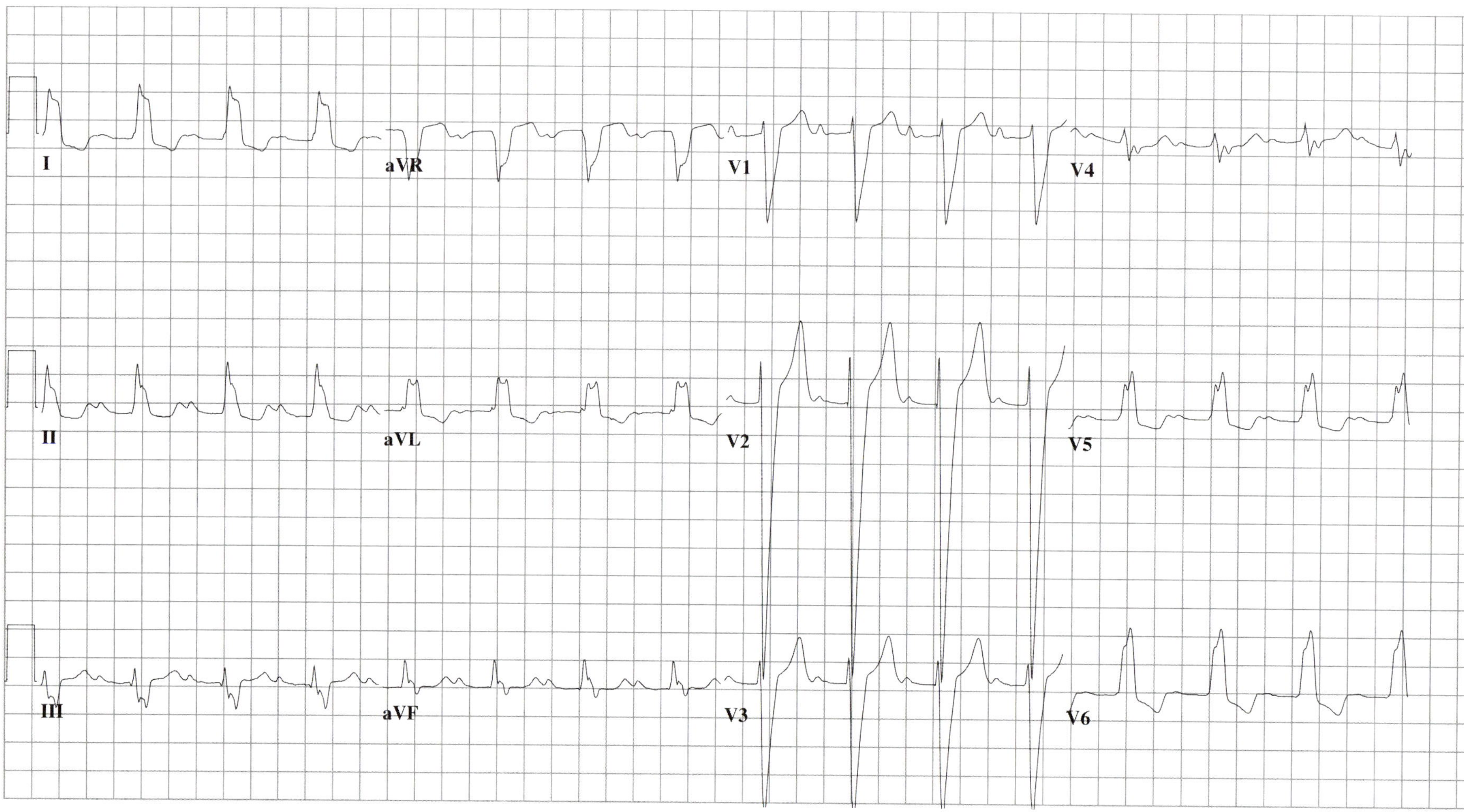

QUESTION

53-1. What does the ECG show?

83
P2-4AC
15.0 cm MI 0.9
Gen TIs 1.1
[2d] G78/71 d
FA4/P90
HAR/FSI0
[C] G50/0.80 kHz
FA5/F1/8
TDI
Amplitude (V)
S-T
interval
Time (s)
2.5
3
3.5

ANSWER

53-1. What does the ECG show?

There is sinus rhythm at a rate slightly slower than 100 beats/min. The QRS axis is normal. The PR interval is prolonged to greater than 200 milliseconds consistent with AV conduction delay/first-degree AV block. The QRS complex is wide (greater than 120 milliseconds) with a broad S wave in lead V1 and a broad, notched R wave in leads I, aVL, and V6 diagnostic of left bundle branch block. There are ST-segment elevations in leads V1 through V3, which are normal in the setting of a left bundle branch block. Similarly, the ST-segment depressions and T-wave inversions in leads V5 through V6, I, and aVL are normal features of left bundle branch block. In general, the ST segment and T wave should be directed opposite to the major polarity of the QRS complex when left bundle branch block is present.

Case #54. A 68-year-old patient post-op from thyroidectomy presents with muscle cramps; Chvostek's and Trousseau's signs are noted on examination.

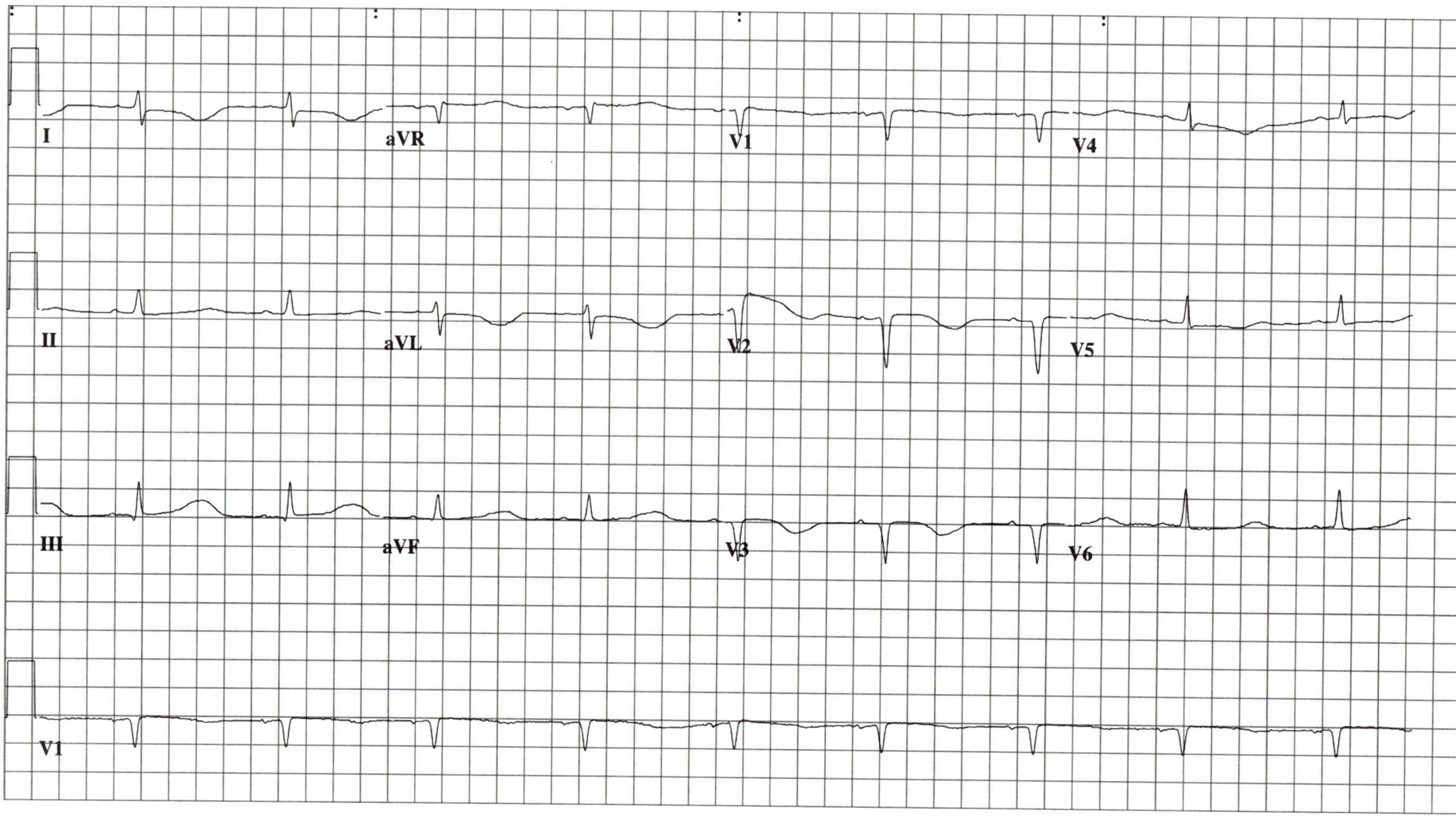

QUESTIONS

54-1. Interpret this ECG.

54-2. What electrolyte is most likely deranged, and what ECG findings are typical of this diagnosis?

83
P2-4AC
15.0 cm MI 0.9
Gen Tls 1.1
[2d] G78/71 d
FA4/P90
HAR/FS10
[C] G50/0.80 kHz
FA5/F1/8
TDI

ANSWERS

54-1. Interpret this ECG.

The rate is bradycardic at 54 beats/min. The rhythm is regular with a narrow QRS and normal-appearing sinus P waves are seen. Axis is normal. The QT interval is very prolonged to more than 600 milliseconds with a long, isoelectric ST segment (best seen in lead V6) and T-wave inversions in leads I, aVL, and V1 through V5. There are Q waves in leads V1 through V3 consistent with anteroseptal myocardial infarction of indeterminate age.

54-2. What electrolyte is most likely deranged, and what ECG findings are typical of this diagnosis?

The clinical history coupled with ECG findings of a long QT and isoelectric ST segment are classic for hypocalcemia. If left untreated, hypocalcemia can progress to tetany and cardiovascular collapse. The long QT interval and sinus bradycardia predispose this patient to torsades de pointes.

Case #55. A 67-year-old smoker presents with chest pain and palpitations on postoperative day 2 after cholecystectomy.

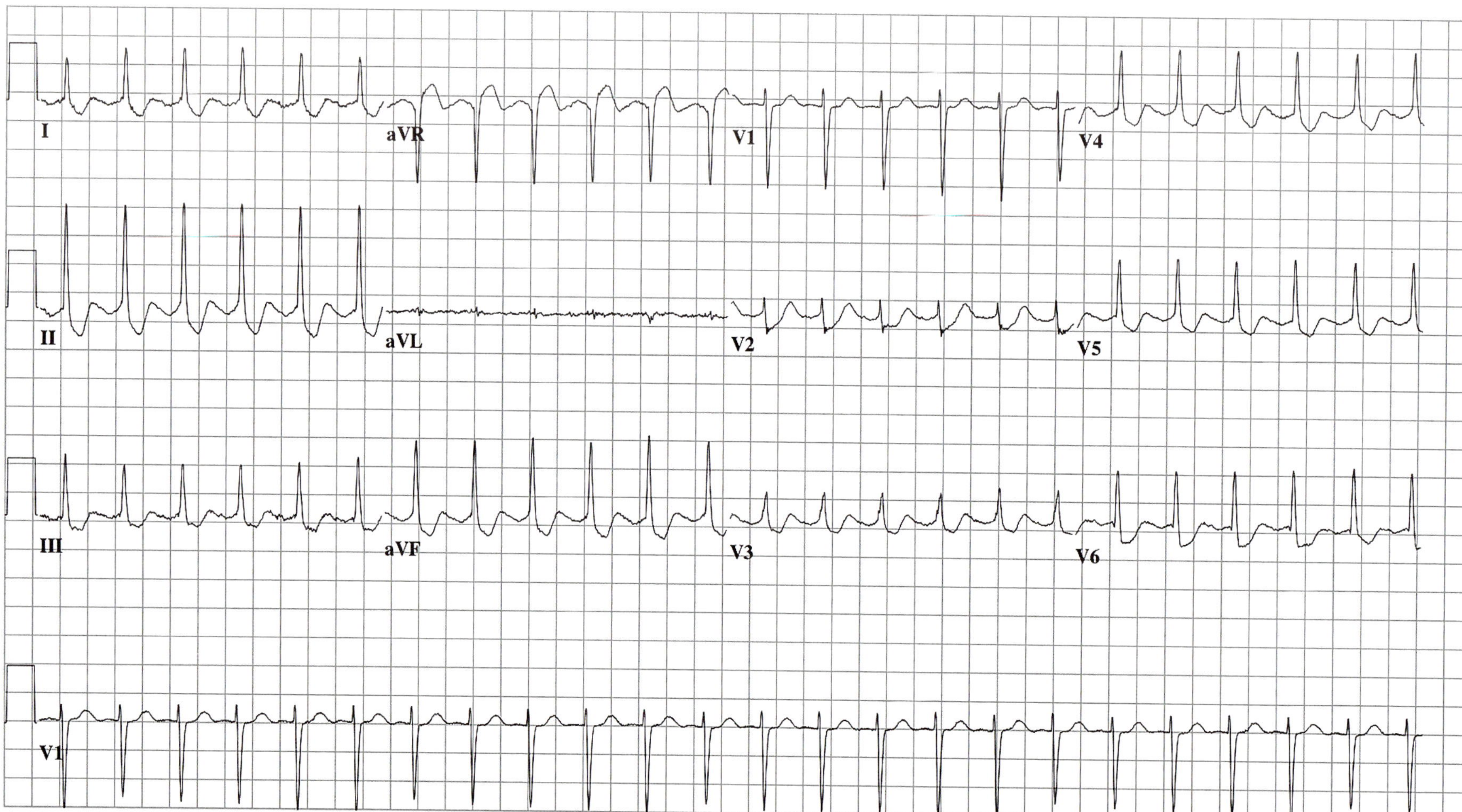

QUESTIONS

55-1. Interpret this tracing.

55-2. What would you do next?

83
P2-4AC
15.0 cm MI 0.9
Gen Tls 1.1
[2d] G78/71 d
FA4/P90
HAR/FSI0
[C] G50/0.80 kHz
FA5/F1/8
TDI
S-T
interval
2.5
3
3.5
Time (s)

ANSWERS

55-1. Interpret this tracing.

There is a narrow-complex, regular tachycardia at a rate of approximately 150 beats/min. No clear atrial activity is evident; hence, this should be classified as a supraventricular tachycardia (SVT). The differential diagnosis includes sinus tachycardia, atrial tachycardia, AVNRT, and atrial flutter. A vagal maneuver or adenosine administration could serve as both a diagnostic and therapeutic maneuver. The QRS axis is normal. No chamber enlargement is noted. There are profound, horizontal, and downsloping ST-segment depressions in nearly all leads with ST-segment elevations in lead aVR.

55-2. What would you do next?

This patient presents with SVT and significant ischemia on the ECG. The first step should be to decrease myocardial oxygen demand by controlling the heart rate. The findings of global ST-segment depression with ST-segment elevation in lead aVR may suggest critical left main coronary stenosis or severe 3-vessel coronary disease. This patient was taken to cardiac catheterization where coronary angiogram revealed a 95% left main coronary stenosis. He was referred for coronary artery bypass grafting.

Case #56. An 18-year-old woman with a "seizure disorder" diagnosed in childhood, who has been event-free on phenytoin.

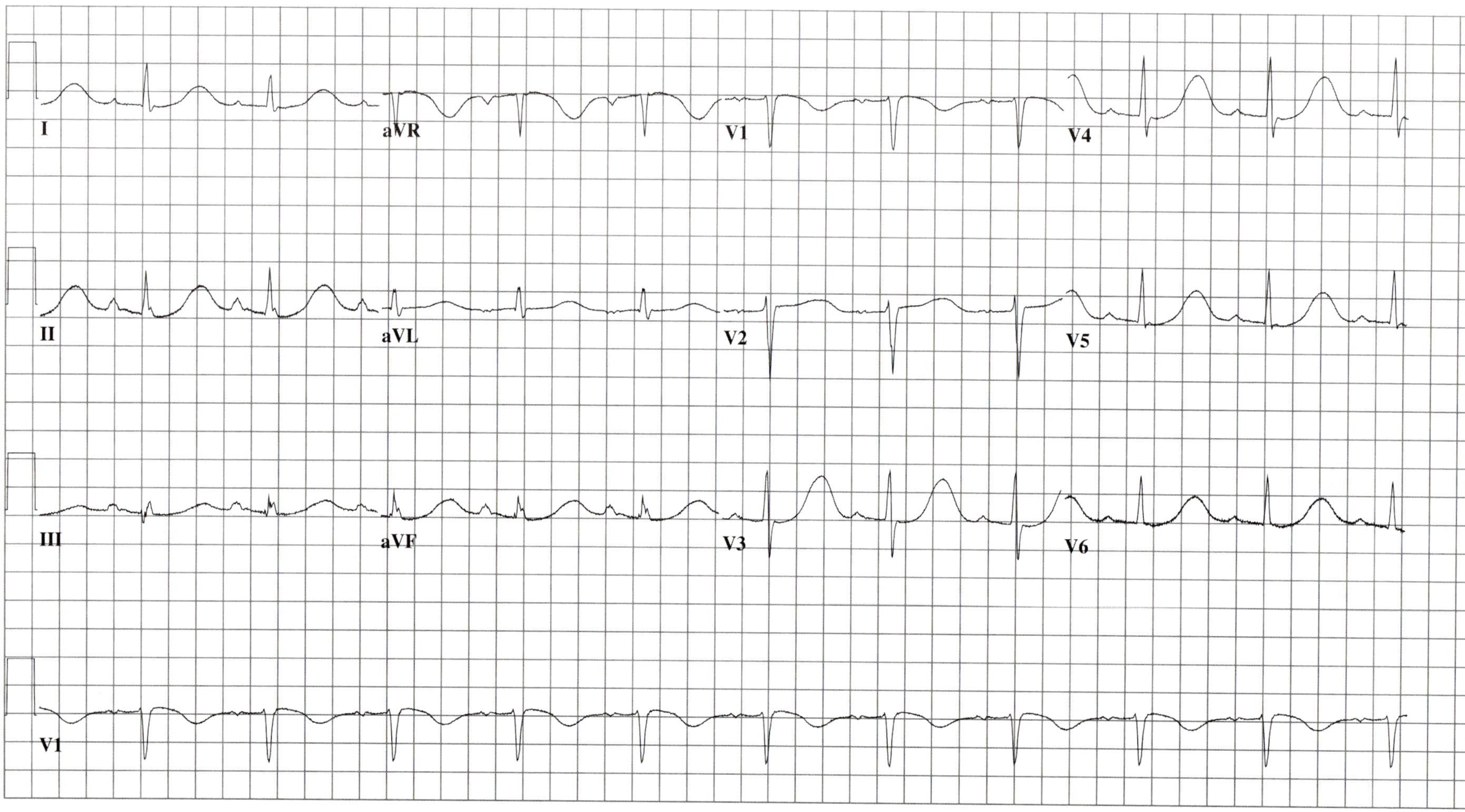

QUESTIONS

56-1. Interpret this tracing: what are the major abnormalities?

56-2. Do you agree with the diagnosis of seizure disorder?

56-3. Why has she been event-free on phenytoin?

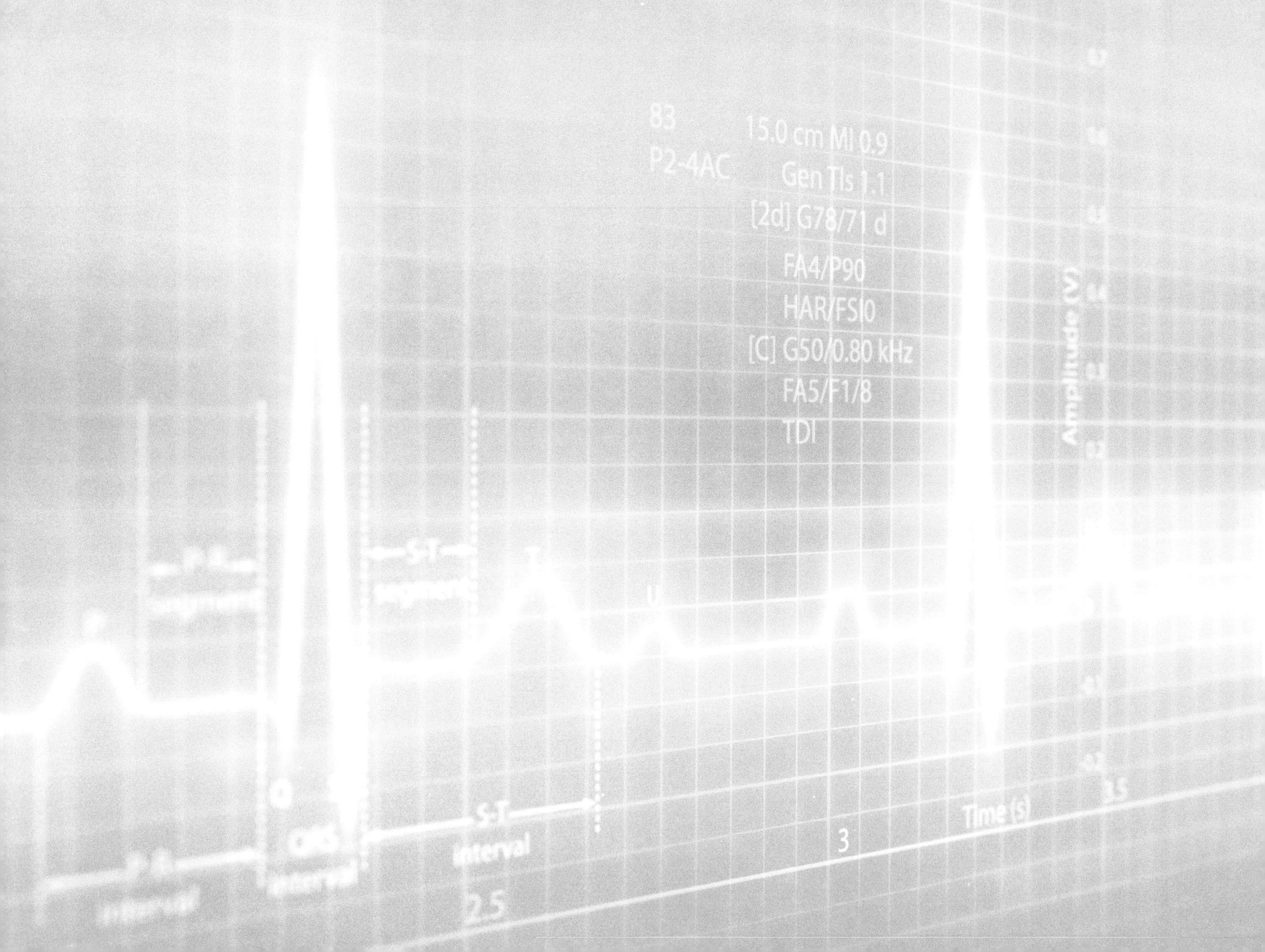
83
P2-4AC
15.0 cm MI 0.9
Gen TIs 1.1
[2d] G78/71 d
FA4/P90
HAR/FSI0
[C] G50/0.80 kHz
FA5/F1/8
TDI
Amplitude (V)
S-T
segment
T
U
S-T
interval
QRS
interval
2.5
3
Time (s)
3.5

ANSWERS

56-1. Interpret this tracing: what are the major abnormalities?

The heart rate is 66 beats/min. Sinus rhythm is present with a first-degree AV block. QRS axis is normal. There is no evidence of chamber enlargement and no evidence of ischemia. The most striking finding is a very prolonged QT interval with broad-based T waves.

56-2. Do you agree with the diagnosis of seizure disorder?

In a young, otherwise healthy patient on no medications with normal electrolytes and a prolonged QT interval on the ECG, the diagnosis of familial long-QT syndrome should be entertained. There are reports of patients with long-QT syndrome presenting with "spells," which can mimic seizures when in fact the "spells" are secondary to arrhythmic syncope.

56-3. Why has she been event-free on phenytoin?

Phenytoin is classified as a Vaughn-Williams class IB antiarrhythmic agent and has been shown to suppress arrhythmia in this clinical situation, although it is rarely used for its antiarrhythmic effect because many better choices are available. β-Blockers and placement of an implantable cardioverter-defibrillator can be considered to treat the long QT syndrome.[1]

[1]Roden DM. Long-QT syndrome. *N Engl J Med* 2008; 358: 169-176.

Case #57. A 45-year-old gentleman presents with dyspnea.

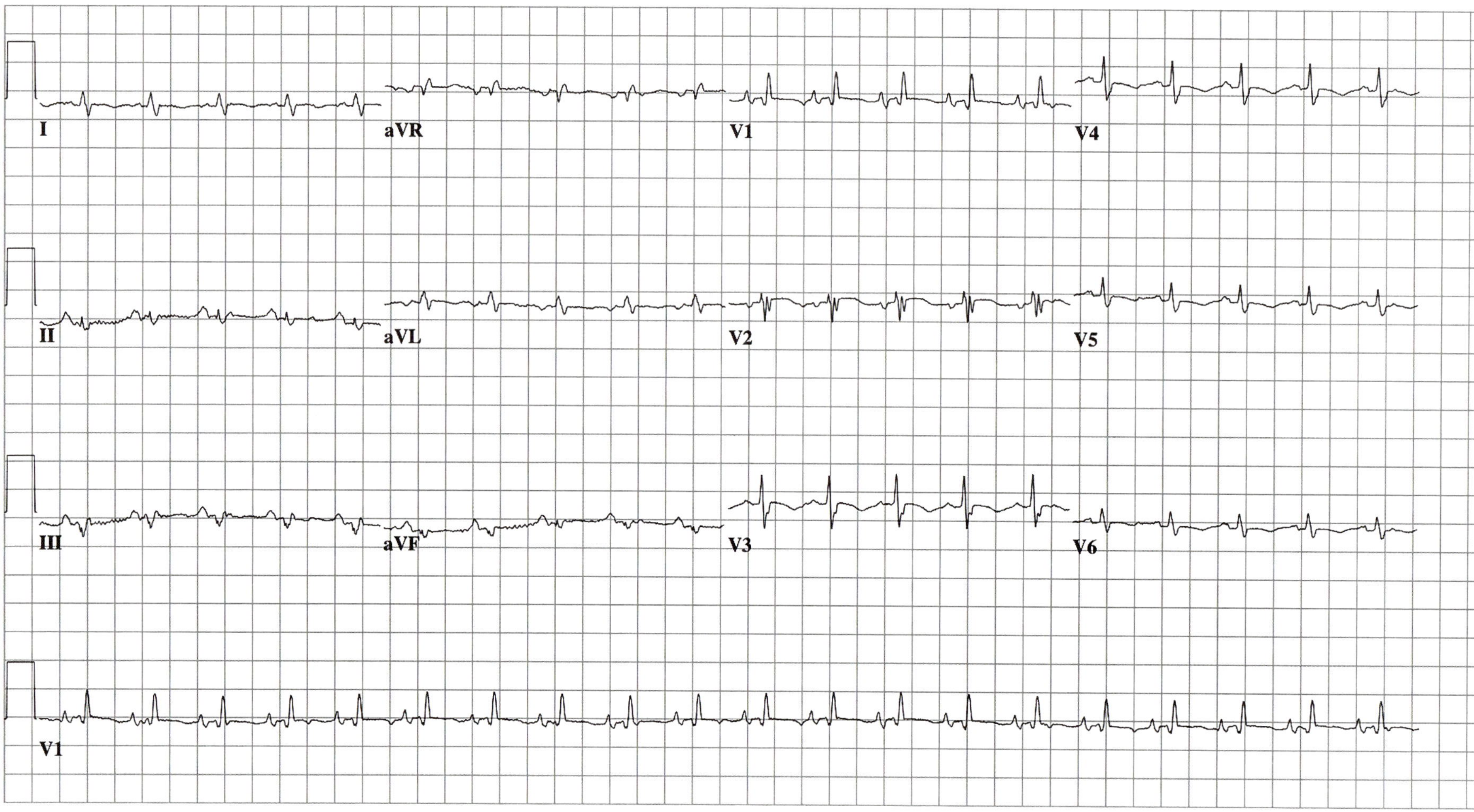

QUESTIONS

57-1. What findings are present on this ECG?

57-2. What are the criteria for low electrocardiogram voltage? What is the differential diagnosis?

83
15.0 cm MI 0.9
P2-4AC
Gen TIs 1.1
[2d] G78/71 d
FA4/P90
HAR/FS0
[C] G50/0.80 kHz
FA5/F1/8
TDI
Amplitude (V)
Time (s)
2.5
3
3.5

ANSWERS

57-1. What findings are present on this ECG?

This tracing demonstrates sinus tachycardia at 120 beats/min. The axis is indeterminate. The QT interval is prolonged. The QRS complex has a right bundle branch morphology with a QRS duration less than 120 milliseconds. This can be referred to as an incomplete right bundle branch block. There is low voltage in the limb and precordial leads. There are T-wave inversions through the precordium, best described as nonspecific T-wave abnormalities.

57-2. What are the criteria for low electrocardiogram voltage? What is the differential diagnosis?

The criteria for low voltage include total QRS amplitude less than 5 mV in all limb leads and less than 10 mV in all precordial leads. The differential diagnosis includes anything that can interrupt current flow from the cardiac conduction system to the ECG electrodes on the skin. Moving outward to inward, therefore, the differential includes poor-quality electrode placement, subcutaneous edema and anasarca, obesity, pleural effusions or pneumothorax, pericardial effusion, pulmonary hyperinflation such as with emphysema, myocardial injury and edema, or infiltrative disease of the myocytes themselves such as amyloidosis and hemochromatosis. This patient was suffering from acute rejection of an orthotopic heart transplant causing profound intramyocardial edema.

Case #58. A 74-year-old woman with a distant history of rheumatic fever presents with dyspnea, hemoptysis, palpitations, and a murmur.

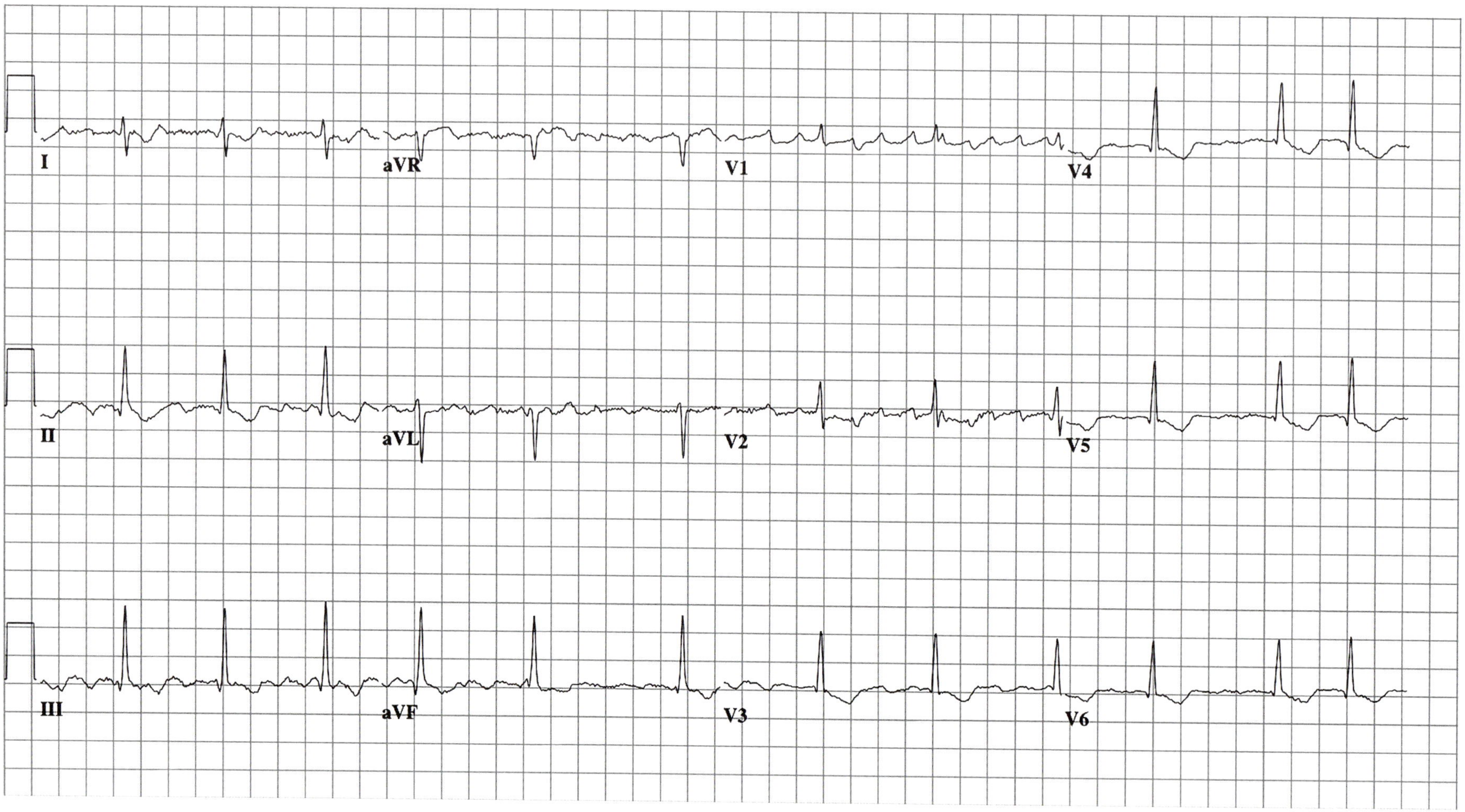

QUESTIONS

58-1. Interpret this ECG.

58-2. What is the likely diagnosis?

58-3. What would you expect to hear on cardiac auscultation?

83
P2-4AC
15.0 cm MI 0.9
Gen TIs 1.1
[2d] G78/71 d
FA4/P90
HAR/FSI0
[C] G50/0.80 kHz
FA5/F1/8
TDI
S-T
Interval
2.5
3
Time (s)
Amplitude (V)

ANSWERS

58-1. Interpret this ECG.

The heart rate is 72 beats/min. There is no organized atrial activity, and the rhythm is "irregularly irregular" most consistent with coarse atrial fibrillation. Although one may be tempted to diagnose atrial flutter on the basis of "flutter waves" in lead V1, the inferior leads do not demonstrate the classic sawtooth pattern of atrial flutter. Further supporting the diagnosis of coarse atrial fibrillation, the rhythm is highly irregular with each R–R interval different from the next. The axis is rightward. Coupled with a tall R wave in V1, this finding suggests right ventricular hypertrophy. Finally, there are diffuse downsloping ST segments with inverted T waves. The morphology of these ST-T waves can be characterized as "sagging" or "scooped" and looks quite distinct from myocardial ischemia. The ST-segment and T-wave abnormality seen here is consistent with digoxin effect.

58-2. What is the likely diagnosis?

The findings of atrial fibrillation and right ventricular hypertrophy in the setting of prior rheumatic fever suggest mitral stenosis.

58-3. What would you expect to hear on cardiac auscultation?

Classic physical findings of mitral stenosis include a loud first heart sound secondary to the increased pressure gradient between left atrium and left ventricle at onset of ventricular systole, an opening snap in early diastole, and a diastolic rumbling murmur. The murmur of mitral stenosis is best heard with the patient positioned in the left lateral decubitus position using the bell of the stethoscope positioned directly over the point of maximal impulse.

Case #59. A 70-year-old gentleman with history of distant myocardial infarction and systolic dysfunction complaining of palpitations and dizziness.

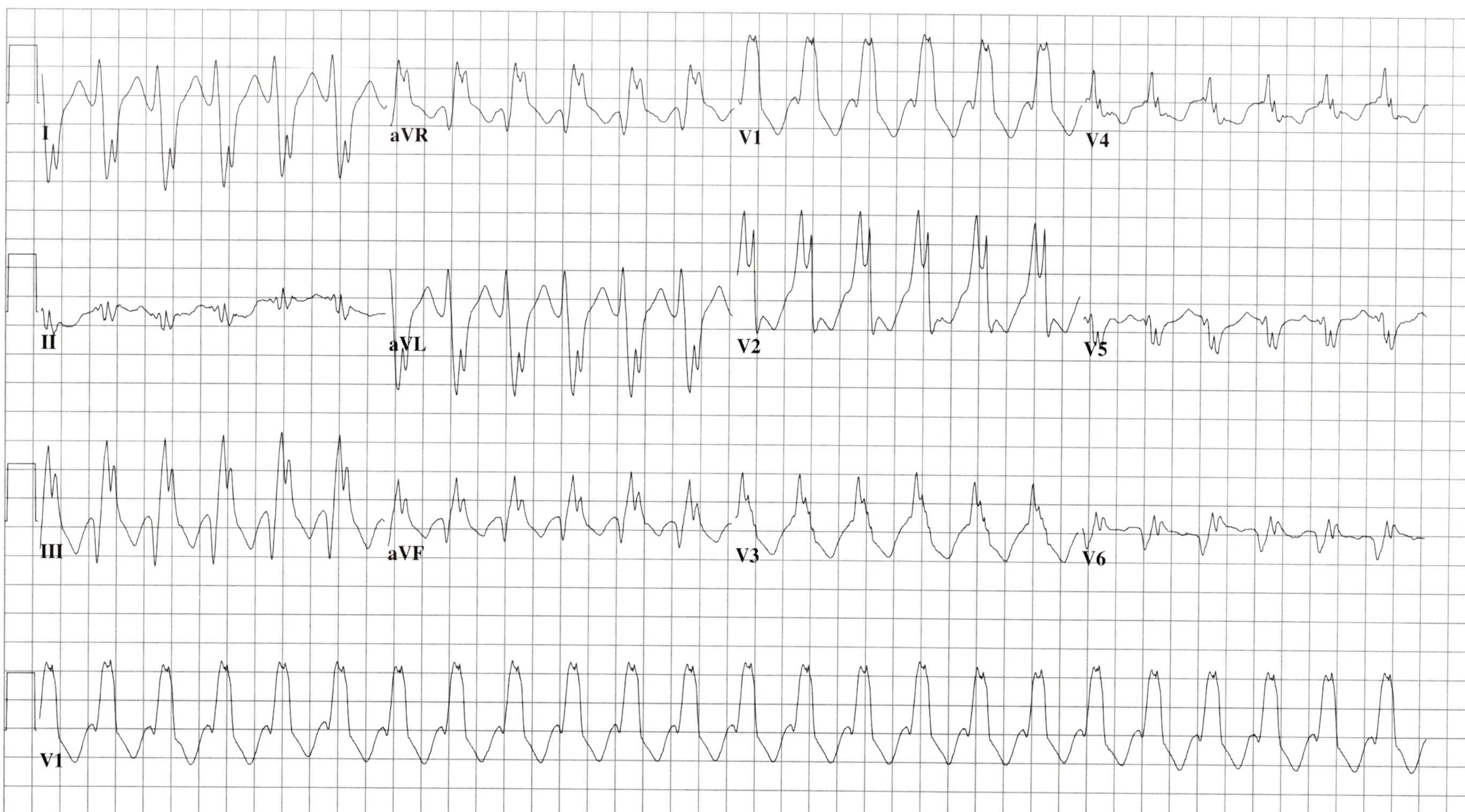

QUESTION

59-1. Interpret this ECG: what is the diagnosis?

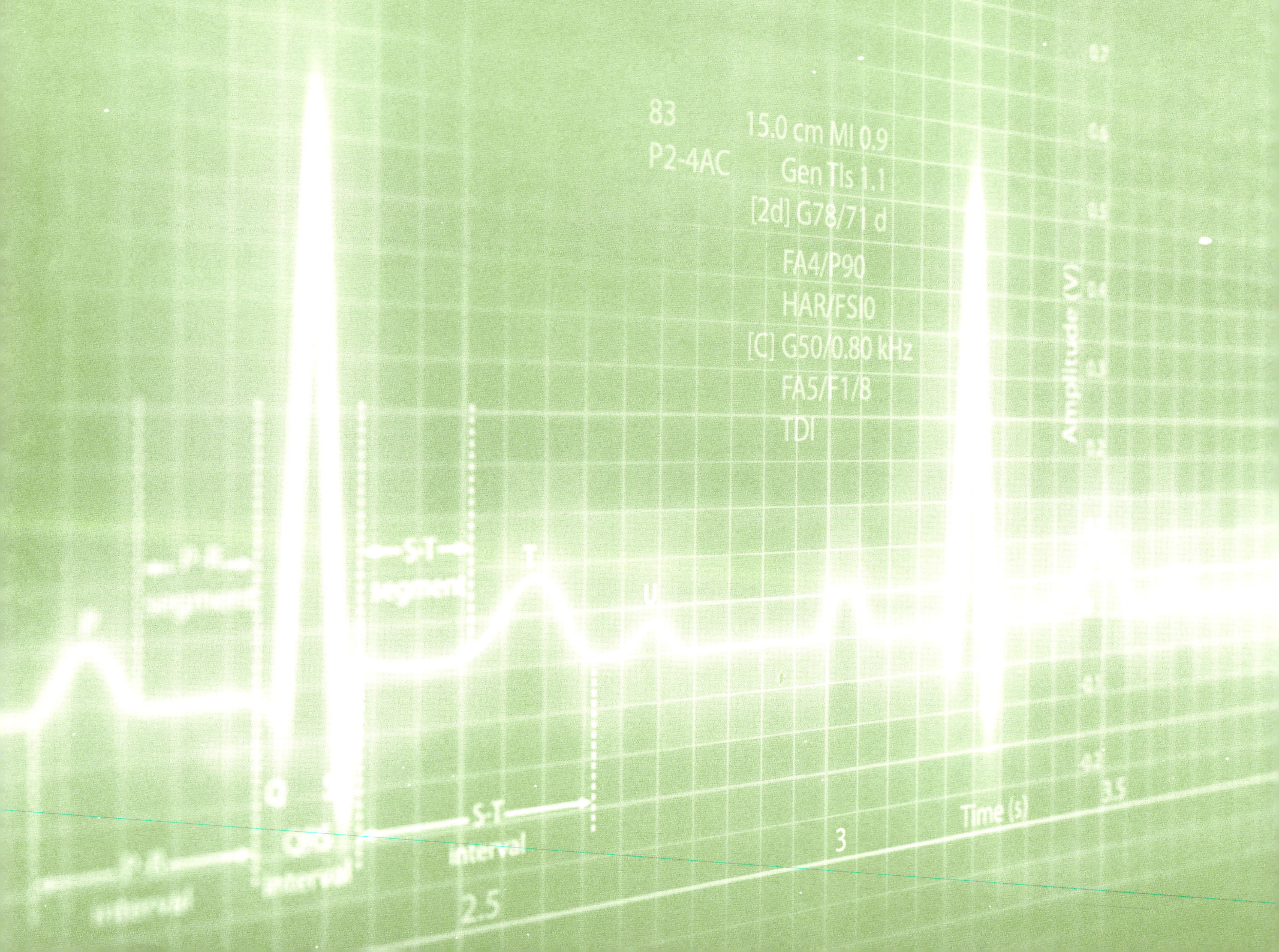
83
P2-4AC
15.0 cm MI 0.9
Gen Tls 1.1
[2d] G78/71 d
FA4/P90
HAR/FSI0
[C] G50/0.80 kHz
FA5/F1/8
TDI
S-T
segment
T
U
S-T
interval
QRS
interval
2.5
3
3.5
Time (s)
Amplitude (V)

ANSWER

59-1. Interpret this ECG: what is the diagnosis?

This is a wide complex tachycardia at 140 beats/min. The morphology is wide and bizarre, not typical of either classic right or left bundle branch block. The tachycardia can be classified as having "right bundle morphology" due to the upright polarity in lead V1. The differential diagnosis includes ventricular tachycardia and supraventricular tachycardia with aberrant conduction. Characteristics favoring ventricular tachycardia over supraventricular tachycardia include the presence of preexisting heart disease, a very broad QRS complex (defined specifically as QRS duration greater than 140 milliseconds if right bundle morphology is present or greater than 160 milliseconds if left bundle morphology is present), a shift in frontal plane axis from the baseline ECG, and the presence of atrioventricular dissociation. This tracing represents ventricular tachycardia. This is a monomorphic ventricular tachycardia: all QRS complexes have similar shape, in contrast to polymorphic tachycardia in which the QRS morphology is variable.

There are several schema to distinguish ventricular tachycardia from supraventricular tachycardia including the Brugada criteria[1,2] and the Verecki criteria.[3]

[1]Brugada P, Brugada J, Mont L, et al. A new approach to the differential diagnosis of a regular tachycardia with a wide QRS complex. *Circulation* 1991; 83: 1649-1659.
[2]Pava LF, Perafan P, Badiel M, et al. R-wave peak time at DII: a new criterion for differentiating between wide complex QRS tachycardias. *Heart Rhythm* 2010; 7: 922-926.
[3]Vereckei A, Duray G, Szenasi G, et al. Application of a new algorithm in the differential diagnosis of wide QRS complex tachycardia. *Eur Heart J* 2007; 28: 589-600.

Case #60. A 56-year-old man presents to a small community hospital with severe left shoulder and arm pain. There is no catheterization lab on site.

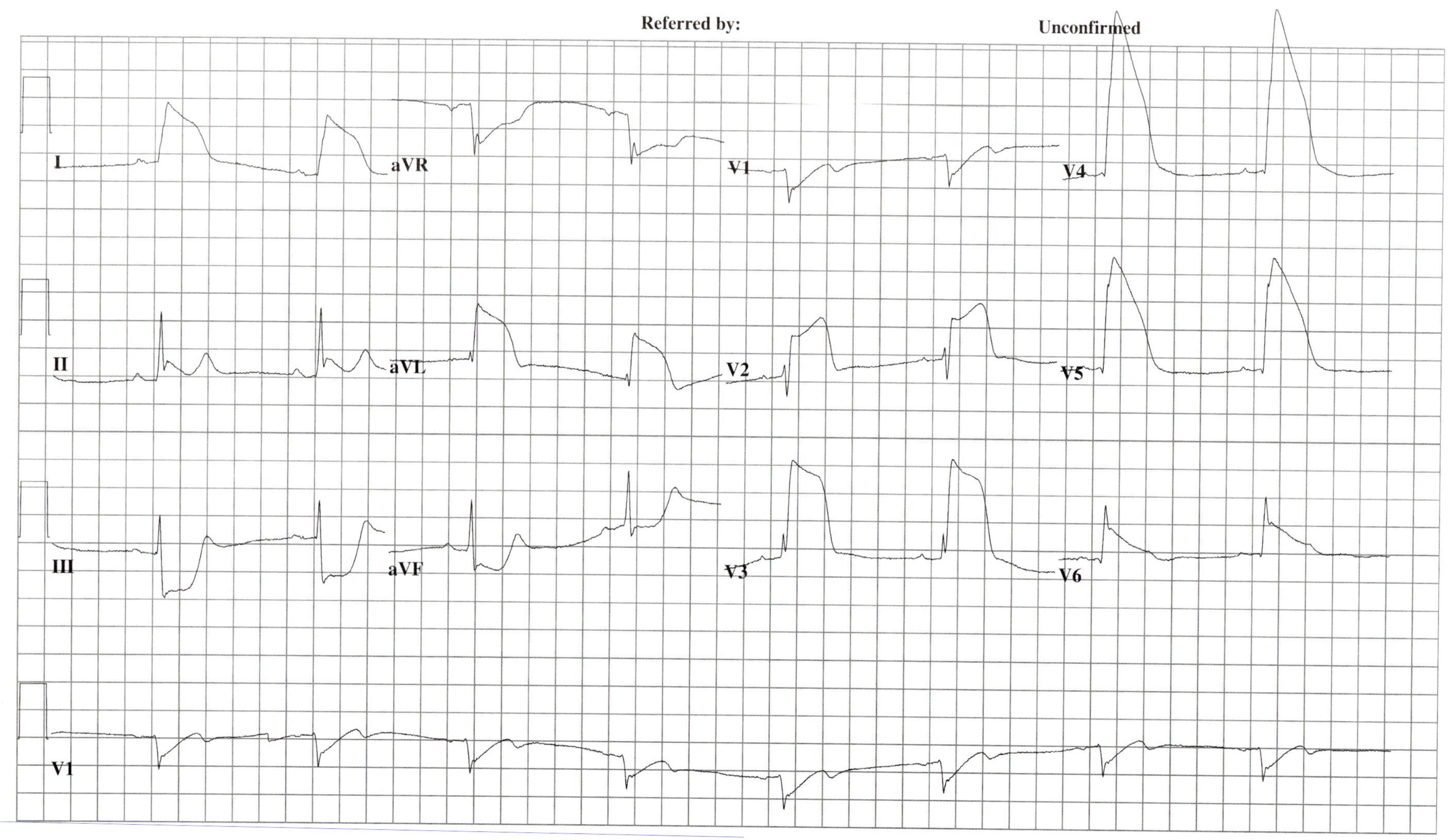

QUESTIONS

60-1. What is the diagnosis?

60-2. How would you manage this patient?

83
P2-4AC
15.0 cm MI 0.9
Gen TIs 1.1
[2d] G78/71 d
FA4/P90
HAR/FSI0
[C] G50/0.80 kHz
FA5/F1/8
TDI
Amplitude (V)
S-T
interval
Time (s)
2.5
3
3.5

ANSWERS

60-1. What is the diagnosis?

Despite the obvious abnormalities, it is important to interpret the tracing systematically so that important findings are not overlooked. Sinus bradycardia is present at a rate of 50 beats/min. The axis and intervals are normal. Massive ST-segment elevation is present in leads I, aVL, and V2 through V6 with reciprocal ST-segment depression in leads III and aVF is consistent with acute myocardial ischemia in the anterolateral territory, most likely due to occlusion of the left anterior descending artery. This tracing demonstrates the "tombstone" appearance of the ST segment and QRS complex sometimes seen in the setting of acute ST-segment myocardial infarction.

60-2. How would you manage this patient?

Urgent coronary revascularization should be arranged. In this case where no catheterization lab is on site, options for therapy include transfer for cardiac catheterization and percutaneous coronary intervention (PCI) or administration of intravenous thrombolytic therapy. Factors impacting the decision of thrombolytic therapy versus transfer for PCI include the anticipated time until reperfusion occurs. If pharmacologic thrombolysis is chosen as a reperfusion strategy, goal is for administration within 30 minutes of arrival, for a "door to needle time" of 30 minutes or less. If PCI is chosen as the reperfusion strategy, the time from patient's arrival to opening of the artery, or the "door to balloon time" should be 90 minutes or less. Transfer to a PCI center could be considered if the "door to balloon time" minus the "door to needle time" is less than 1 hour. Another important factor to consider in choosing a reperfusion strategy for this patient is whether contraindications to thrombolytics are present; contraindications to pharmacologic thrombolysis include recent surgery, history of intracranial hemorrhage, thrombocytopenia, recent stroke, uncontrolled hypertension, or arterial puncture at a noncompressible site. The presence of these factors would favor transfer for PCI.[1]

---

[1]Antman EM, Anbe DT, Armstrong PW, et al. ACC/AHA guidelines for the management of patients with ST-segment myocardial infarction—executive summary. *Circulation* 2004; 110: 588-636.

Case #61. A 23-year-old man presents with "neck pounding" that occurs without warning about once each month.

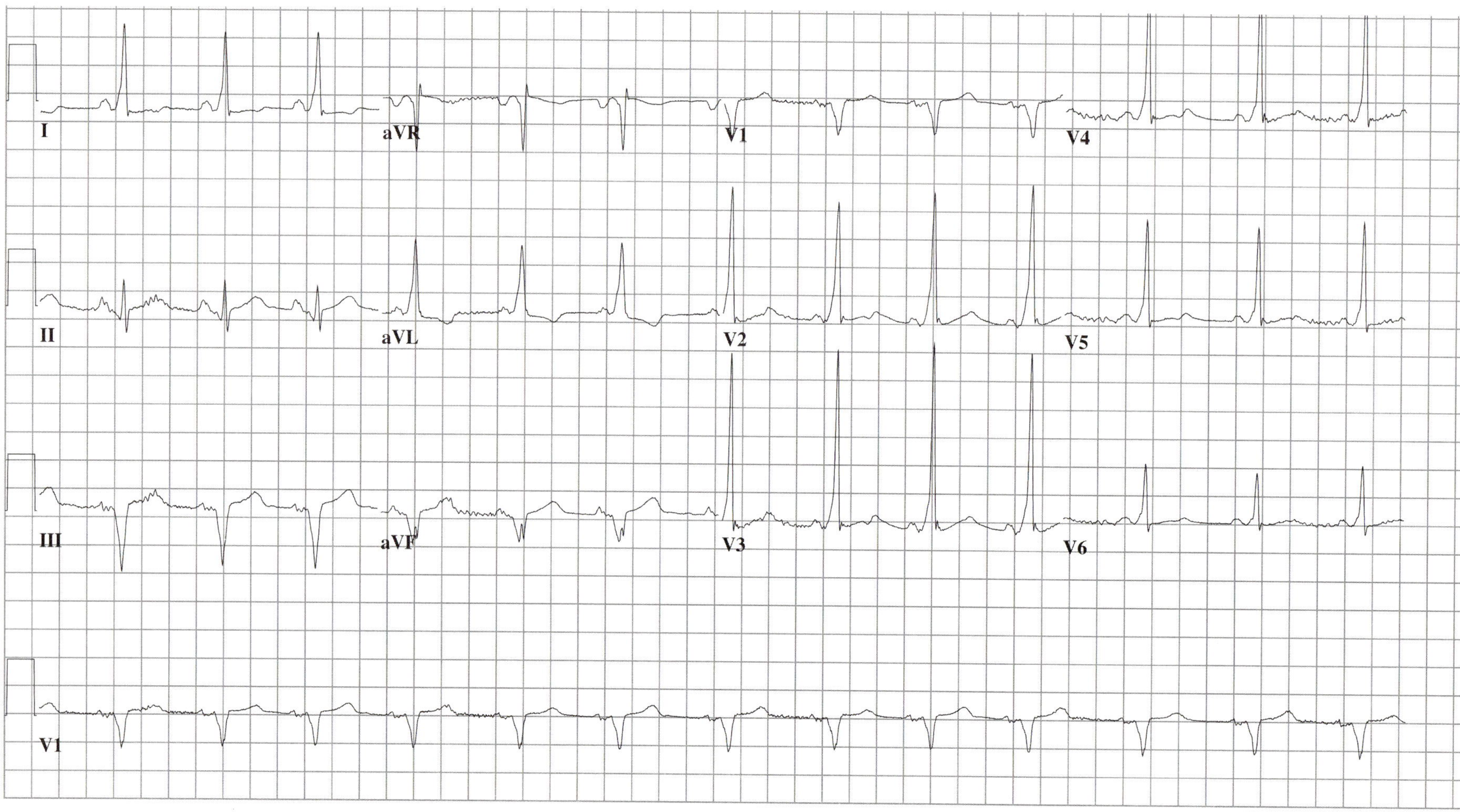

QUESTIONS

61-1. Interpret this ECG.

61-2. What would you do next?

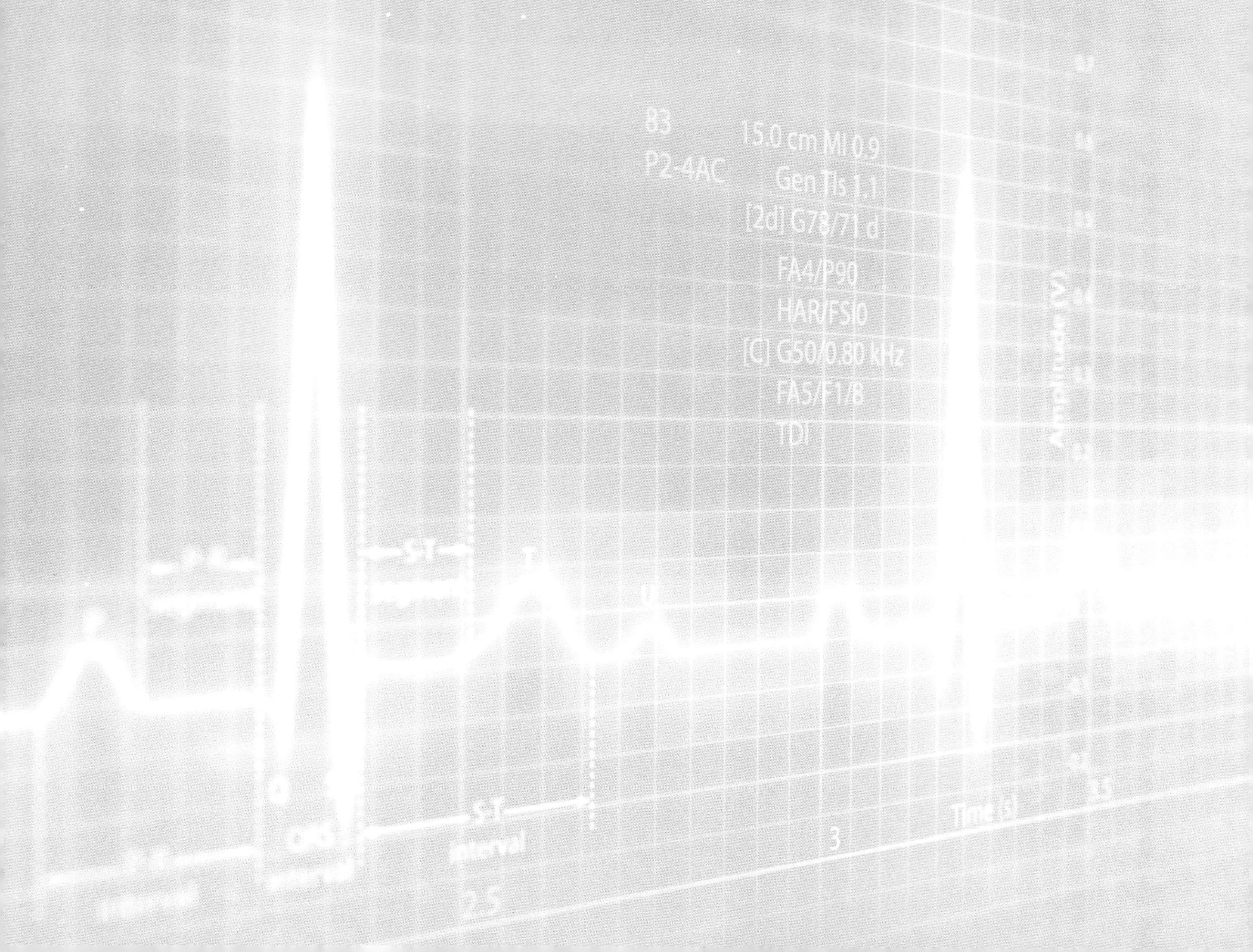
83
P2-4AC
15.0 cm MI 0.9
Gen TIs 1.1
[2d] G78/71 d
FA4/P90
HAR/FSI0
[C] G50/0.80 kHz
FA5/F1/8
TDI
Amplitude (V)
S-T
T
S-T
interval
2.5
3
Time (s)

ANSWERS

61-1. Interpret this ECG.

This tracing demonstrates sinus rhythm at a rate of 80 beats/min. The axis is normal. The PR interval is shortened to less than 120 milliseconds, and the QRS is widened with a slurred upstroke, the so-called delta wave, as shown in the figure. There is a tall R wave in lead V2 consistent with an early R-wave transition in the precordial leads. There are inferior Q waves and T-wave inversions in leads I and aVL. The combination of a short PR interval, delta wave, and clinical information suggestive of intermittent supraventricular tachycardia suggests a diagnosis of the Wolff-Parkinson-White (WPW) syndrome. Patients with WPW may have abnormalities of the QRS complex, ST segment, and T waves, including Q waves and repolarization abnormalities. In this case, the early R-wave transition and inferior Q waves are caused by preexcitation and the delta waves rather than ischemia.

A short PR interval of less than 120 milliseconds coupled with a slurred upstroke to the QRS called a delta wave suggests a Wolff-Parkinson-White ECG pattern.

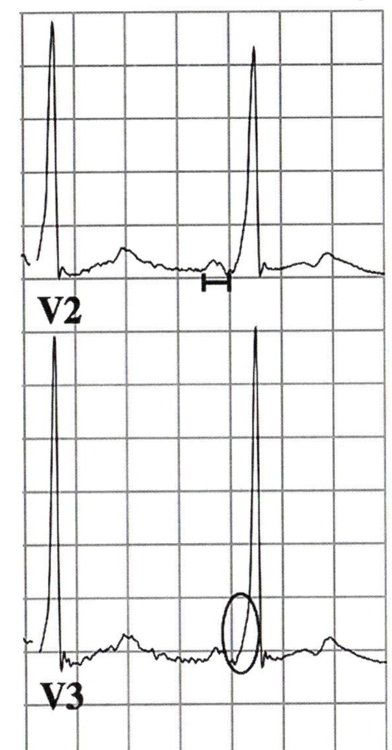

61-2. What would you do next?

Neck pounding is suggestive of intermittent supraventricular tachycardia, and the patient should be further investigated with an electrophysiology study. If the expected accessory pathway is confirmed, radiofrequency ablation is curative in the vast majority of cases.

Case #62. A 21-year-old runner presents for a preparticipation physical examination. This ECG is obtained because of an irregular heart rhythm.

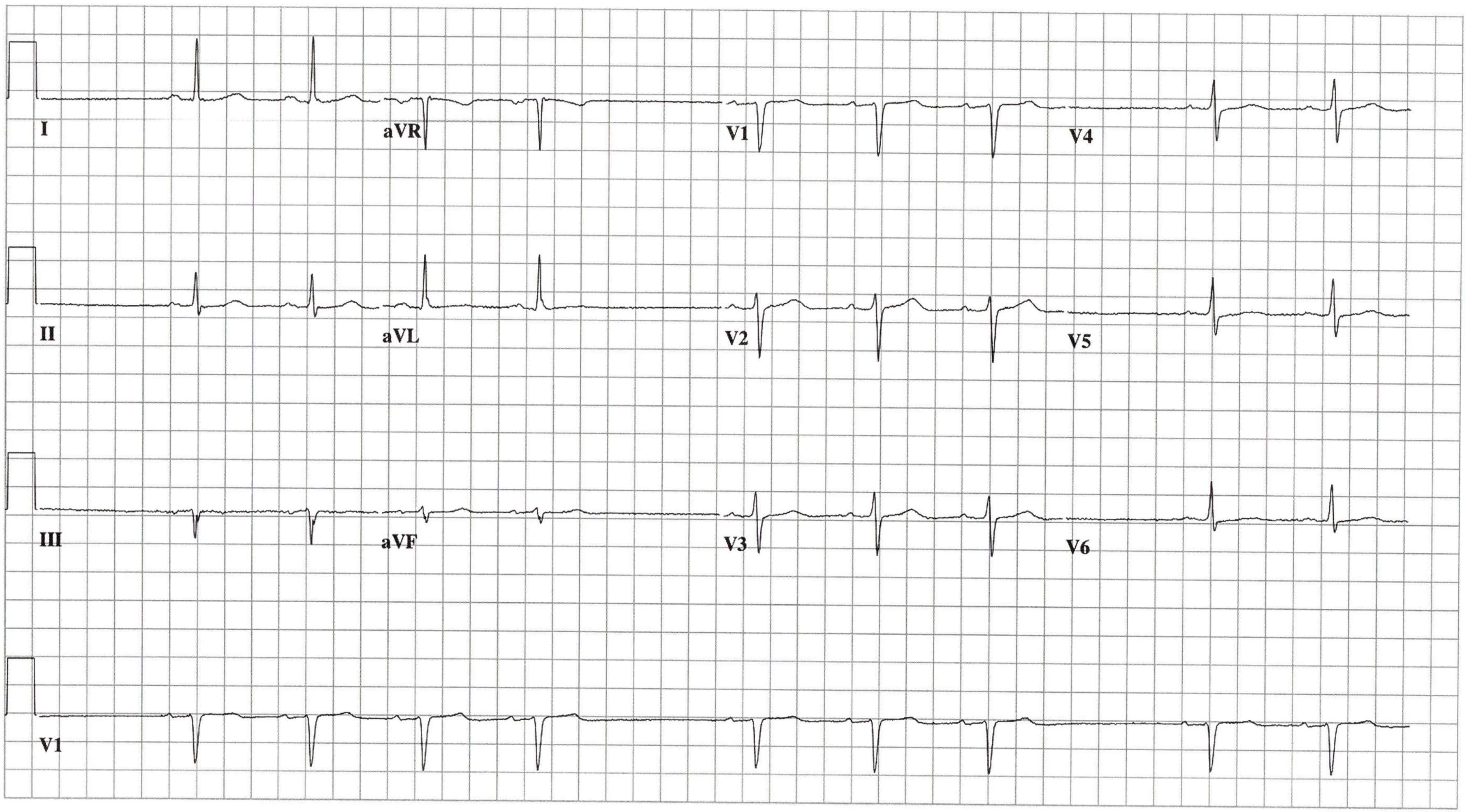

QUESTIONS

62-1. Interpret this ECG.

62-2. What other ECG findings are common in young athletes?

83
P2-4AC
15.0 cm MI 0.9
Gen TIs 1.1
[2d] G78/71 d
FA4/P90
HAR/FSI0
[C] G50/0.80 kHz
FA5/F1/8
TDI
Amplitude (V)
Time (s)
3
2.5

ANSWERS

62-1. Interpret this ECG.

Sinus rhythm is present with normal-appearing P waves preceding each QRS complex, although the rhythm is markedly irregular. There is no evidence of AV block. The variation in the R–R interval is phasic, seemingly with respiration, and is consistent with sinus arrhythmia. Sinus arrhythmia is evidence of high vagal tone, common in highly conditioned athletes and young individuals. Otherwise, the axis and intervals are normal and there is no evidence of chamber hypertrophy or ischemia.

62-2. What other ECG findings are common in young athletes?

Sinus bradycardia, junctional rhythms, and AV block can all be seen in athletes, particularly when asleep. These rhythms are not pathologic but rather reflect heightened vagal tone in these patients. All of these arrhythmias resolve with increase in activity or sympathetic tone.

ECG 1:

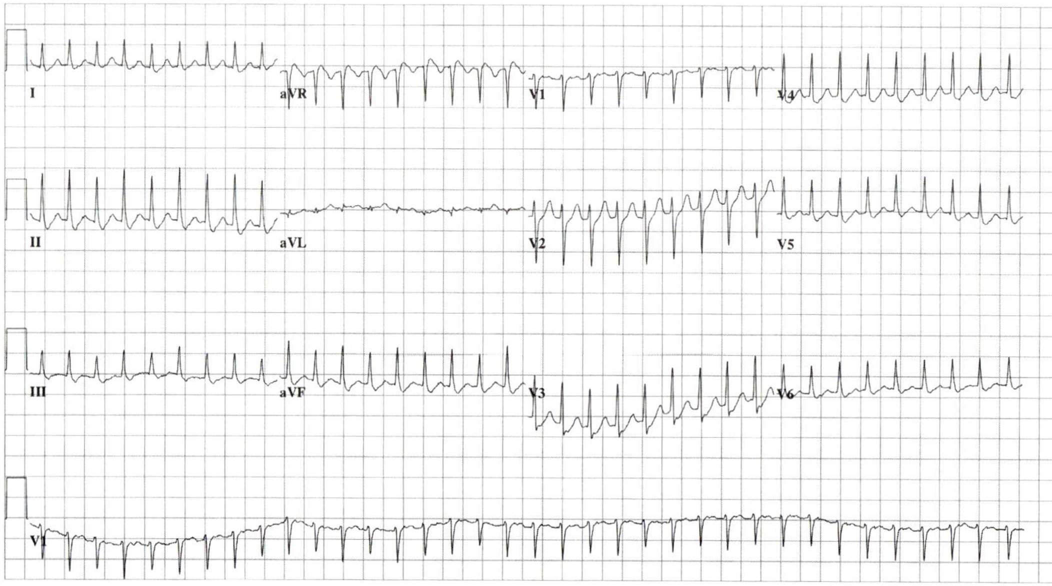

ECG 2:

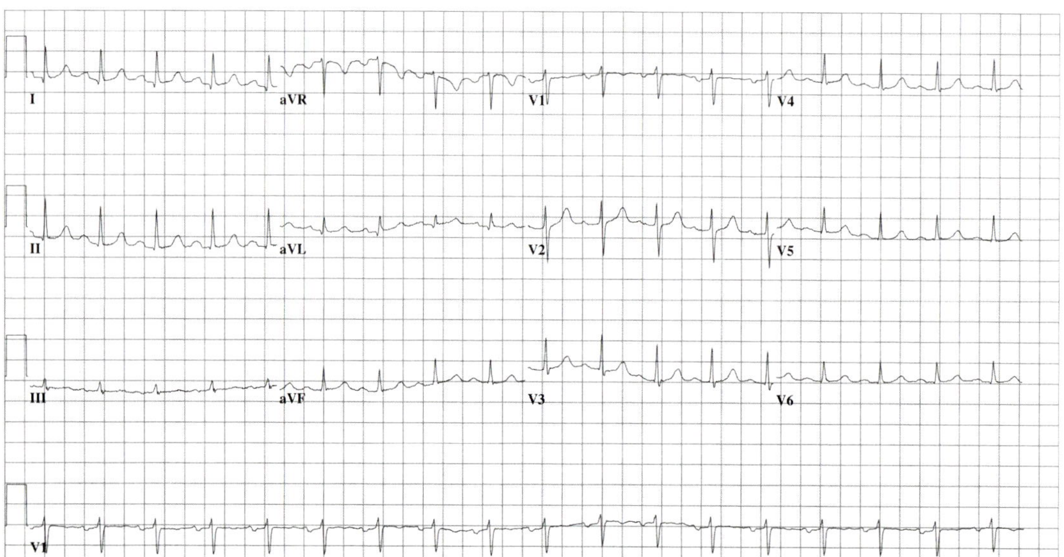

Case #63. A 47-year-old woman presents to the emergency department with palpitations and the initial ECG. Carotid sinus massage is performed, after which the second ECG is recorded.

QUESTIONS

63-1. Interpret both the pre- and post-treatment ECGs. What is the diagnosis?

63-2. Describe the physiologic effect of carotid sinus massage.

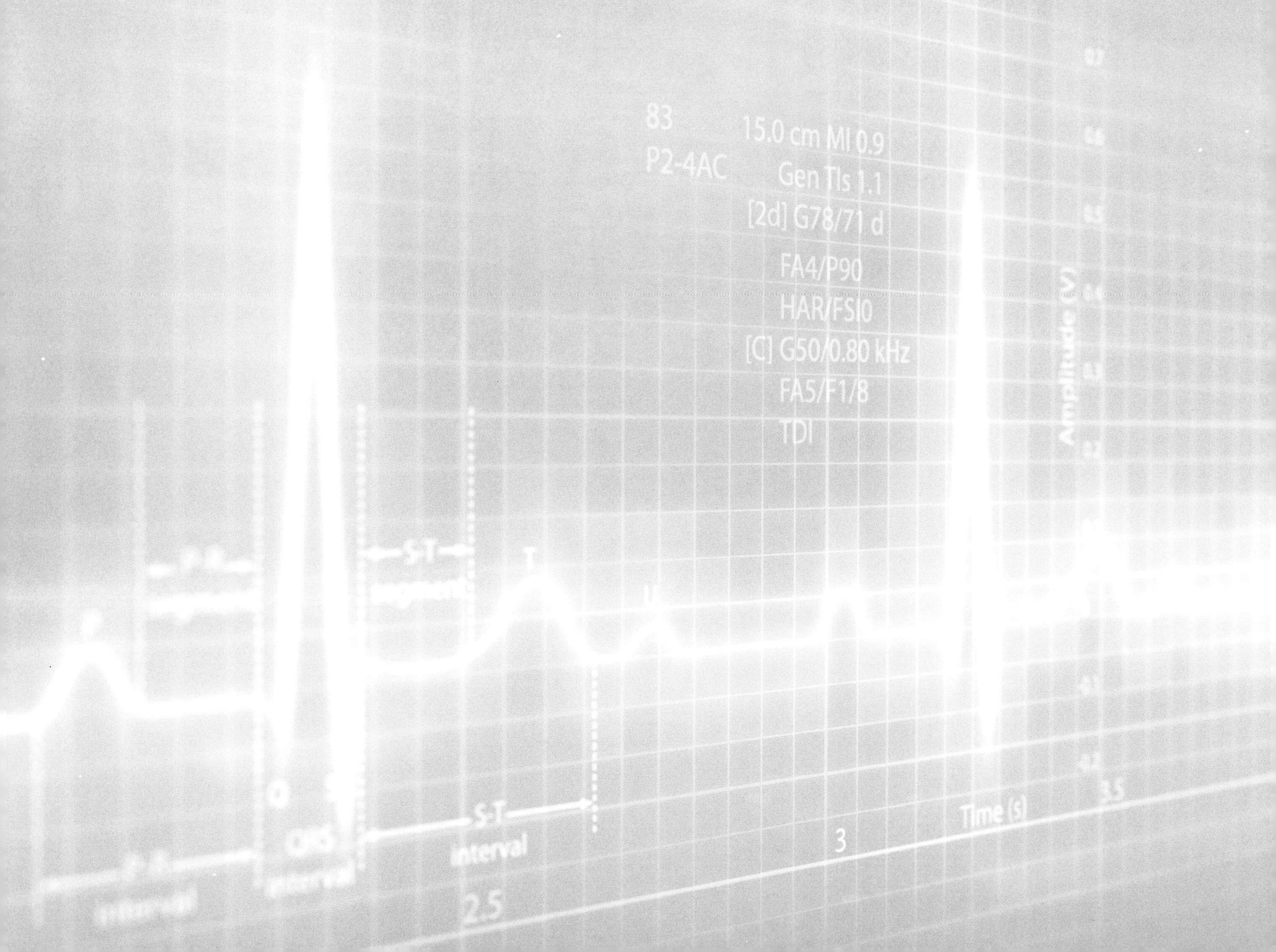
83
P2-4AC
15.0 cm MI 0.9
Gen TIs 1.1
[2d] G78/71 d
FA4/P90
HAR/FSI0
[C] G50/0.80 kHz
FA5/F1/8
TDI
Amplitude (V)
T
S-T
S-T
interval
2.5
3
Time (s)
3.5

ANSWERS

63-1. Interpret both the pre- and post-treatment ECGs. What is the diagnosis?

The initial ECG reveals a narrow complex, regular tachycardia with a very rapid rate. There are 36 QRS complexes in the 10-second rhythm strip, yielding an estimated heart rate of 216 beats/min. The differential diagnosis of a regular narrow complex tachycardia includes sinus tachycardia, atrial tachycardia, atrial flutter with constant AV block, AVNRT and AVRT, and junctional tachycardias, which are rare. A careful search for atrial activity will help distinguish among these dysrhythmias. On first glance, no clear P waves are seen in the presentation tracing. However, rounded "S waves" are present at the terminal portion of the QRS complex in leads II, III, and aVF. Comparing the QRS complex in these leads to the same leads in the post-treatment tracing (when sinus rhythm is present), one appreciates that the "S waves" are present only during tachycardia, clearly shown in the figure. Hence, this finding represents retrograde atrial activation, or a so-called "pseudo S wave," and is consistent with AVNRT. The remainder of the presentation tracing reveals baseline artifact, a normal QRS axis, and no evidence of chamber enlargement or ischemia. The tracing after carotid sinus pressure reveals sinus tachycardia at approximately 100 beats/min. The axis and intervals are normal, and there is no evidence of chamber enlargement or ischemia. There is slight baseline artifact present.

63-2. Describe the physiologic effect of carotid sinus massage.

The carotid sinus contains baroreceptors that provide regulation of heart rate and vascular tone by modulating the sympathetic and parasympathetic nervous systems. Application of carotid sinus pressure causes increased vagal tone relative to sympathetic tone; the effects on the cardiac conduction system include sinus node slowing and increased AV node refractoriness. In the cases of arrhythmias that are "AV node dependent," which include arrhythmias with a reentrant mechanism where the AV node is included in the circuit, the change in AV nodal conduction properties can result in termination of the arrhythmia, as was observed in this case.

ANSWERS (Cont.)

Circles illustrate the rounded terminal deflections present in tachycardia but not in sinus rhythm, which represent retrograde P waves.

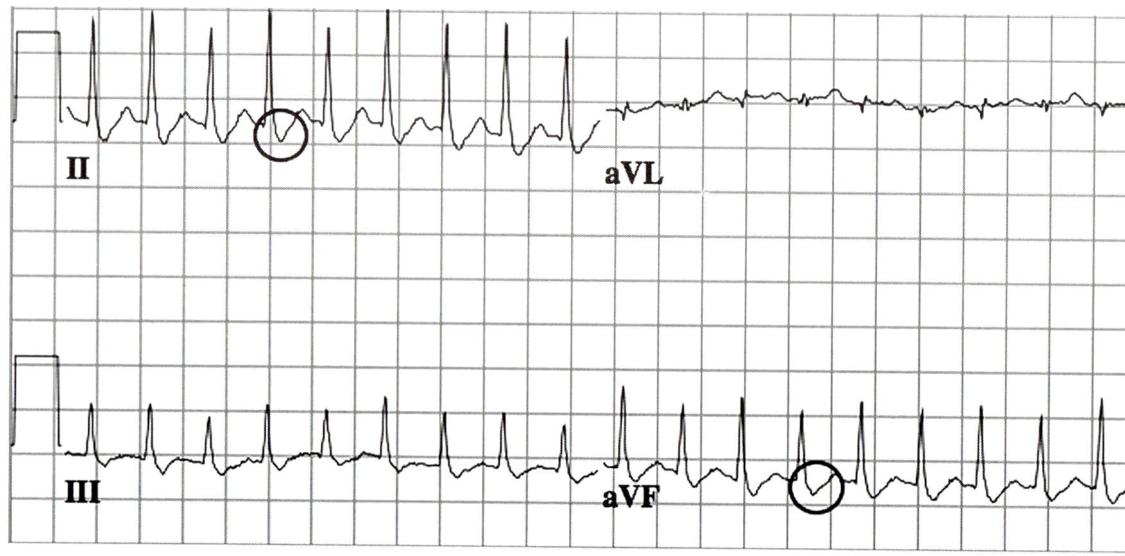

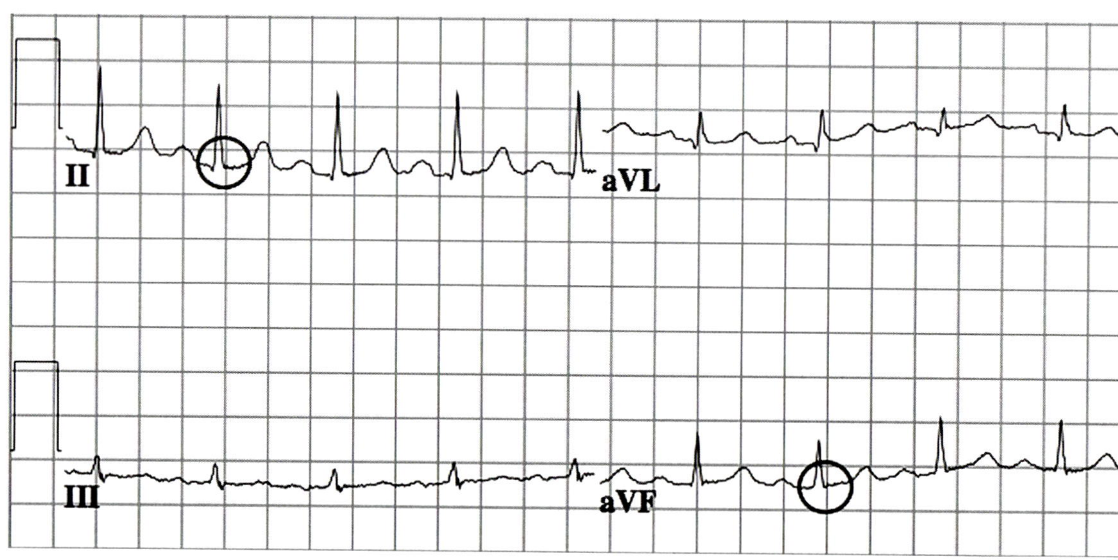

Case #64. A 76-year-old man with a history of coronary disease presents with palpitations.

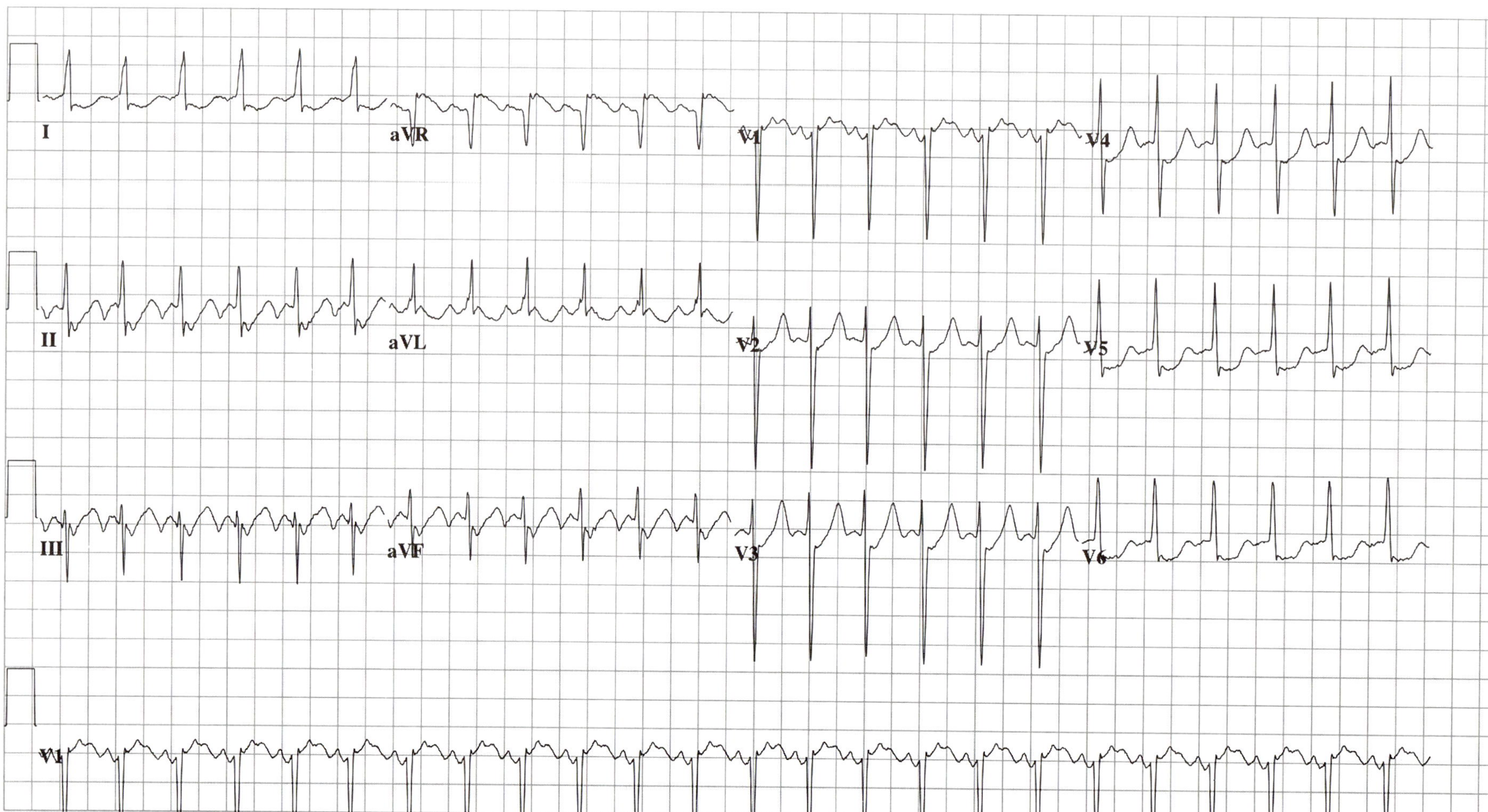

QUESTIONS

64-1. What is the rhythm?

64-2. What other abnormalities are present?

64-3. What is the differential diagnosis for the ST-segment abnormalities?

83
P2-4AC
15.0 cm MI 0.9
Gen TIs 1.1
[2d] G78/71 d
FA4/P90
HAR/FSI0
[C] G50/0.80 kHz
FA5/F1/8
TDI
Amplitude (V)
S-T
T
S-T
Interval
Time (s)
2.5
3
3.5

ANSWERS

64-1. What is the rhythm?

This tracing reveals a narrow complex tachycardia at 150 beats/min. In analyzing narrow complex tachycardia, first determine if the rhythm is regular or irregular.[1] In this case, QRS complexes occur at regular intervals. Next, perform a careful search for atrial activity and note the relationship of the atrial to the ventricular depolarization. In lead V1, a deflection precedes each QRS complex and a second deflection is buried in each ST segment; the rate of this atrial activity is 300 beats/min. Inspecting lead II, one appreciates that the atrial activity has a classic "sawtooth" morphology. These abnormalities suggest a diagnosis of atrial flutter with 2 to 1 atrioventricular conduction. Atrial flutter should be considered in the differential diagnosis of any supraventricular tachycardia with a ventricular rate approximating 150 beats/min.

64-2. What other abnormalities are present?

The axis is normal. The sum of the R-wave amplitude in aVL and the S-wave amplitude in V3 is just greater than 28 mV, suggesting left ventricular hypertrophy. There are horizontal ST-segment depressions in the anterior and lateral leads, most prominent in leads V4, V5, and V6. In addition, there are ST-segment depressions in the inferior leads II, III, and aVF that are of a different morphology and are most likely secondary to superimposed atrial flutter waves.

64-3. What is the differential diagnosis for the ST-segment abnormalities?

The differential diagnosis for ST-segment depression includes artifact, repolarization changes from ventricular hypertrophy, subendocardial ischemia due to the rupture of a coronary plaque with nonocclusive thrombus, and subendocardial ischemia due to conditions that increase myocardial oxygen demand or decrease myocardial oxygen supply. In this case, it is possible that the ischemic-appearing ST changes in V4, V5, and V6 are due to increased myocardial oxygen demand from tachycardia. A repeat ECG once the patient's heart rate normalizes would be indicated.

[1] Fox DJ, Tischenko A, Krahn AD, et al. Supraventricular tachycardia: diagnosis and management. *Mayo Clin Proc* 2008; 83: 1400-1411.

Case #65. A 22-year-old young woman with profound weight loss and poor oral intake.

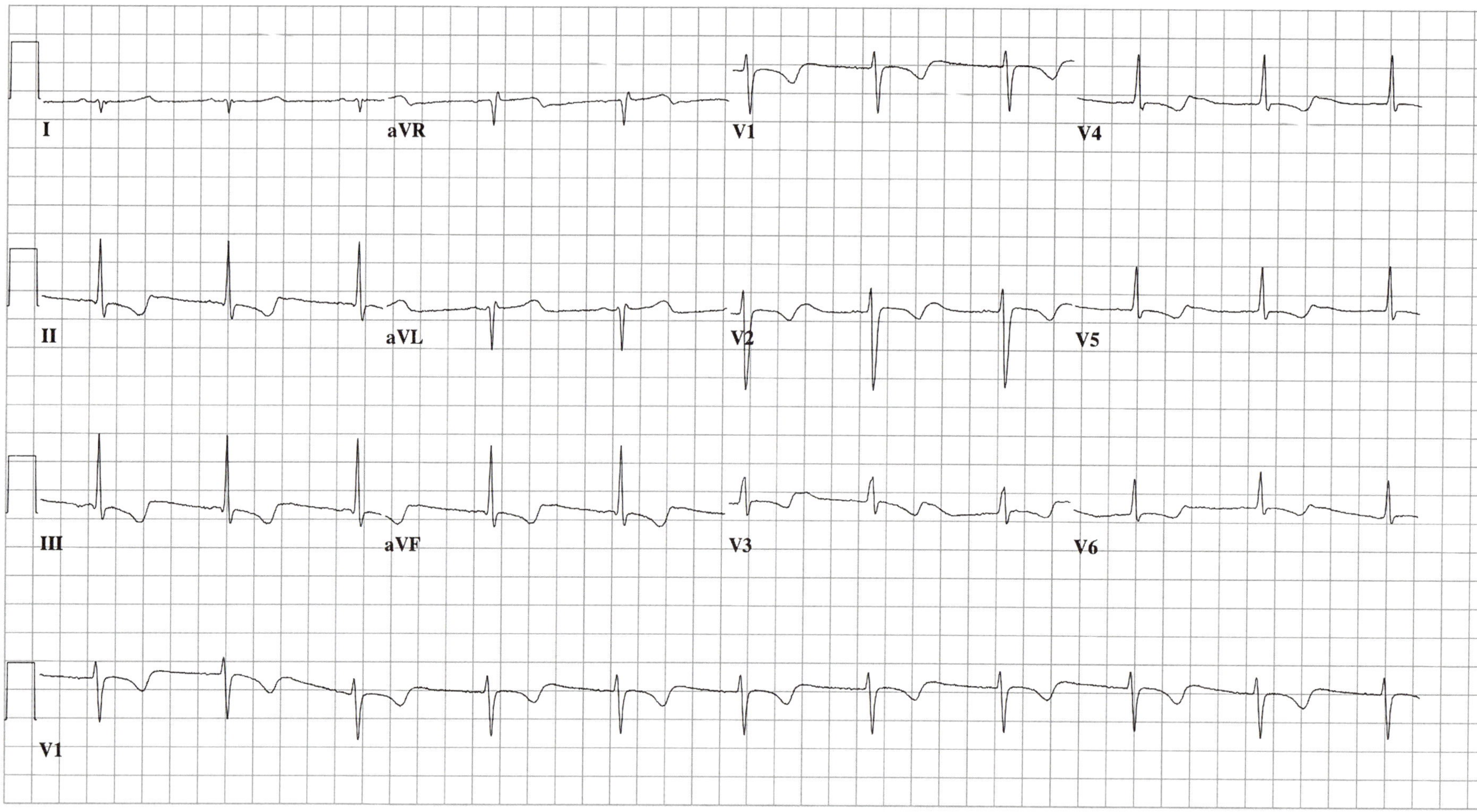

QUESTIONS

65-1. What are the findings?

65-2. What do you expect the laboratory studies to demonstrate?

83
P2-4AC
15.0 cm MI 0.9
Gen TIs 1.1
[2d] G78/71 d
FA4/P90
HAR/FSI0
[C] G50/0.80 kHz
FA5/F1/8
TDI
S-T
interval
QRS
interval
2.5
3
Time (s)
Amplitude (V)

ANSWERS

65-1. What are the findings?

The heart rate is 66 beats/min and sinus rhythm is present as evidenced by low-amplitude, otherwise normal-appearing P waves in lead I. The axis is rightward. There is no evidence of chamber enlargement. There are diffuse ST-segment depressions with inverted T waves. Best seen in lead V2 is a large U wave merging with the T wave (positive deflection at the terminal portion of the T wave), as shown in the figure.

65-2. What do you expect the laboratory studies to demonstrate?

The presence of U waves and the diffusely abnormal ST segments coupled with the clinical history suggest hypokalemia. In fact, this patient presented with lethargy, malnutrition, and multiple electrolyte abnormalities including a potassium of 1.8.

U waves are noted with arrows, seen as a large positive deflection merging with the T wave.

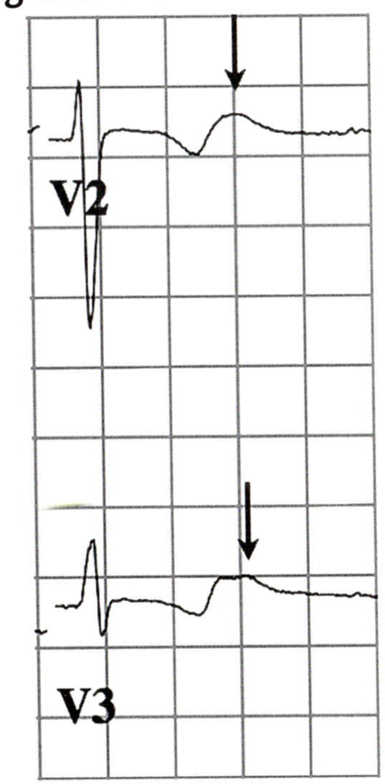

Case #66. A 72-year-old woman presents for routine follow-up.

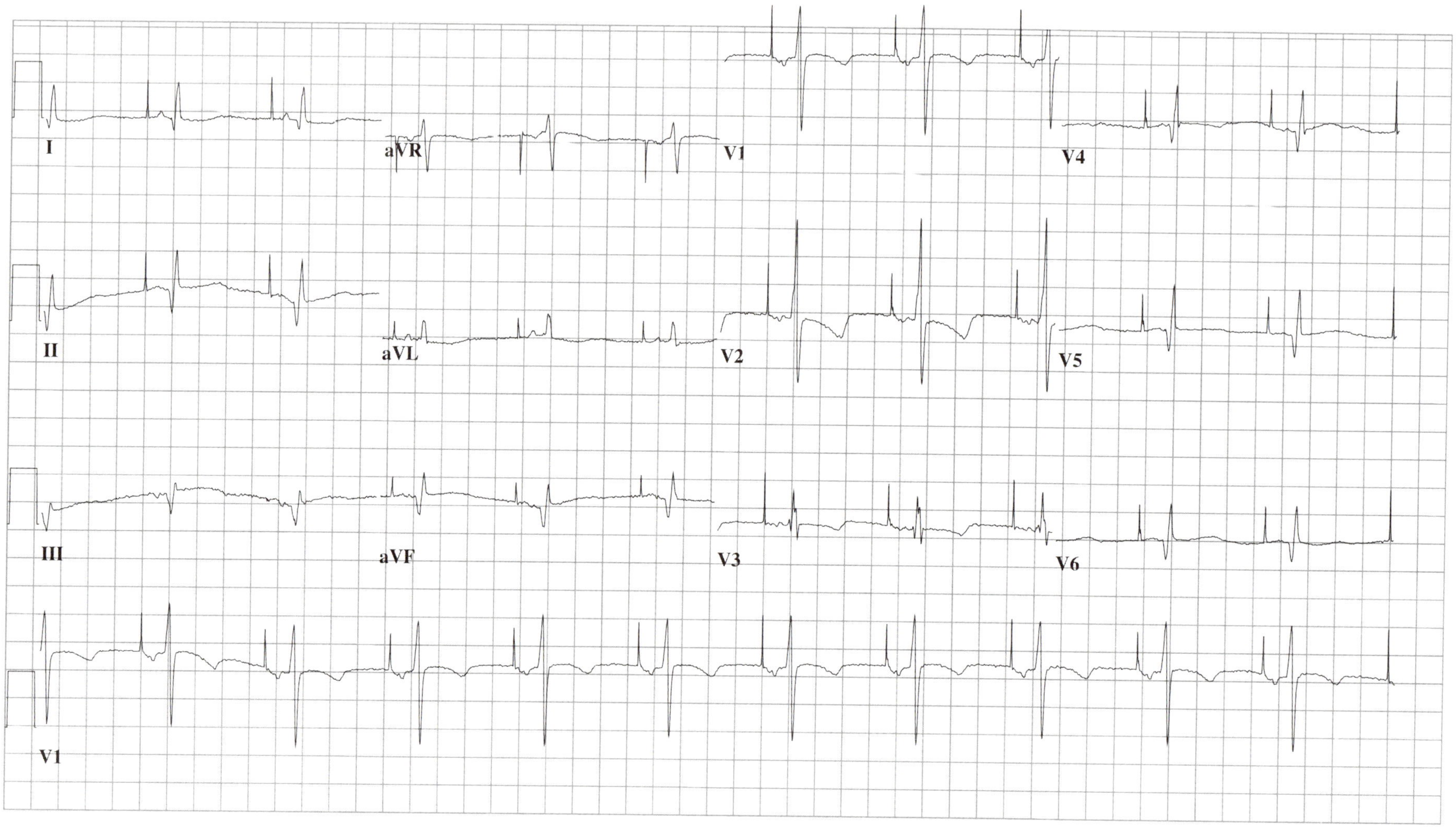

QUESTIONS

66-1. Interpret this ECG.

66-2. What past medical history can you surmise on the basis of this tracing?

83
P2-4AC
15.0 cm MI 0.9
Gen TIs 1.1
[2d] G78/71 d
FA4/P90
HAR/FSI0
[C] G50/0.80 kHz
FA5/F1/8
TDI
Amplitude (V)
S-T
interval
2.5
3
Time (s)
3.5

ANSWERS

66-1. Interpret this ECG.

The heart rate is 65 beats/min. Atrial pacing is present—the P waves have a different morphology than sinus P waves and are preceded by pacing impulses. The QRS axis is normal. There are no signs of chamber enlargement or hypertrophy. There are Q waves in the inferior leads II, III, and aVF and the anterolateral leads V4, V5, V5, and lead I. Finally, there is a tall R wave in lead V1 and V2, which is abnormal. A tall R wave in leads V1 and V2, when considered in the context of inferior Q waves, likely corresponds to posterior wall infarction. Finally, there are T-wave inversions in leads V1 through V3 with ST-segment depression most notable in lead V2, which may be consistent with ischemia in the right clinical context.

66-2. What past medical history can you surmise on the basis of this tracing?

This patient has Q waves in the inferoposterior and anterolateral distribution consistent with myocardial infarction of indeterminate age and bespeaks a significant coronary history. Note that some patients present without describing prior history of myocardial infarction but with Q waves on the ECG. These patients are sometimes said to have suffered a "silent myocardial infarction." The presence of pacemaker stimuli on this tracing suggests a history of symptomatic bradycardia or sick sinus syndrome.

Case #67. A 67-year-old man presents with 2 days of dizziness and lightheadedness.

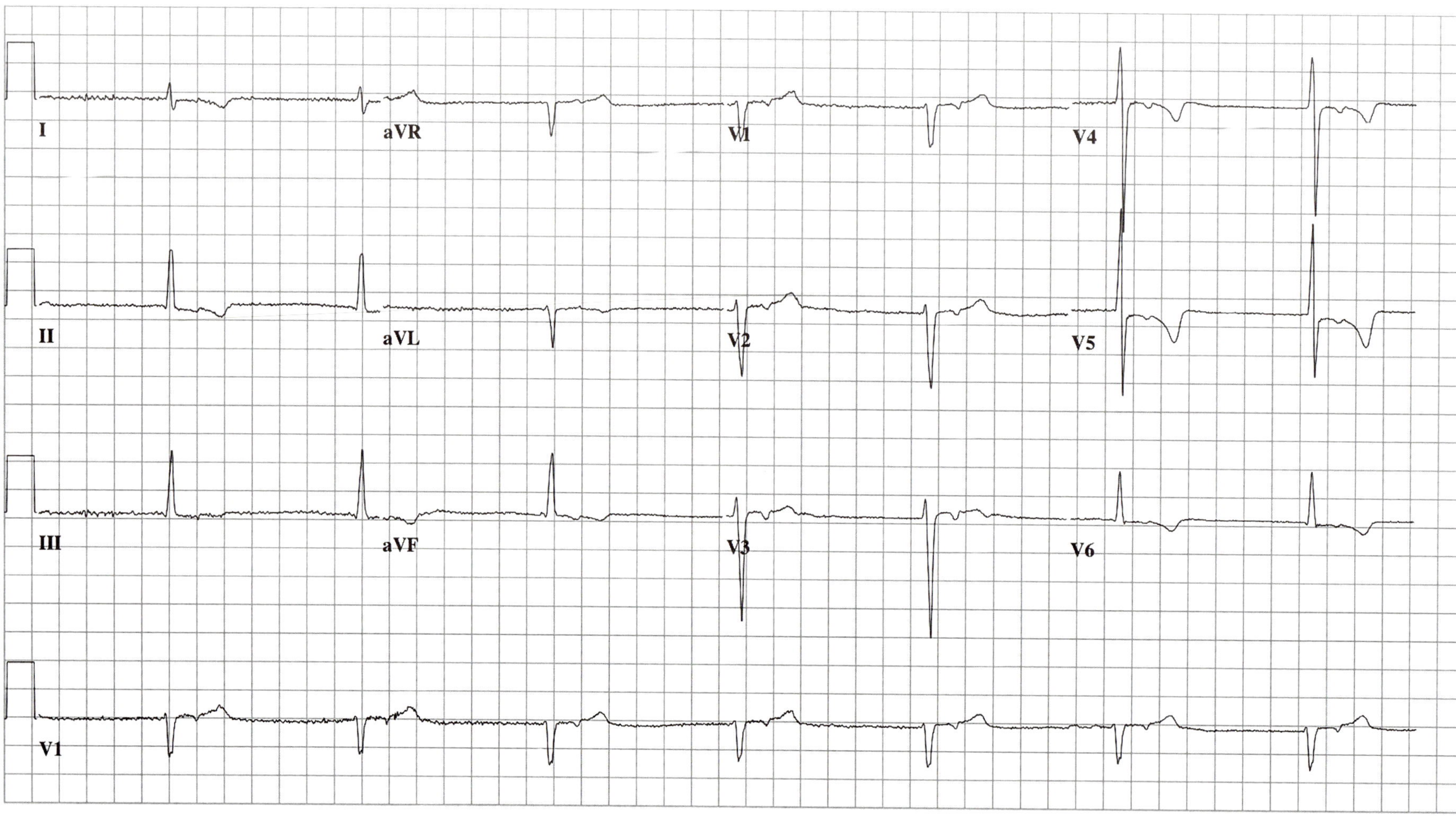

QUESTIONS

67-1. Interpret this ECG. What abnormalities are present on this tracing?

67-2. What intervention would you recommend?

83
P2-4AC
15.0 cm MI 0.9
Gen TIs 1.1
[2d] G78/71 d
FA4/P90
HAR/FS|0
[C] G50/0.80 kHz
FA5/F1/8
TDI
S-T
S-T
interval
2.5
3
Time (s)

ANSWERS

67-1. Interpret this ECG. What abnormalities are present on this tracing?

This tracing demonstrates a regular bradycardia at 45 beats/min. There are no P waves evident before each QRS complex, but approximately 160 milliseconds after each QRS complex there are sharply inscribed deflections within the T wave that are consistent with P waves. These P waves likely represent retrograde atrial activation, as they occur after the QRS complex, are associated with each QRS complex by an interval that is constant, and are negative in the inferior leads and positive in lead aVR, as would be expected if the P wave was traveling up from the AV node toward the SA node (opposite to the normal atrial depolarization). The QRS axis is borderline rightward at approximately +90 degrees. The QRS complex is narrow at 100 milliseconds, and the QT interval is normal. There are T-wave inversions in the inferior and lateral leads. The most likely diagnosis is junctional bradycardia with retrograde atrial activation. The T-wave abnormalities may represent ischemia.

67-2. What intervention would you recommend?

The patient has symptomatic bradycardia and would therefore be a candidate for pacemaker implantation. Prior to placing a pacemaker, however, one should rule out reversible causes of bradycardia such as an overdose of β-blockers or calcium channel blockers or myocardial ischemia (especially given the diffuse T-wave inversions noted on the ECG).

Case #68. A 60-year-old man with diabetes presents with increasing lower-extremity edema and effort intolerance.

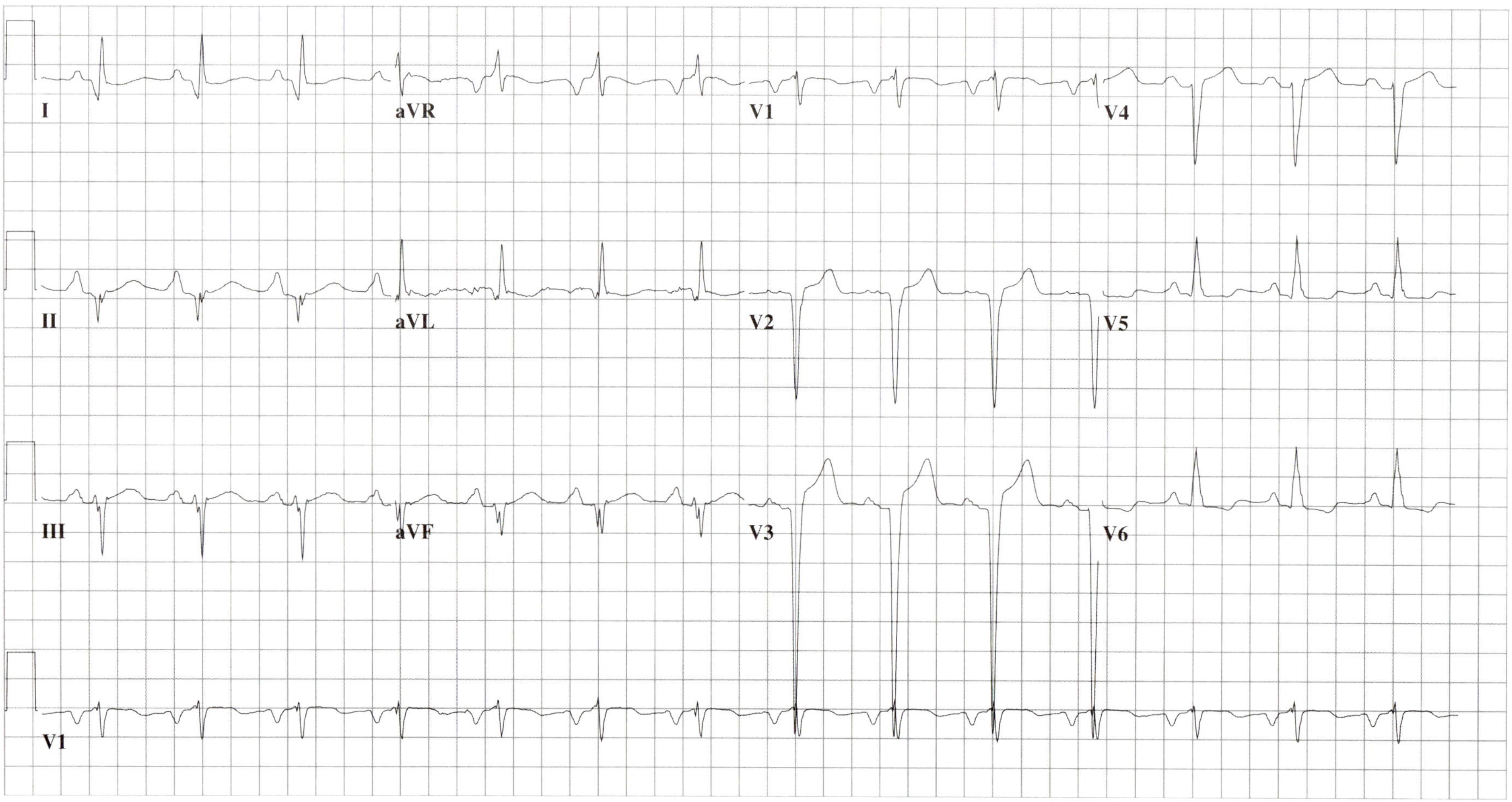

QUESTIONS

68-1. What does the ECG show?

68-2. What is the most likely diagnosis?

83
P2-4AC
15.0 cm MI 0.9
Gen TIs 1.1
[2d] G78/71 d
FA4/P90
HAR/FSI0
[C] G50/0.80 kHz
FA5/F1/B
TDI

ANSWERS

68-1. What does the ECG show?

Sinus rhythm is present at 84 beats/min. The axis is leftward. The PR and QT intervals and QRS duration are normal. Left ventricular hypertrophy is present: the sum of the S wave in lead V3 and the R wave in lead aVL is greater than 28 mV. In addition, there is left atrial abnormality, given that the negative deflection of the P wave in lead V1 is deeper than 1 mV and broader than 1 millisecond. There is right atrial abnormality as well, given the height of the P wave in lead II is greater than 2.5 mV. In summary, there is biatrial abnormality and left ventricular hypertrophy. With regard to ischemic changes, there are pathologic Q waves present in leads I and aVL, suggesting prior myocardial infarction of an undetermined age. There is a Q wave in lead II and an intermittent Q wave in lead aVF, suggesting inferior myocardial infarction of undetermined age. Finally, there are large Q waves present in leads V2 and V3 with only a tiny R wave present in lead V4, suggesting anterior myocardial infarction of undetermined age. There are T-wave inversions and ST-segment abnormalities in the lateral leads, which are nonspecific, and there is 2 mm of ST-segment elevation in leads V2 and V3, which may be secondary to the left ventricular hypertrophy.

68-2. What is the most likely diagnosis?

This patient presents with symptoms of heart failure and an electrocardiogram suggesting prior myocardial infarctions in multiple coronary territories. An echocardiogram would be indicated to evaluate left ventricular function and wall motion abnormalities, suggesting prior infarction. The most likely overall diagnosis is ischemic cardiomyopathy.

Case #69. A 70-year-old woman with known multiple myeloma presents with increasing fatigue and confusion. Two tracings are shown.

Presentation:

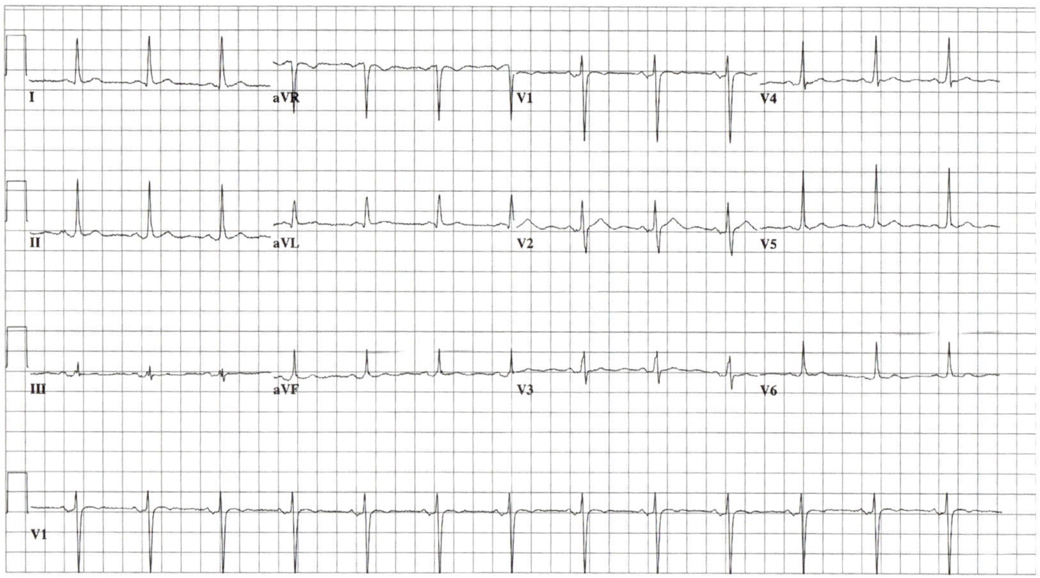

Baseline:

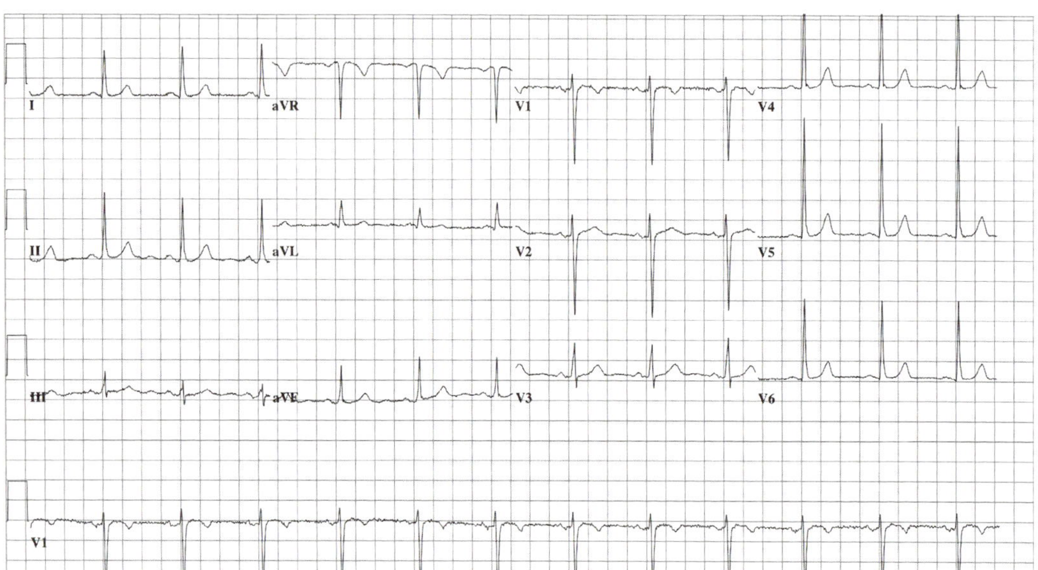

QUESTIONS

69-1. Interpret these tracings.

69-2. What is the differential diagnosis for the observed abnormality?

83
P2-4AC
15.0 cm MI 0.9
Gen TIs 1.1
[2d] G78/71 d
FA4/P90
HAR/FS|0
[C] G50/0.80 kHz
FA5/F1/8
TDI

ANSWERS

69-1. Interpret these tracings.

The initial ECG shows normal sinus rhythm at approximately 80 beats/min with normal QRS axis and a relatively short QT interval (320 milliseconds, corrected to 367 milliseconds for heart rate). There is suggestion of a U wave in leads V2 through V4. Compared to the baseline tracing, the ST segment is shorter. Furthermore, the morphology of the ST segment has changed such that the T wave appears to arise directly from the J point with absence of the isoelectric ST segment. See the figure for a direct comparison of the T wave and ST segment between the baseline and presentation tracings.

69-2. What is the differential diagnosis for the observed abnormality?

QT-interval shortening may be congenital or acquired. Congenital short QT syndrome can be associated with sudden cardiac death. Acquired shortening of the QT interval may result from digitalis, hyperkalemia, and, most classically, hypercalcemia. This patient's calcium was markedly elevated consistent with her clinical syndrome.

ANSWERS (Cont.)

Presentation and baseline tracings are shown, demonstrating interval shortening and change in morphology of the ST segment.

Presentation

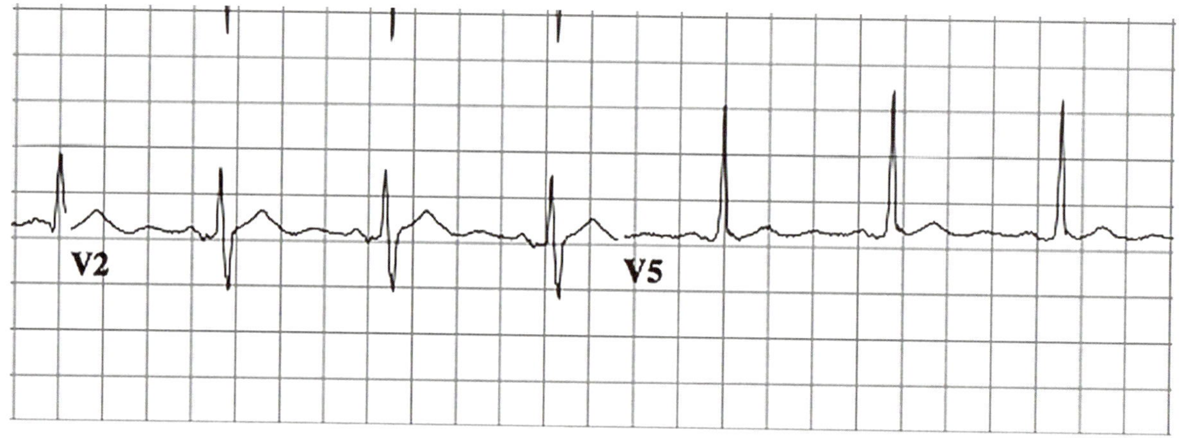

Baseline

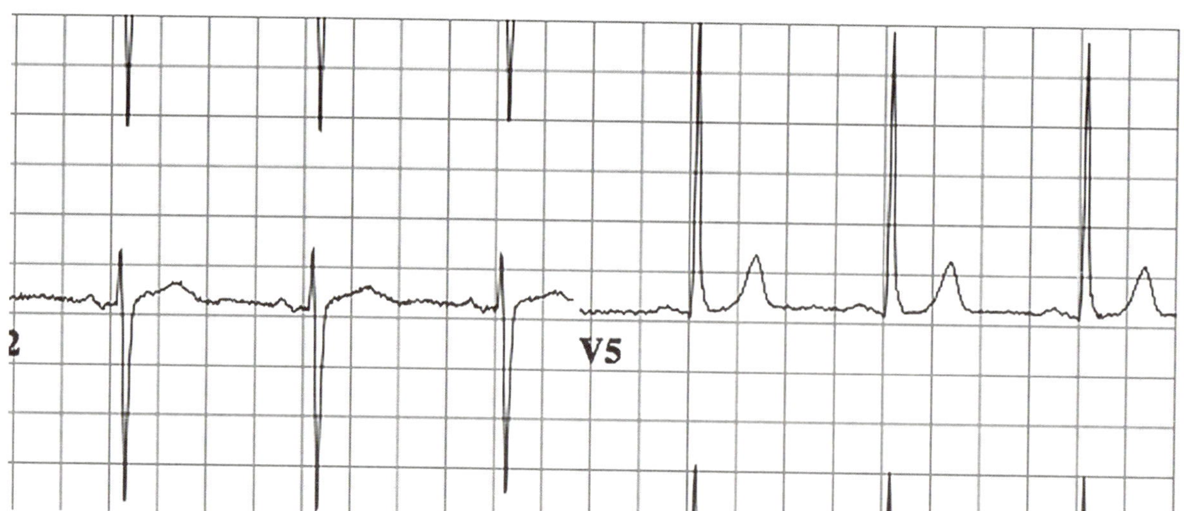

Case #70. A 58-year-old woman presents with a syndrome of alcohol withdrawal.

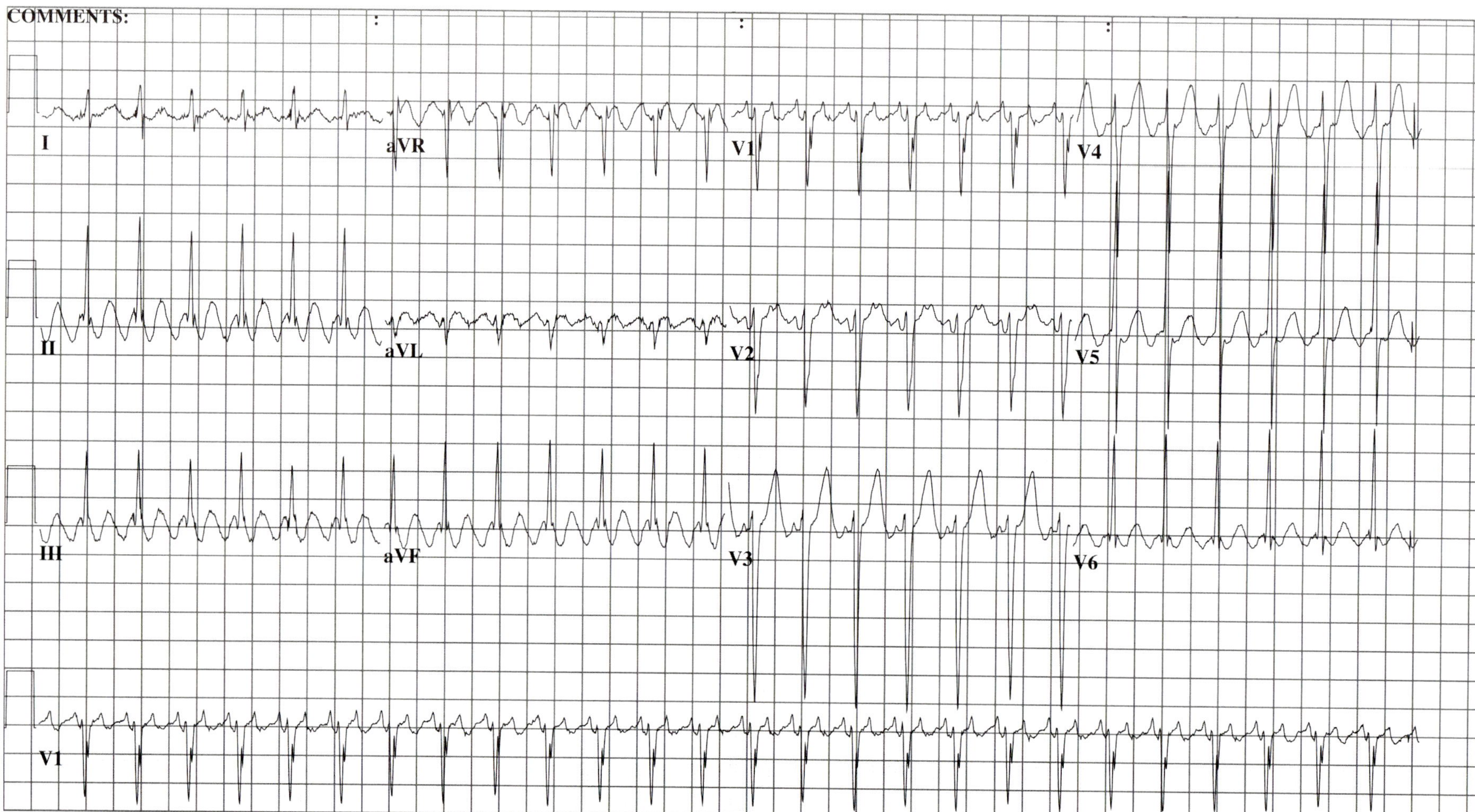

QUESTIONS

70-1. Interpret this ECG.

70-2. What factors predispose to this arrhythmia?

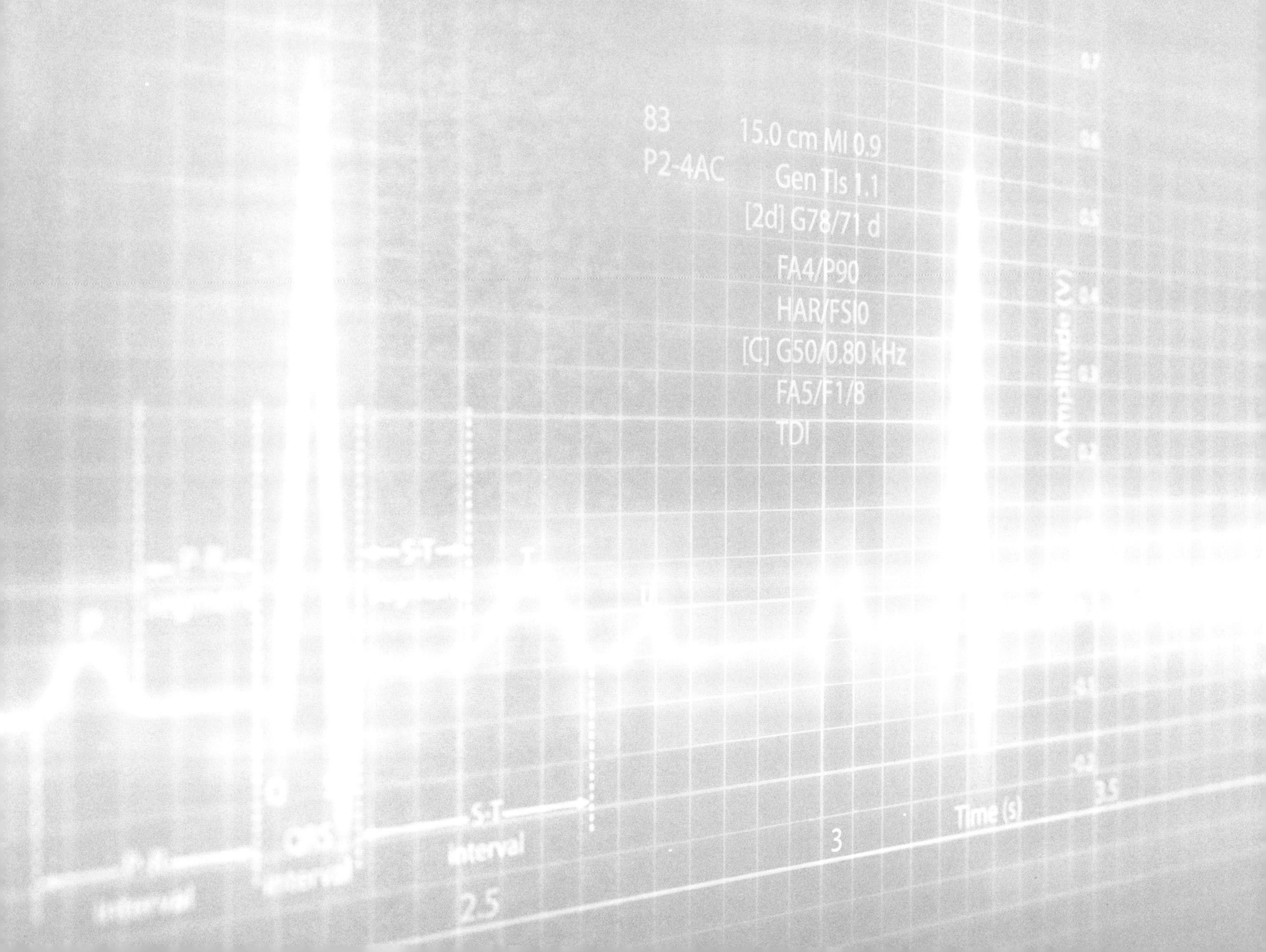
83
P2-4AC
15.0 cm MI 0.9
Gen TIs 1.1
[2d] G78/71 d
FA4/P90
HAR/FS|0
[C] G50/0.80 kHz
FA5/F1/8
TDI
Amplitude (V)
S-T
S-T
interval
2.5
3
3.5
Time (s)

ANSWERS

70-1. Interpret this ECG.

This ECG reveals a regular narrow complex tachycardia at a rate of 150 beats/min. Coarse sawtooth waves are seen best in the inferior leads diagnostic of atrial flutter with 2 to 1 AV conduction. Whenever a supraventricular tachycardia at a rate of close to 150 beats/min is present, the diagnosis of atrial flutter should be considered. The QRS axis is normal, and there is no clear evidence of ischemia. There is left ventricular hypertrophy by voltage criteria, examining the precordial leads.

70-2. What factors predispose to this arrhythmia?

Typical atrial flutter is caused by a macro-reentrant circuit in the right atrium, involving the tricuspid annulus. Structural heart disease, intrinsic lung disease, and states of increased sympathetic tone can all predispose to this arrhythmia. The phenomenon of atrial arrhythmia after alcohol intake is also well described and is germane to this case.

Case #71. An 82-year-old woman presents with fatigue and syncope.

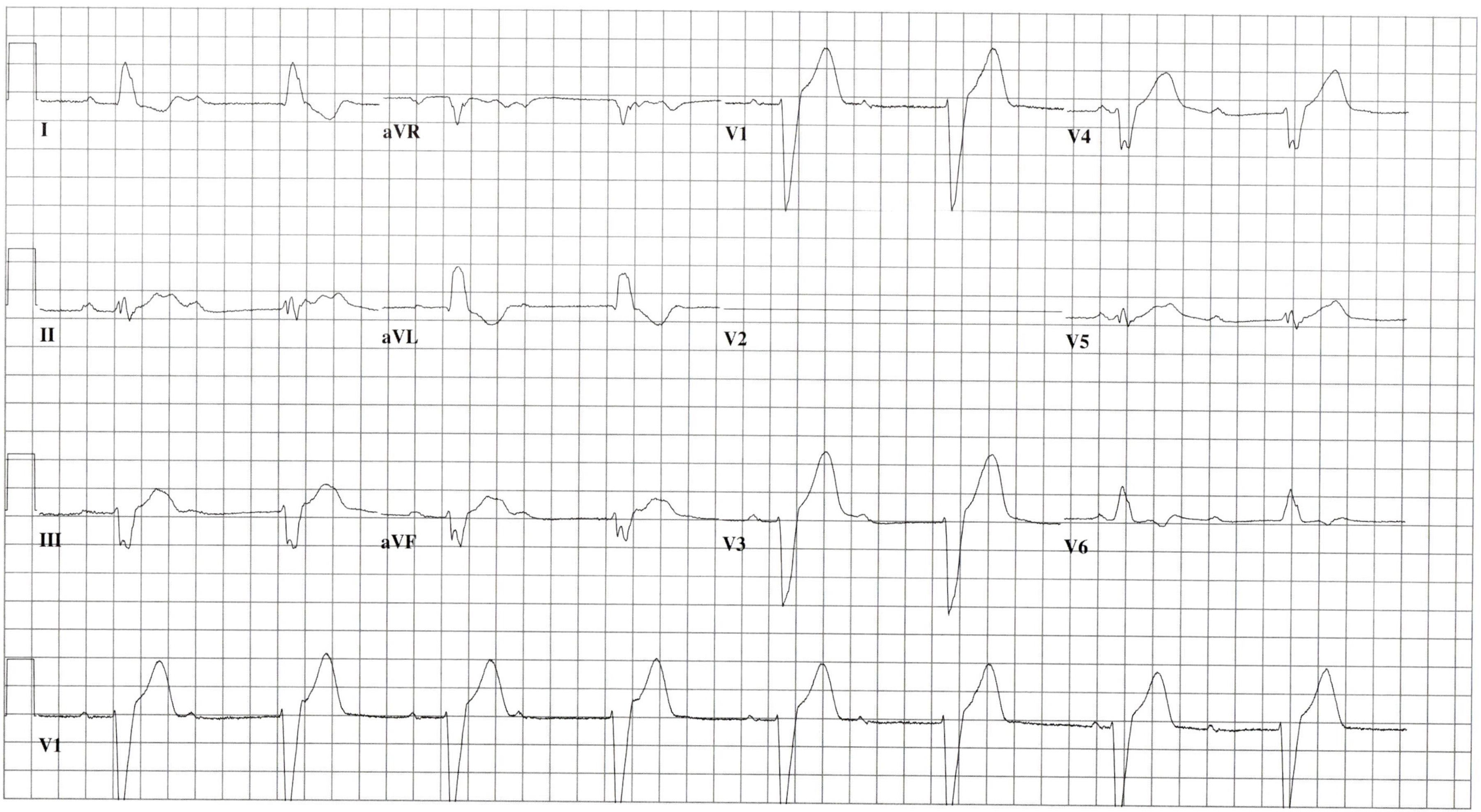

QUESTIONS

71-1. Interpret this ECG. What abnormalities are present on this tracing?

71-2. What physical exam findings might you appreciate on this patient's physical exam?

83
P2-4AC
15.0 cm MI 0.9
Gen TIs 1.1
[2d] G78/71 d
FA4/P90
HAR/FSI0
[C] G50/0.80 kHz
FA5/F1/8
TDI
Amplitude (V)
S-T
segment
S-T
interval
QRS
interval
interval
Time (s)
2.5
3
3.5

ANSWERS

71-1. Interpret this ECG. What abnormalities are present on this tracing?

This tracing demonstrates a regular wide complex bradycardia at 50 beats/min. There are P waves but no clear relationship between the P waves and QRS complexes (AV dissociation is present). The P waves march out at a rate of 75 beats/min (some are hidden within the QRS complexes and T waves), whereas the QRS complexes march out at a rate of 50 beats/min. Because the atrial activity is independent of and faster than ventricular activity, the rhythm is complete heart block. The QRS complex is widened at 160 milliseconds with a left bundle branch morphology, and, in the setting of complete heart block, represents an escape mechanism. Lead V2 is absent.

71-2. What physical exam findings might you appreciate on this patient's physical exam?

Complete heart block results in dyssynchrony between the atria and the ventricles. If the right atrium contracts against a closed tricuspid valve during ventricular systole, large venous pulsations can be observed when inspecting the internal jugular veins. These periodic, large-amplitude venous pulsations in the neck due to right atrial contraction against a closed tricuspid valve are called "cannon a-waves" and can be observed in the setting of complete heart block, ventricular tachycardia, or any other disease where the atrial and ventricular depolarizations are not synchronized.

Case #72. A 52-year-old man with no history of previous medical care presents with hypothermia, somnolence, and an abnormal deep tendon reflex.

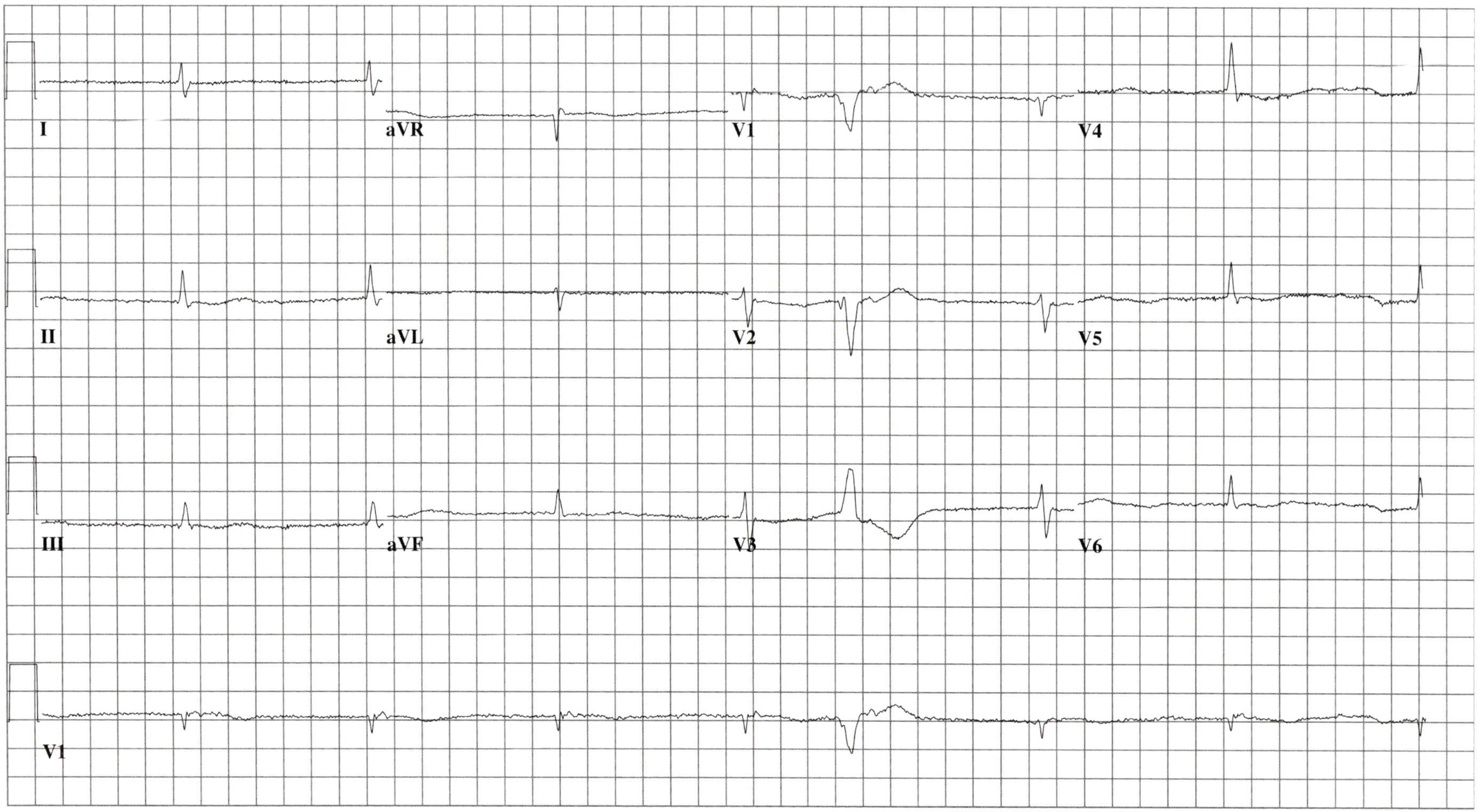

QUESTIONS

72-1. What are the ECG findings?

72-2. What is the most likely diagnosis?

72-3. What cardiac findings are classically seen in this condition?

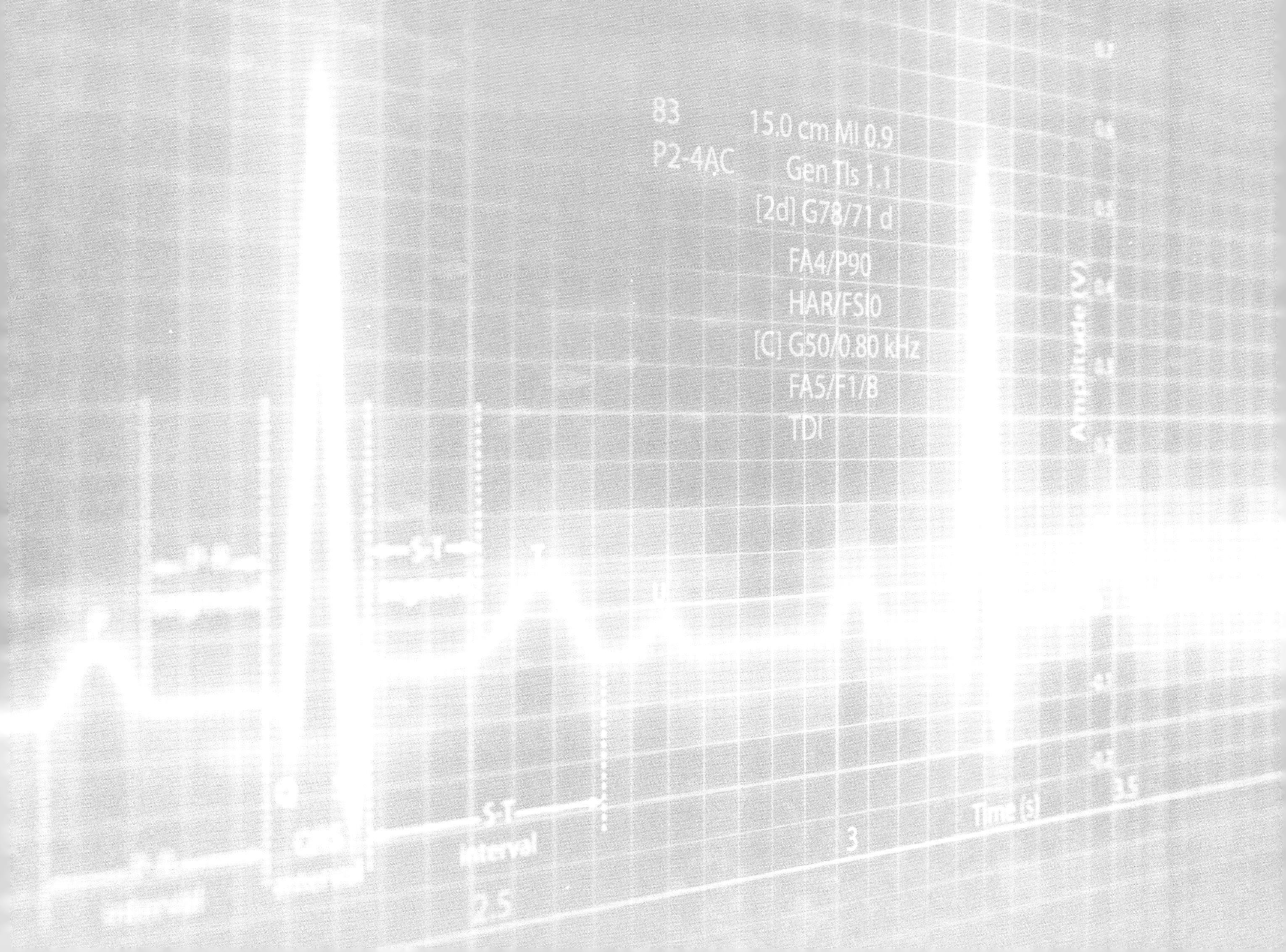
83
P2-4AC
15.0 cm MI 0.9
Gen TIs 1.1
[2d] G78/71 d
FA4/P90
HAR/FSI0
[C] G50/0.80 kHz
FA5/F1/8
TDI
Amplitude (V)
S-T
S-T
interval
2.5
3
Time (s)
3.5

ANSWERS

72-1. What are the ECG findings?

The patient is bradycardic with a ventricular rate of 42 beats/min. There are subtle P waves seen in lead V1 that are just after each QRS complex within the ST segment (figure). This rhythm is a junctional bradycardia with retrograde ventriculoatrial conduction. In addition, there is a single premature ventricular contraction also with retrograde V-A conduction (figure). Other findings include low voltage and diffuse T-wave flattening with prolonged QT interval.

Junctional bradycardia with retrograde P waves marked by arrows. The final beat of this strip is a premature ventricular contraction.

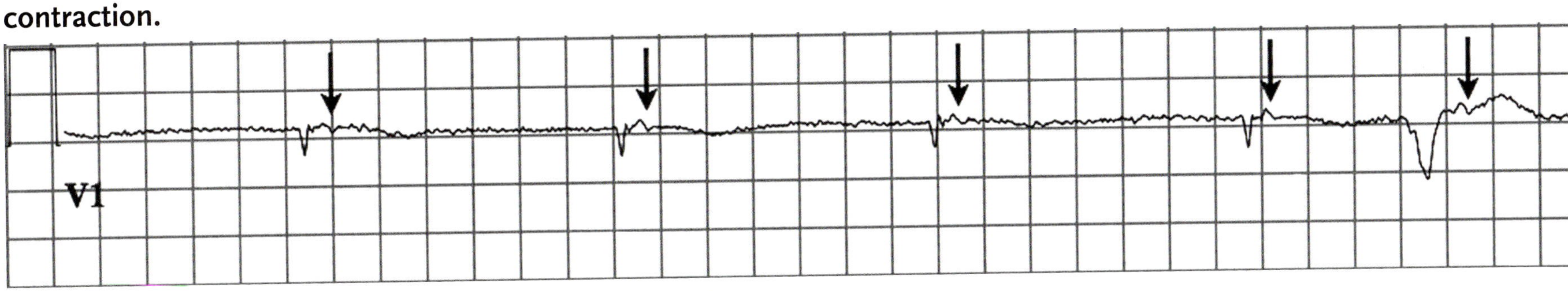

ANSWERS (Cont.)

72-2. What is the most likely diagnosis?

The differential diagnosis for low voltage includes any condition impeding transmission of electrical impulses from the myocytes to the ECG electrodes including infiltrative myocardial disease, myocardial edema, pericardial effusion, emphysema, pleural effusion, pneumothorax, subcutaneous edema, or obesity. The combination of bradycardia, low ECG voltage, and the clinical history strongly suggests hypothyroidism in this case.

72-3. What cardiac findings are classically seen in this condition?

The cardiac findings associated with hypothyroidism include depressed systolic function and cardiomyopathy, bradycardia, and pericardial effusion. These findings can fully resolve with thyroid replacement therapy.

Case #73. A 79-year-old gentleman presents with 1 hour of chest pain and an episode of syncope.

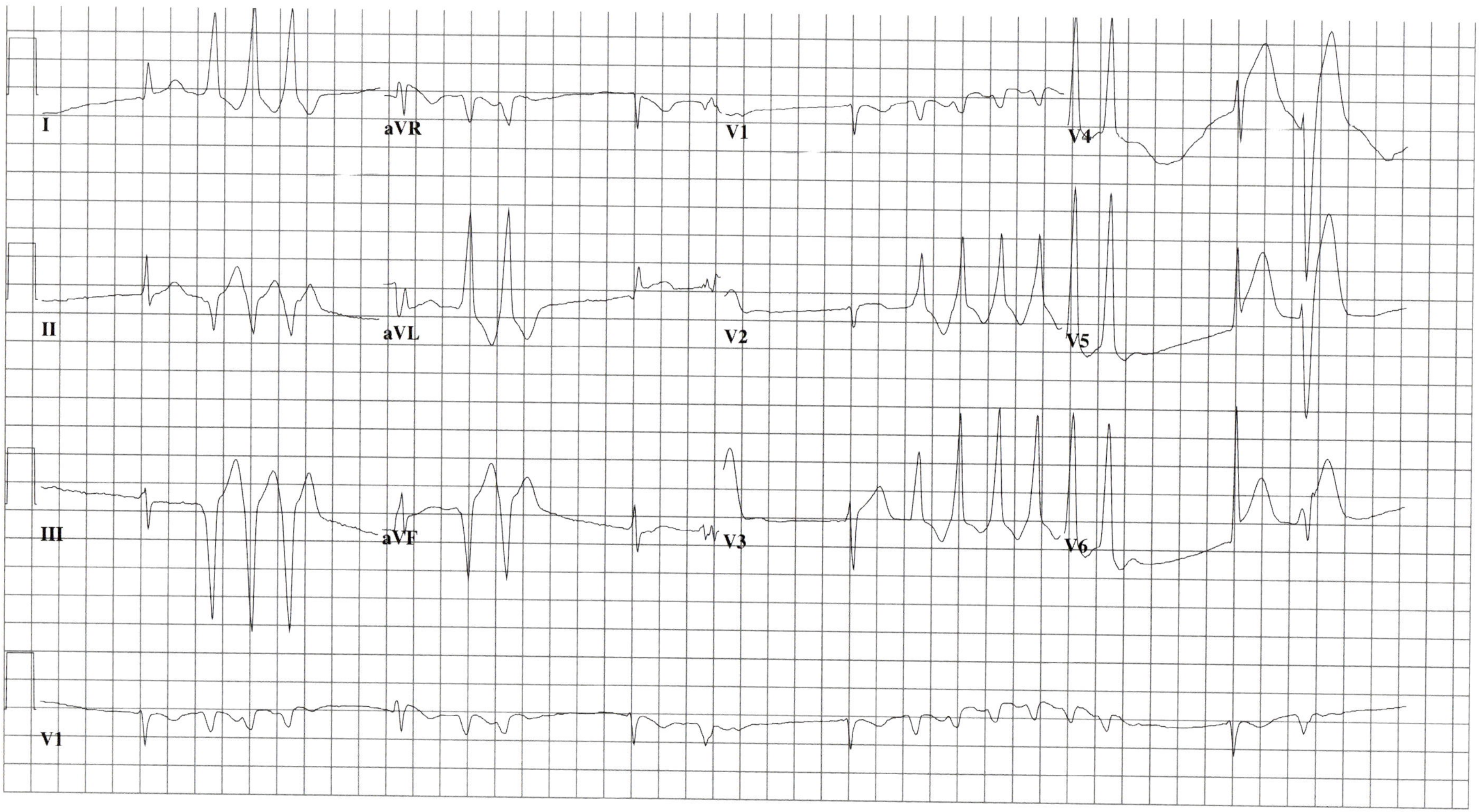

QUESTIONS

73-1. What is the diagnosis?

73-2. How would you manage this patient acutely?

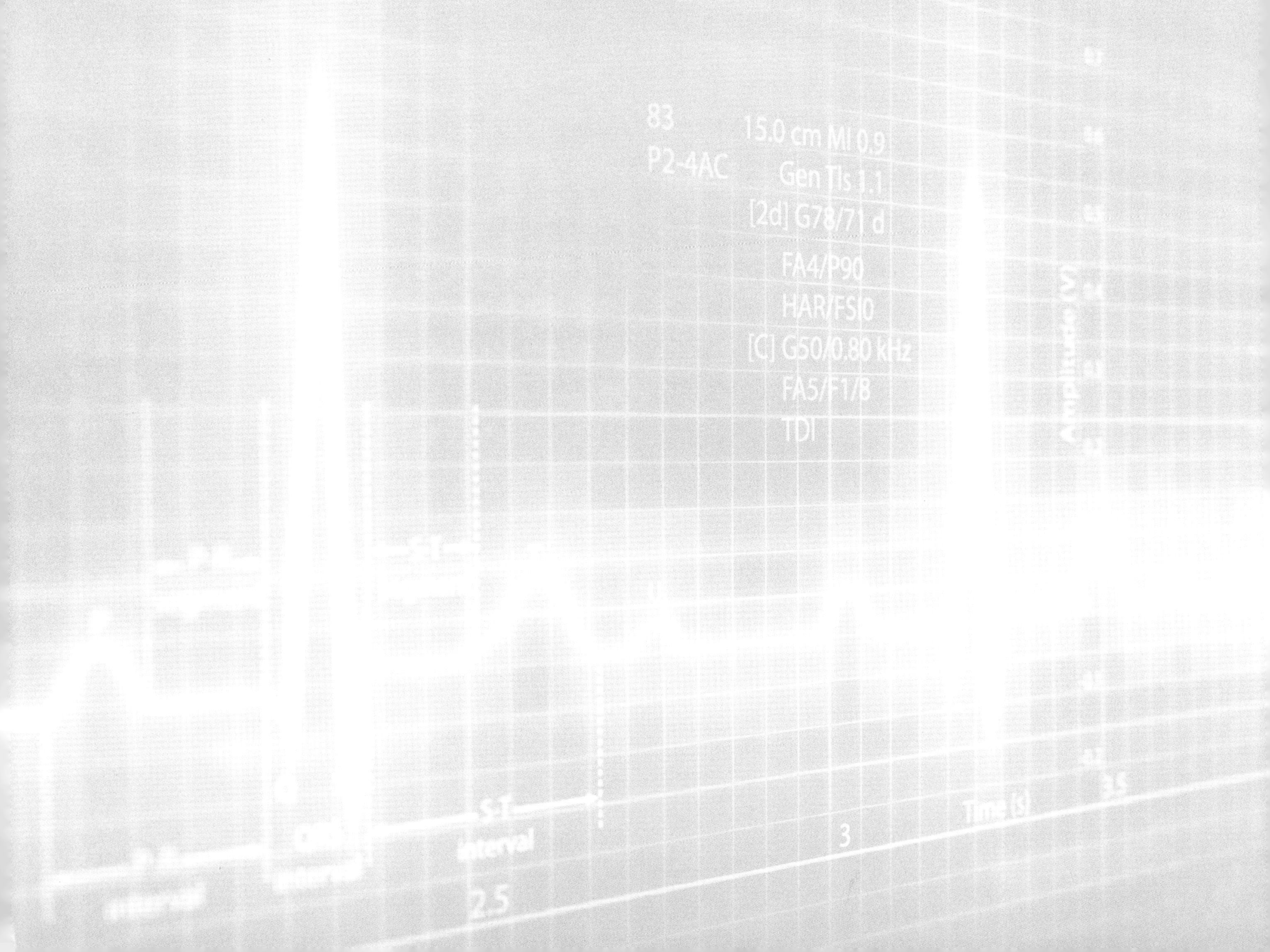
83
P2-4AC
15.0 cm MI 0.9
Gen TIs 1.1
[2d] G78/71 d
FA4/P90
HAR/FS0
[C] G50/0.80 kHz
FA5/F1/B
TDI
Amplitude (V)
S-T
interval
2.5
3
Time (s)
3.5

ANSWERS

73-1. What is the diagnosis?

This tracing demonstrates narrow QRS complexes interspersed with bursts of a nonsustained wide complex tachycardia. No organized atrial activity is present and the rhythm is irregular consistent with atrial fibrillation as the atrial rhythm. Next, focusing on the narrow QRS complexes for analysis: The narrow QRS complexes demonstrate normal axis and ST-segment elevation with tall, broad-based T waves in leads I, aVL, and V4 through V6. No Q waves are present. Overall, these findings suggest early transmural ischemia in a lateral distribution. Regional ST-segment elevation without Q-wave formation is termed acute myocardial injury without infarction. Now, focusing on the nonsustained wide complex tachycardia: The bursts of wide complex tachycardia demonstrate a rate of approximately 190 beats/min. The axis is shifted leftward as compared to the narrow complex beats. This is most likely ventricular tachycardia in the setting of acute myocardial ischemia. Baseline artifact is present, a common finding on ECGs performed on critically ill patients, and it is important to interpret the salient ECG findings despite this artifact.

73-2. How would you manage this patient acutely?

For the acute myocardial ischemia, urgent reperfusion with either percutaneous coronary intervention or thrombolytic therapy should be arranged. Adjunct pharmacotherapy should include aspirin and clopidogrel, statin therapy, and nitrates if the blood pressure allows and there is ongoing chest pain. If sustained ventricular tachycardia occurs, antiarrhythmic therapy with amiodarone or lidocaine could be used with urgent defibrillation and other ACLS measures as needed.

Case #74. You are asked to see this 73-year-old hospitalized patient for evaluation of a new arrhythmia.

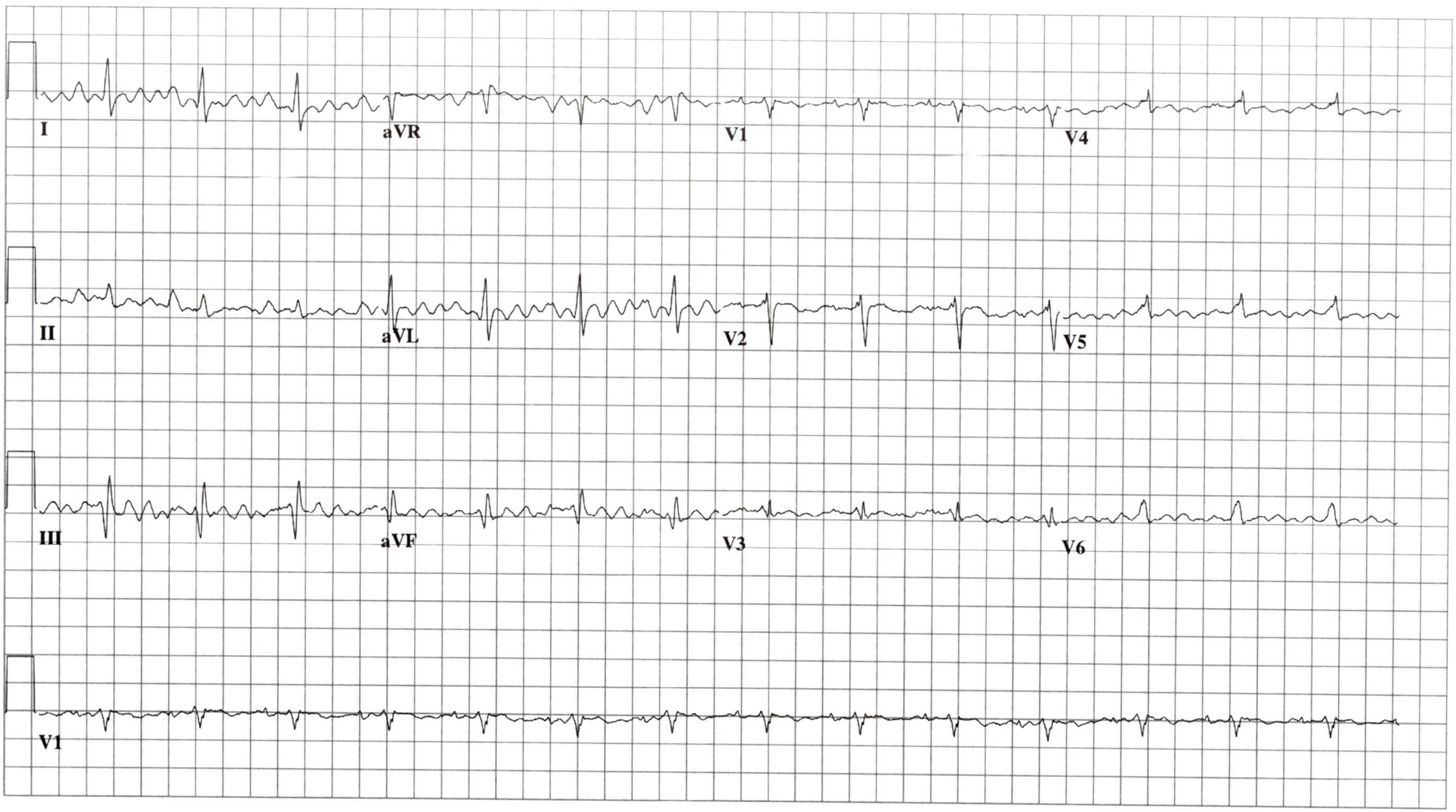

QUESTIONS

74-1. What are the findings? What is the rhythm?

74-2. What do you recommend?

83
P2-4AC
15.0 cm MI 0.9
Gen TIs 1.1
[2d] G78/71 d
FA4/P90
HAR/FSI0
[C] G50/0.80 kHz
FA5/F1/8
TDI
S-T
interval
2.5
3
Time (s)
3.5
Amplitude (V)

ANSWERS

74-1. What are the findings? What is the rhythm?

The rhythm is regular at approximately 80 beats/min. At first glance, there appears to be fibrillation waves suggesting atrial fibrillation; however, the R–R interval is regular rather than irregular as would be expected if atrial fibrillation were present. Looking closely, P waves precede each QRS complex best seen in lead V1, suggesting the diagnosis of prominent baseline motion artifact and sinus rhythm rather than atrial arrhythmia.

74-2. What do you recommend?

A repeat ECG should be performed with attempts to minimize baseline artifact.

Case #75. A 27-year-old gentleman with fever and rash after a camping trip.

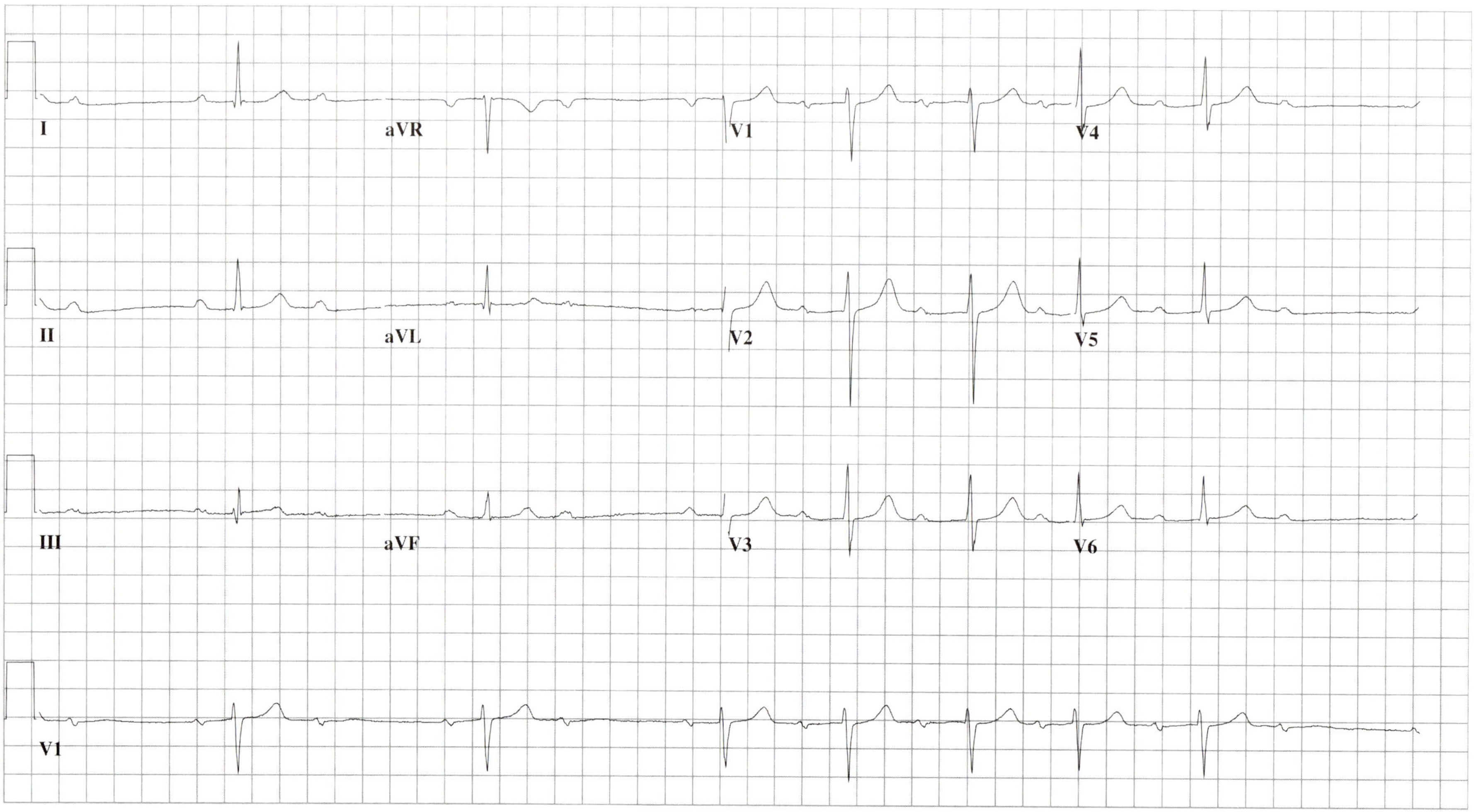

QUESTIONS

75-1. Interpret this ECG.

75-2. What is the differential diagnosis for his presentation?

83
P2-4AC
15.0 cm MI 0.9
Gen TIs 1.1
[2d] G78/71 d
FA4/P90
HAR/FS10
[C] G50/0.80 kHz
FA5/F1/8
TDI
Amplitude (V)

ANSWERS

75-1. Interpret this ECG.

There is sinus rhythm with an atrial rate of approximately 60 beats/min. Some P waves are not followed by QRS complexes consistent with AV block. The rhythm strip starts with a nonconducted P wave followed by 2 cycles of 2 to 1 AV conduction. This is followed by a cycle of 5 P waves that conduct with progressive PR prolongation. The rhythm strip terminates with a nonconducted P wave. AV block with progressive prolongation of the PR interval prior to a nonconducted P wave is diagnostic of Mobitz type I, or Wenckebach second-degree heart block. The frontal plane axis is normal, and there are no abnormalities of the ST segment or T waves. There is no evidence of chamber enlargement or hypertrophy.

75-2. What is the differential diagnosis for his presentation?

Fever, rash, and heart block have a broad differential diagnosis including viral myocarditis, endocarditis, Lyme disease, rheumatic fever, sarcoidosis, and lupus. This patient presenting just after camping was subsequently diagnosed with Lyme disease.

Case #76. A 44-year-old man with a long history of substance abuse used cocaine 2 days prior and presents with 48 hours of unremitting chest pain.

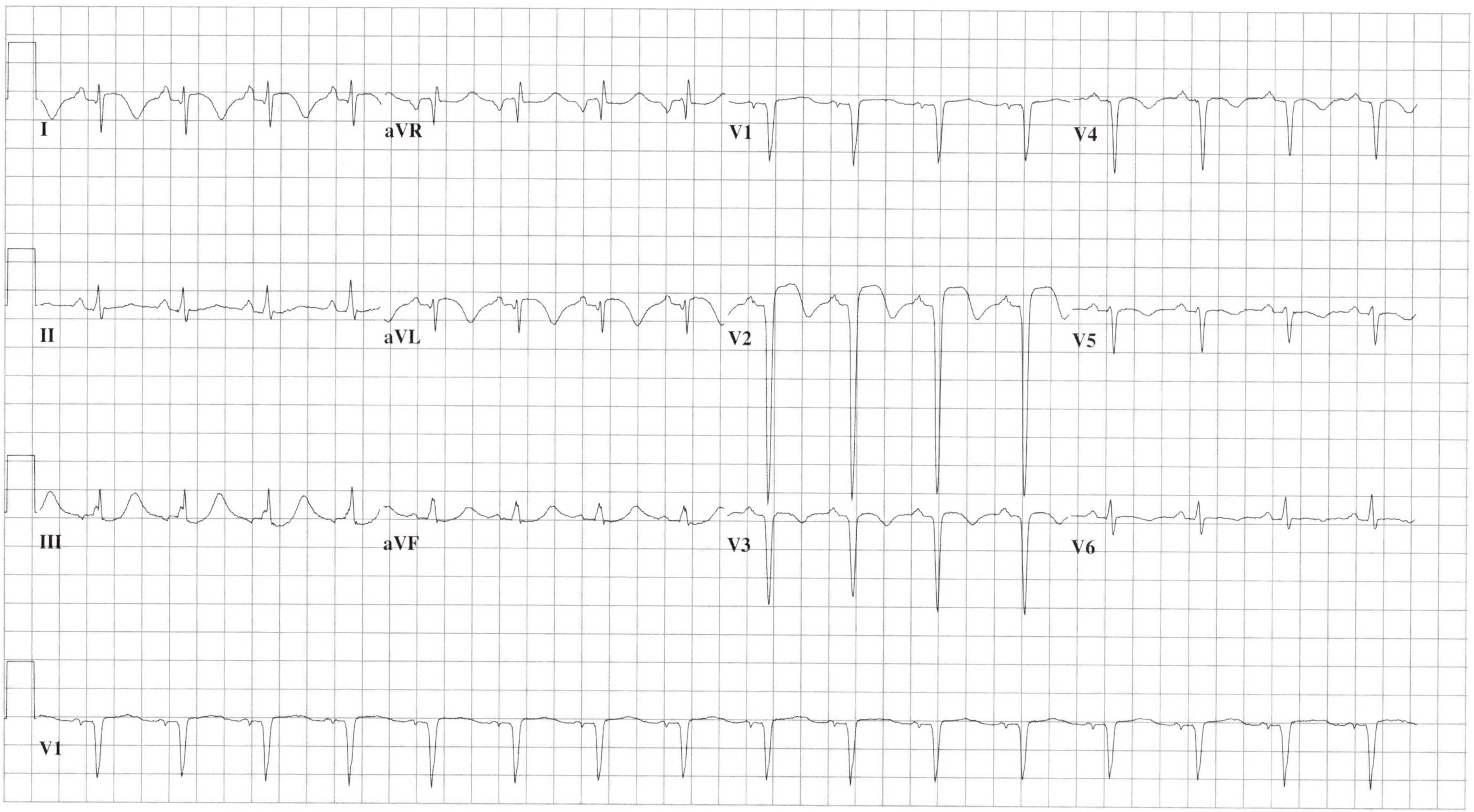

QUESTIONS

76-1. Interpret this ECG: where is the lesion?

76-2. What is the typical time course and sequence of ECG changes in ST-segment elevation MI?

76-3. What are the major complications of the disease demonstrated in this tracing?

83
P2-4AC
15.0 cm MI 0.9
Gen Tls 1.1
[2d] G78/71 d
FA4/P90
HAR/FS0
[C] G50/0.80 kHz
FA5/F1/8
TDI

ANSWERS

76-1. Interpret this ECG: where is the lesion?

This tracing demonstrates sinus rhythm at slightly slower than 100 beats/min. The axis is rightward. The QT interval is prolonged to greater than half the R–R interval. Deep, wide Q waves are present in leads V1, V2, V3, and V4 and subtle Q waves are present in lead aVL. There is ST-segment elevation most notable in V2 and present to a lesser degree in I, aVL, and V1. Deep, symmetric T-wave inversions are present in the anteroseptal (V1-V5) and high lateral (I and aVL) leads. The clinical history coupled with this ECG suggests that the patient suffered an ST-segment elevation MI starting days ago.

76-2. What is the typical time course and sequence of ECG changes in ST-segment elevation MI?

Within the first 30 minutes of occlusion of an epicardial coronary artery, hyperacute T waves are seen. Shortly thereafter, the ST segment will elevate. Q-wave formation follows, typically occurring within the first 9 hours of ischemia, although some patients manifest Q waves earlier in their course. T waves will begin to invert between 6 and 12 hours of ischemia. Generally, after 12 hours of ischemia, the ST-segment elevation will begin to resolve as the infarct completes.[1] Persistent ST elevation can indicate aneurysm formation or ongoing active ischemia.

76-3. What are the major complications of the disease demonstrated in this tracing?

Major complications of myocardial infarction can be categorized as mechanical, electrical, or thromboembolic. Large, akinetic areas of infarcted myocardium can serve as a nidus for thrombus formation and predispose to embolization to the brain or other organs. Electrical complications include conduction blocks, supraventricular tachycardias, ventricular tachycardia, and ventricular fibrillation leading to sudden cardiac death. Mechanical complications include heart failure, cardiogenic shock, ischemic mitral regurgitation or papillary muscle rupture, ventricular septal defect formation, and left ventricular free wall rupture.

[1]Morris F, Brady WJ. ABC of clinical electrocardiography: acute myocardial infarction—Part 1. *BMJ* 2002; 324: 831-834.

Case #77. An 82-year-old woman presents with syncope and chest pain. She has a distant history of myocardial infarction.

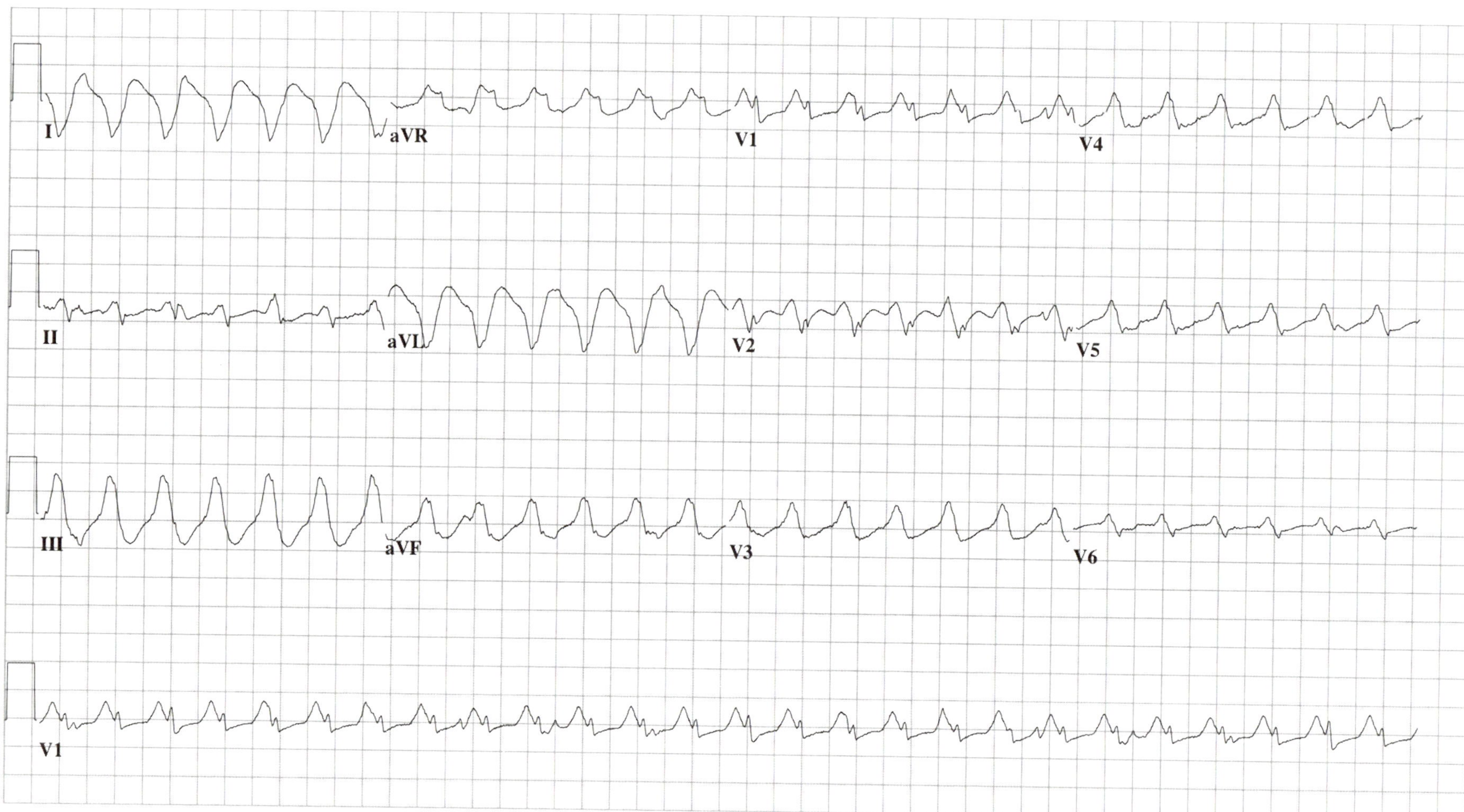

QUESTION

77-1. What is the diagnosis?

83
15.0 cm MI 0.9
P2-4AC
Gen TIs 1.1
[2d] G78/71 d
FA4/P90
HAR/FSI0
[C] G50/0.80 kHz
FA5/F1/8
TDI
S-T
Interval
3
2.5

ANSWER

77-1. What is the diagnosis?

The tracing reveals a wide complex monomorphic tachycardia at a rate of 150 beats/min. The frontal plane QRS axis is negative in lead I and positive in lead aVF, suggesting rightward axis. The QRS complex is positive in lead V1 and hence can be classified as a wide complex tachycardia with "right bundle branch block morphology" (in contrast to the case if the QRS complex were negative in lead V1 in which case the wide complex tachycardia would be classified as having a "left bundle branch block morphology"). The differential diagnosis of wide complex monomorphic tachycardia includes supraventricular tachycardia with aberrancy versus ventricular tachycardia. In this case, there is clear evidence of atrioventricular dissociation as demonstrated in the figure. The QRS rate is faster than the atrial rate, and the atria and ventricles depolarize completely dissociated from each other. A-V dissociation in this case is diagnostic of ventricular tachycardia.

P waves are identified with arrows. The atrial rate is slower than the ventricular rate and the atria, and ventricles depolarize completely dissociated from each other. This is diagnostic of VT in this case.

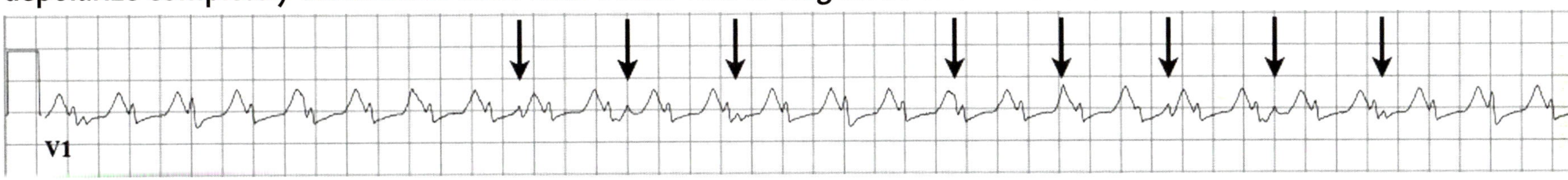

Case #78. A 56-year-old businessman presents with hemoptysis and pleuritic chest pain after returning to Boston from a conference in China.

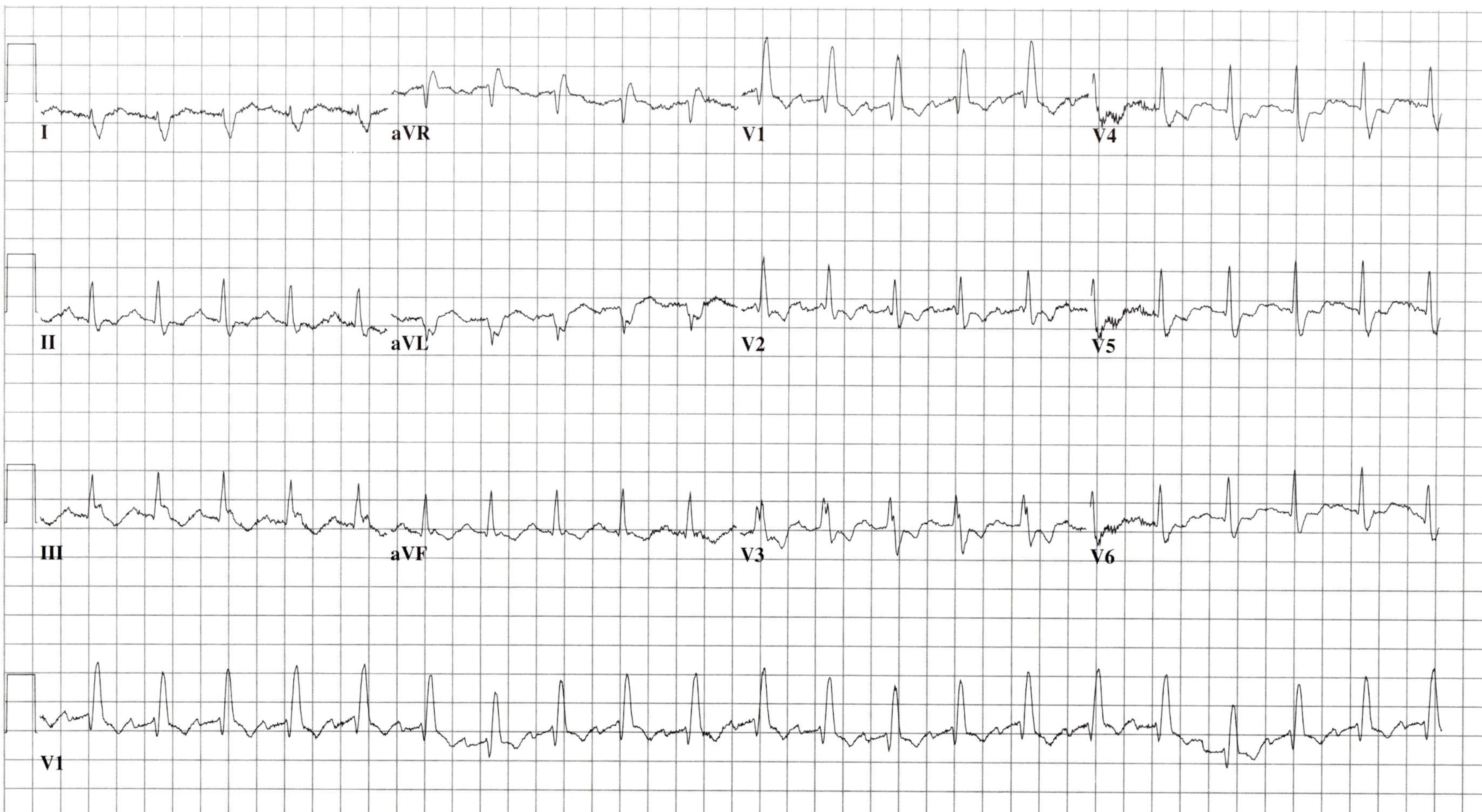

QUESTIONS

78-1. What abnormalities are present on this ECG?

78-2. What is the most likely diagnosis?

78-3. Assuming your diagnosis is correct, what are the potential treatments and how would you choose among them?

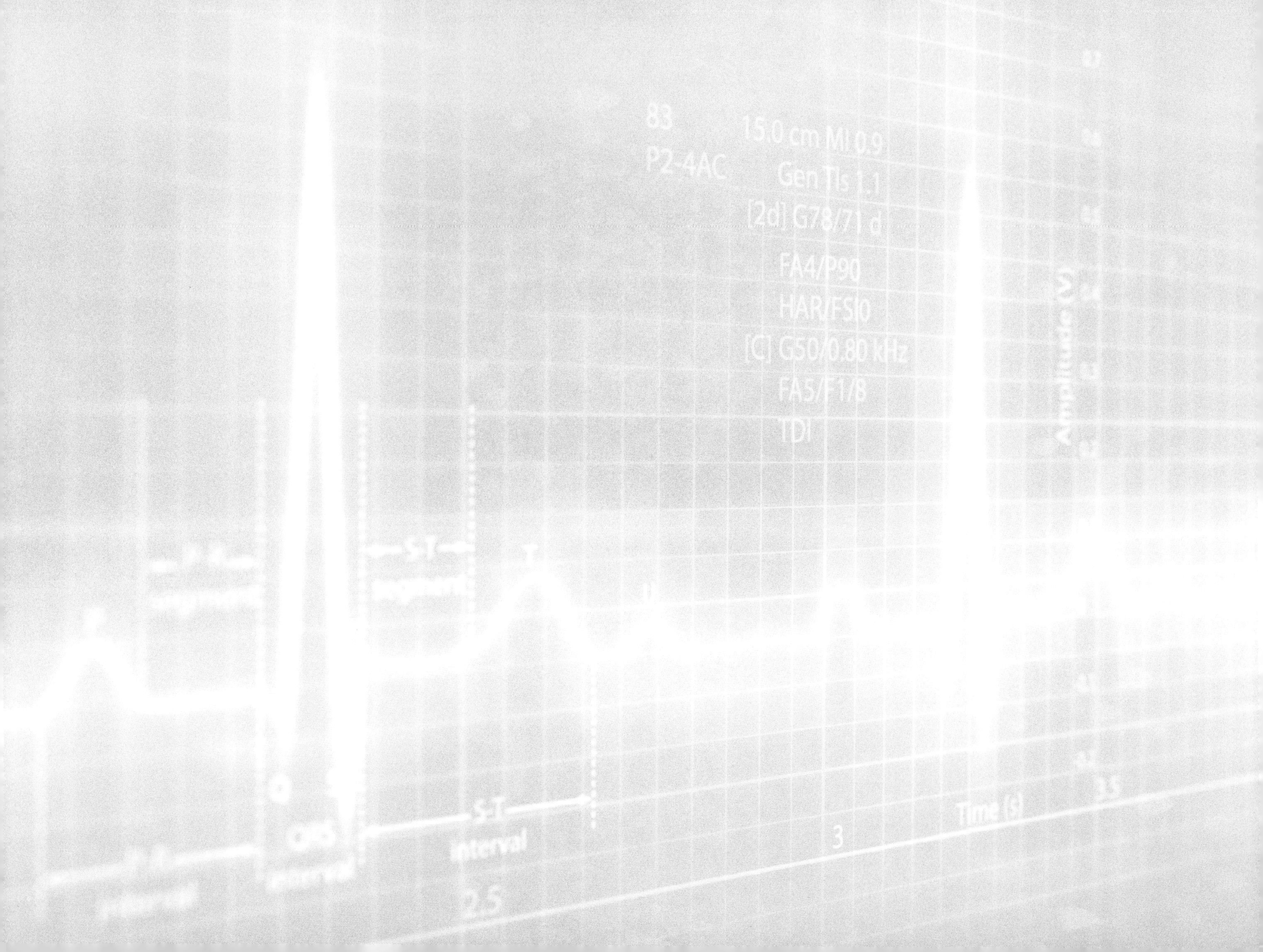
83
P2-4AC
15.0 cm MI 0.9
Gen TIs 1.1
[2d] G78/71 d
FA4/P90
HAR/FSI0
[C] G50/0.80 kHz
FA5/F1/8
TDI
Amplitude (V)
S-T
interval
QRS
interval
2.5
3
3.5
Time (s)

ANSWERS

78-1. What abnormalities are present on this ECG?

This tracing demonstrates sinus tachycardia at a rate of 120 beats/min. Borderline first-degree AV block is present with PR interval of 200 milliseconds. The axis is rightward. A widened QRS with right bundle branch block is present. ST-segment depressions with T-wave inversions are present in leads V1 through V6. Normally, in the setting of a right bundle branch block, ST-segment abnormalities and T-wave inversions are present in leads V1 through V3, so-called "secondary" T-wave changes. In this tracing, those changes persist throughout the precordium.

78-2. What is the most likely diagnosis?

In this patient with hemoptysis after a (presumably) long air flight coupled with sinus tachycardia, rightward axis, and right bundle branch block, pulmonary embolism is a prime concern.

78-3. Assuming your diagnosis is correct, what are the potential treatments and how would you choose among them?

Treatment for pulmonary embolism includes anticoagulation alone or coupled with reperfusion strategies including pharmacologic thrombolysis, catheter-based mechanical thrombolysis, or surgical thrombectomy. "Massive" pulmonary embolism is defined as pulmonary embolism with right heart strain and hypotension, hemodynamic compromise, and shock. "Submassive" pulmonary embolism is defined as a pulmonary embolism without hemodynamic compromise yet with evidence of right heart strain. Right heart strain can be identified as right ventricular enlargement on CT scan or right heart dysfunction on echocardiography. Serum biomarkers of right heart strain include natriuretic peptide measurement (BNP) and markers of cardiac ischemia (troponin). Patients without evidence of right heart strain should be treated with anticoagulation alone. Patients with massive PE should be considered for a reperfusion strategy. The optimal approach to management of submassive PE is controversial.

Case #79. A 44-year-old man presents with palpitations.

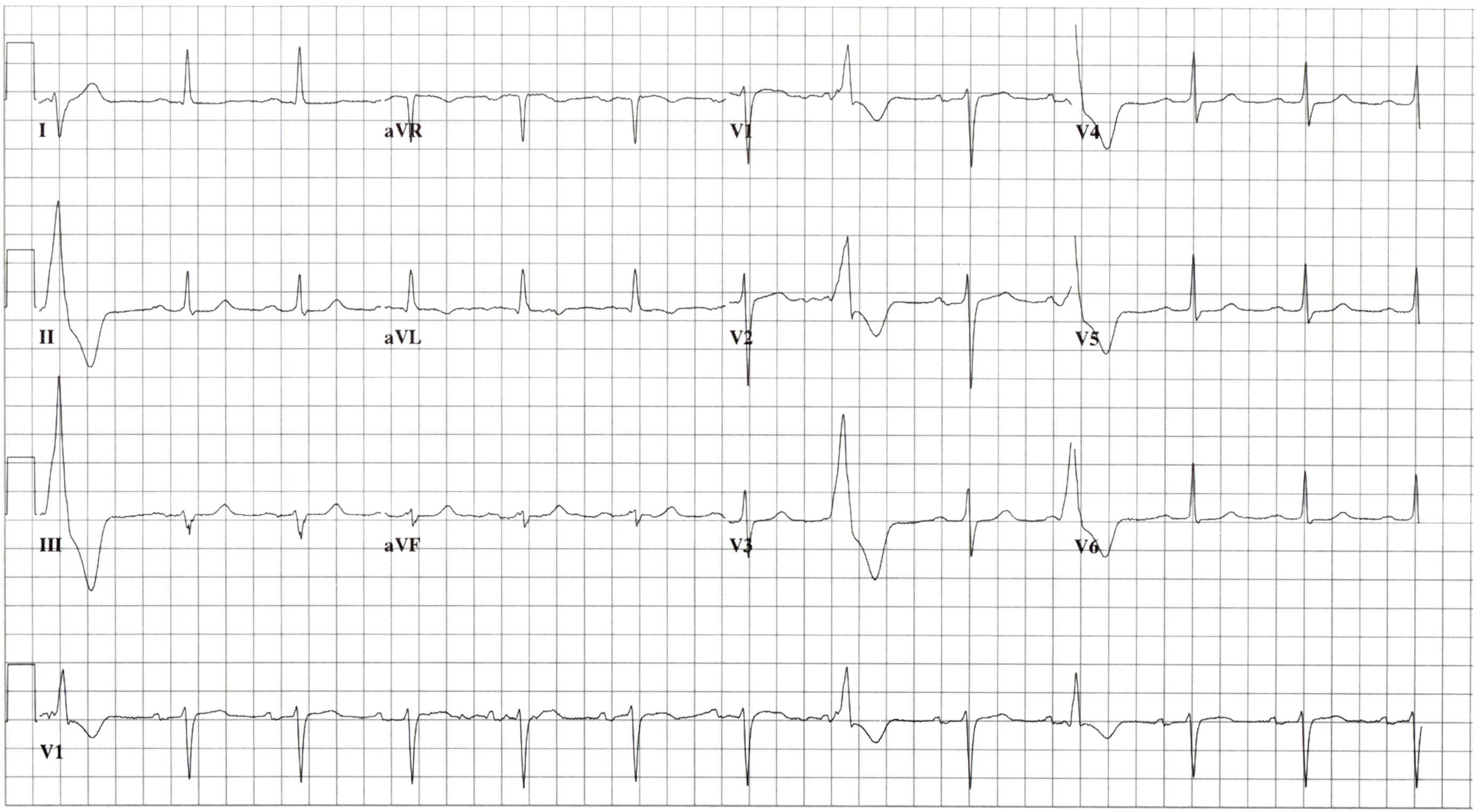

QUESTIONS

79-1. What abnormalities are present on this tracing?

79-2. Explain the differences between the 8th, 9th, and 10th QRS complexes.

83
P2-4AC
15.0 cm MI 0.9
Gen TIs 1.1
[2d] G78/71 d
FA4/P90
HAR/FS0
[C] G50/0.80 kHz
FA5/F1/8
TDI
2.5
3

ANSWERS

79-1. What abnormalities are present on this tracing?

This tracing demonstrates sinus rhythm at 75 beats/min. There is no evidence of chamber enlargement or hypertrophy, and the axis and intervals are normal. There are several premature ventricular contractions (PVCs) present, visible as wide complex beats that occur earlier than the expected natively conducted beat.

79-2. Explain the differences between the 8th, 9th, and 10th QRS complexes.

The eighth QRS complex is a PVC followed by the ninth beat, which is natively conducted. The 10th beat looks somewhat like a PVC but somewhat like a native beat. This is called a fusion complex, a beat indeterminate in morphology between native conduction and ventricular contractions. The fusion beat occurs when supraventricular conduction and the ventricular ectopic beat occur nearly synchronously resulting in "fusion" of the supraventricular (narrow complex) and ventricular ectopic (wide complex) beats. To make the diagnosis of a fusion complex, one must identify a ventricular complex, a supraventricular native complex, and a beat that is indeterminate between the two.

Case #80. A 55-year-old woman with nonischemic cardiomyopathy presents with this wide complex tachycardia.

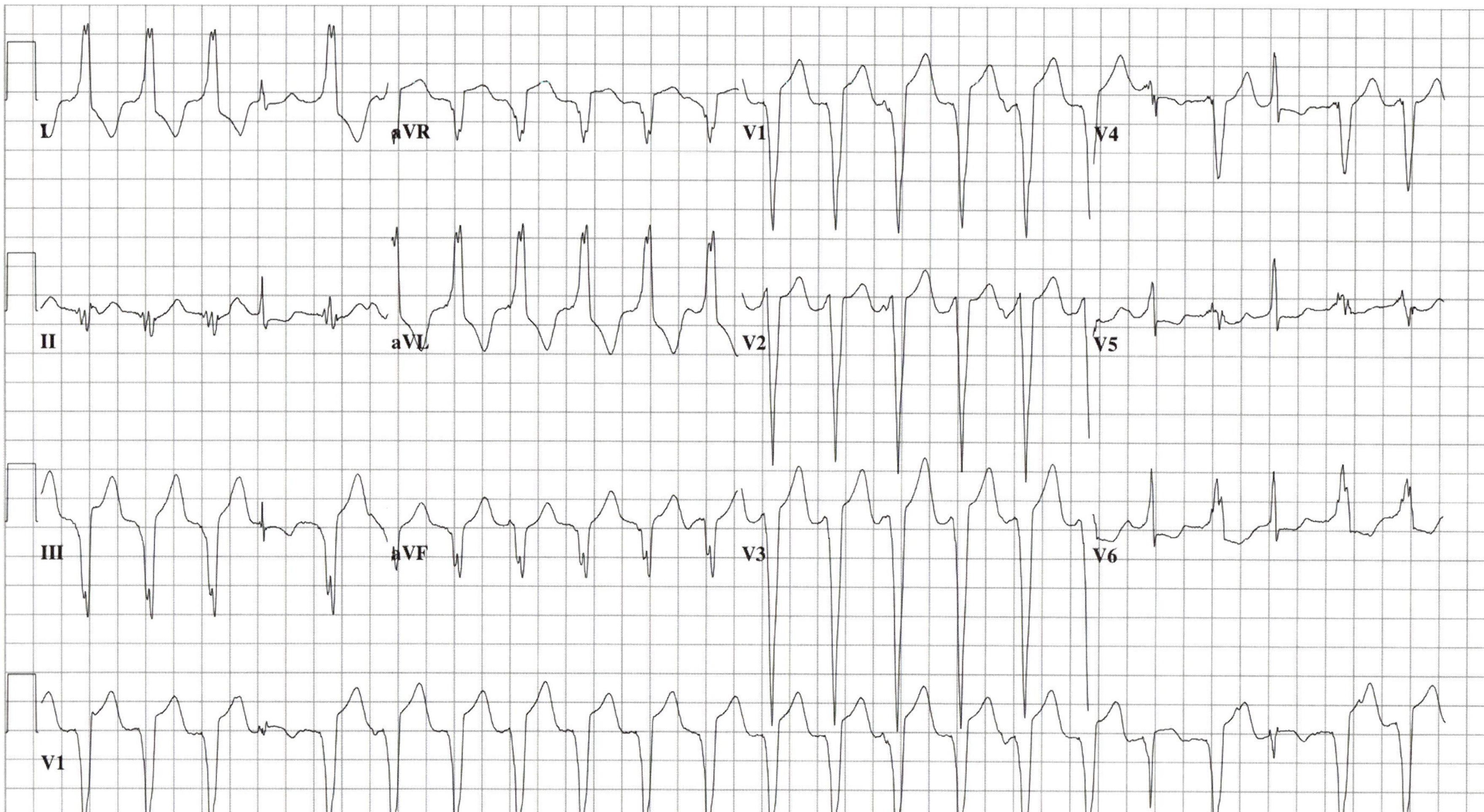

QUESTION

80-1. Interpret this tracing. What is a fusion beat, and are any present? What is a capture beat, and are any present?

83
P2-4AC
15.0 cm MI 0.9
Gen Tls 1.1
[2d] G78/71 d
FA4/P90
HAR/FS|0
[C] G50/0.80 kHz
FA5/F1/B
TDI
3
2.5

ANSWER

80-1. Interpret this tracing. What is a fusion beat, and are any present? What is a capture beat, and are any present?

This tracing reveals a wide complex tachycardia at a rate of approximately 150 beats/min. Most of the ventricular beats have identical morphologies; hence, this is a monomorphic wide complex tachycardia (in contrast to a polymorphic ventricular tachycardia where the majority of the QRS complexes have a varying morphology). The differential diagnosis of a monomorphic wide complex tachycardia includes ventricular tachycardia or supraventricular tachycardia conducted with aberrancy. Several clues in this tracing suggest the diagnosis of ventricular tachycardia.

When ventricular tachycardia occurs, ventricular depolarization does not conduct through the normal His–Purkinje system but rather conducts slowly directly through ventricular myocardium. During some ventricular tachycardias, sinus node depolarization continues unabated, and most of the sinus impulses meet a refractory ventricle due to the dominant ectopic ventricular activity preventing conduction. If, however, a sinus P wave occurred between the ectopic ventricular depolarizations such that the ventricle were not refractory, a narrow-appearing "normal" QRS complex would result interspersed between ventricular beats. This phenomenon is called a "capture beat." If the ventricular depolarization and sinus node were to meet and simultaneously depolarize the ventricle, the resulting QRS complex would be intermediate in morphology between the ventricular beat and the sinus beat. This is called a "fusion beat." Both fusion beats and capture beats are present in this tracing, noted in the figure below with asterisks. Fusion and capture beats connote atrioventricular dissociation, which is a diagnostic hallmark of ventricular tachycardia. P waves dissociated from the QRS complexes are shown in the figure with arrows. In sum, this tracing demonstrates evidence of A-V dissociation with fusion and capture beats diagnostic of ventricular tachycardia.

Monomorphic ventricular tachycardia. Dissociated P waves are marked with arrows. Fusion beats and capture beats are marked with asterisks.

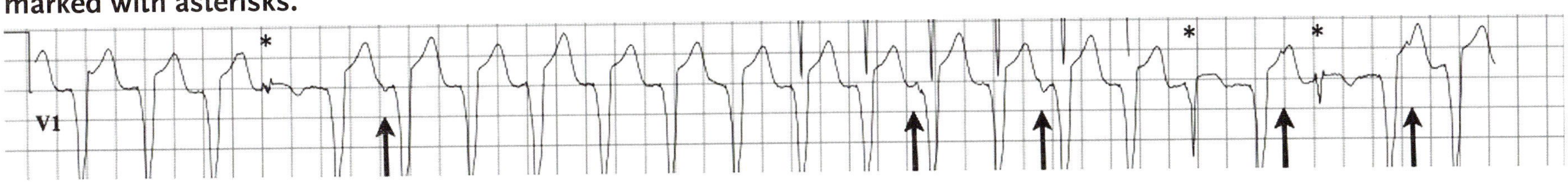

Case #81. A 53-year-old female with shortness of breath presents to her cardiologist. She has a loud second heart sound on examination.

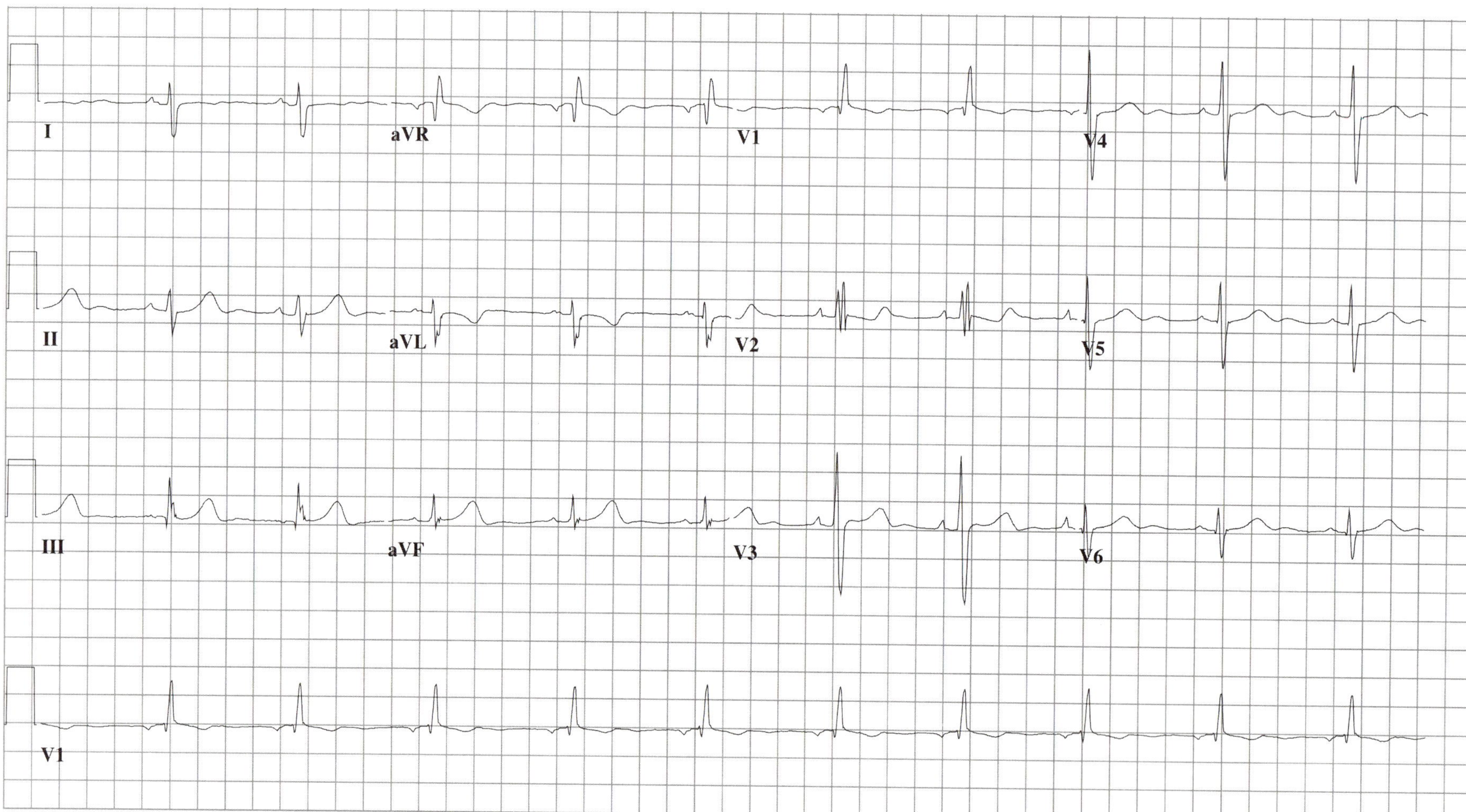

QUESTIONS

81-1. What are the abnormalities?

81-2. What is the differential diagnosis?

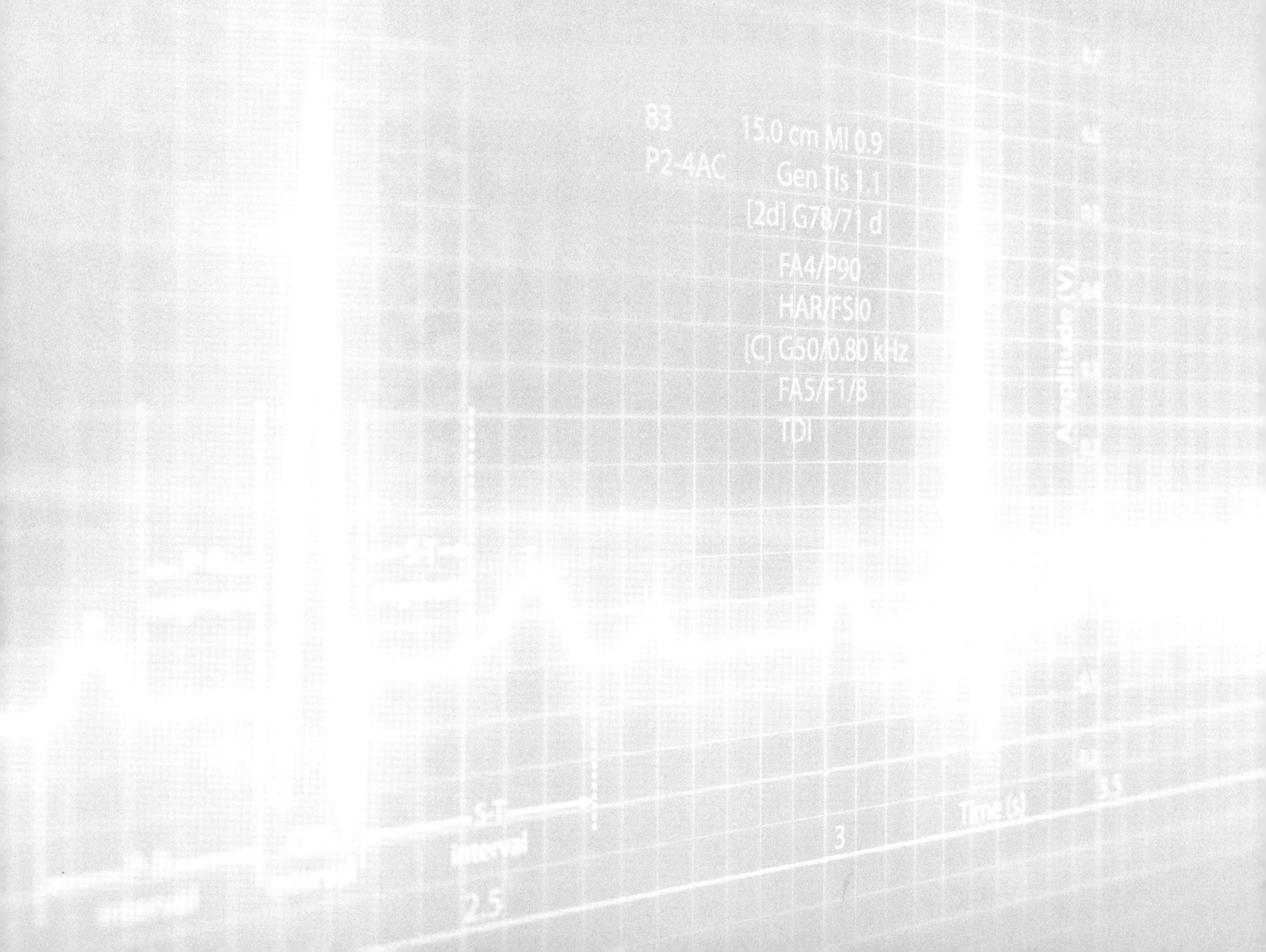
83
P2-4AC
15.0 cm MI 0.9
Gen TIs 1.1
[2d] G78/71 d
FA4/P90
HAR/FSI0
[C] G50/0.80 kHz
FA5/F1/8
TDI
Amplitude (V)
S-T
Interval
2.5
3
3.5
Time (s)

ANSWERS

81-1. What are the abnormalities?

This tracing demonstrates normal sinus rhythm at 60 beats/min. There is right axis deviation. There is evidence of right ventricular hypertrophy on the basis of the rightward axis coupled with a tall R wave in lead V1, which is greater than 7 mV. Criteria for right ventricular hypertrophy, each of which is fairly specific but insensitive, include

- R-wave magnitude greater than S-wave magnitude in lead V1,
- R-wave magnitude greater than 7 mV in lead V1, and
- a decline in the ratio of R-wave magnitude to S-wave magnitude moving across precordial leads from V1 to V6.

Other electrocardiographic findings that can suggest right ventricular hypertrophy (RVH) include right axis deviation, incomplete right bundle branch block, and right atrial abnormality, also called P pulmonale.

81-2. What is the differential diagnosis?

Causes of right ventricular hypertrophy include processes that cause volume or pressure loading of the right ventricle such as pulmonary stenosis, primary pulmonary hypertension, intrinsic lung disease, left heart failure, valvular heart disease, and chronic pulmonary thromboembolic disease.

Case #82. A 77-year-old woman with atrial fibrillation presents with 3 days of fatigue. She is on no AV nodal blocking medications.

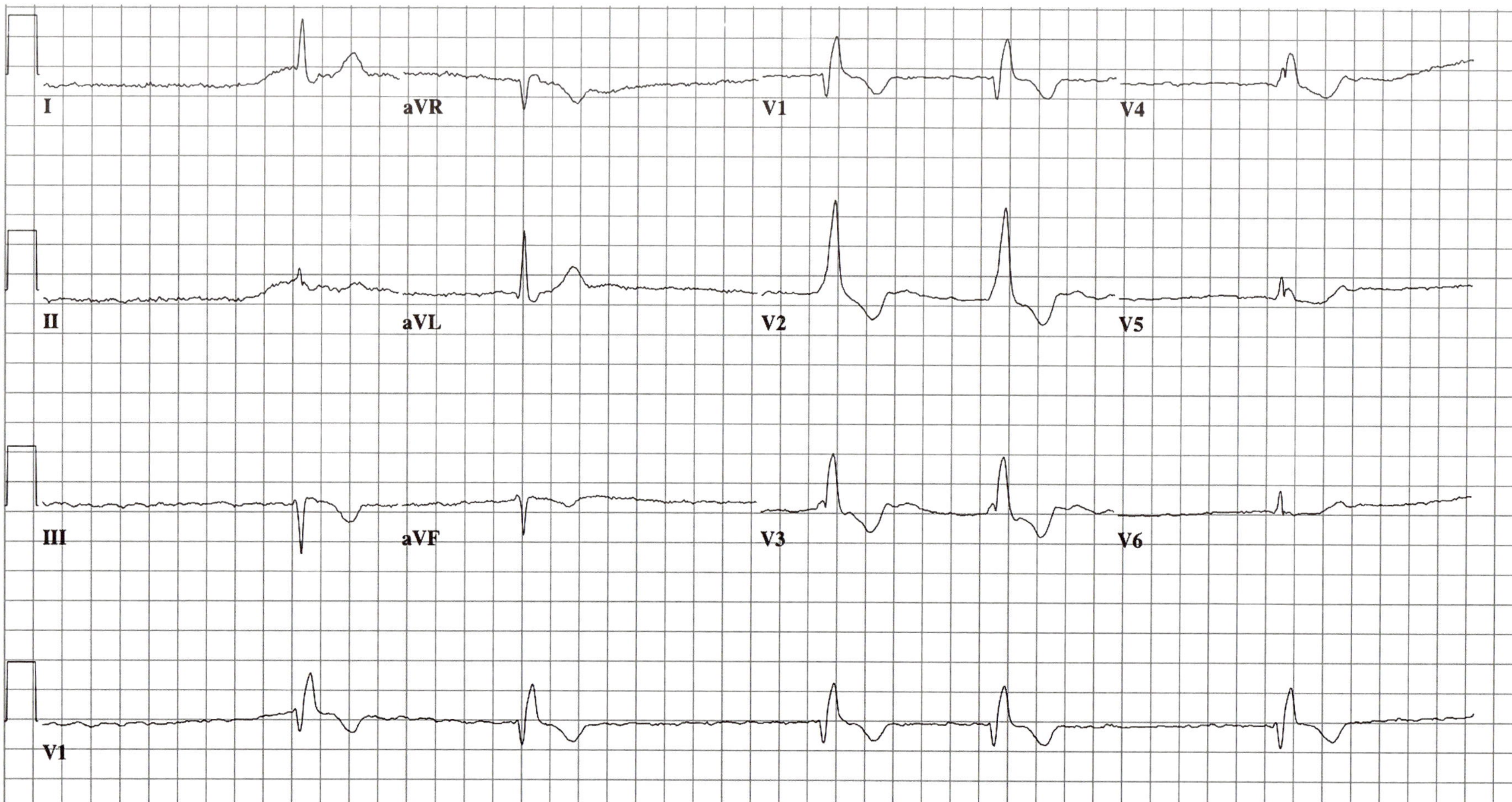

QUESTIONS

82-1. Interpret this ECG. What abnormalities are present?

82-2. What can you surmise about the health of the patient's AV conduction?

83
P2-4AC
15.0 cm MI 0.9
Gen TIs 1.1
[2d] G78/71 d
FA4/P90
HAR/FSI0
[C] G50/0.80 kHz
FA5/F1/B
TDI
S-T
Interval
2.5
3

ANSWERS

82-1. Interpret this ECG. What abnormalities are present?

This tracing shows an irregularly irregular wide complex bradycardia with ventricular rate of 36 beats/min. There is no organized atrial activity visualized consistent with a diagnosis of atrial fibrillation with a slow ventricular response. The QRS axis is normal. The QRS complex is wide with duration of approximately 160 milliseconds and a right bundle branch block. The QT interval is normal. Baseline artifact is present.

82-2. What can you surmise about the health of the patient's conduction system?

The patient likely has significant multilevel conduction system disease. When atrial fibrillation is present, the rate of atrial depolarization is typically 400 to 600 beats/min. When a healthy AV node receives such rapid impulses in the absence of AV nodal blocking medications, the resulting ventricular rate is usually rapid. When ventricular rates in atrial fibrillation are very slow in the absence of AV nodal blocking medications (as in this patient), significant AV nodal disease is usually present. In addition, the patient has right bundle branch block, which also is diagnostic of infranodal conduction system disease.

Case #83. A 31-year-old female with a family history of sudden cardiac death of a brother and a maternal aunt.

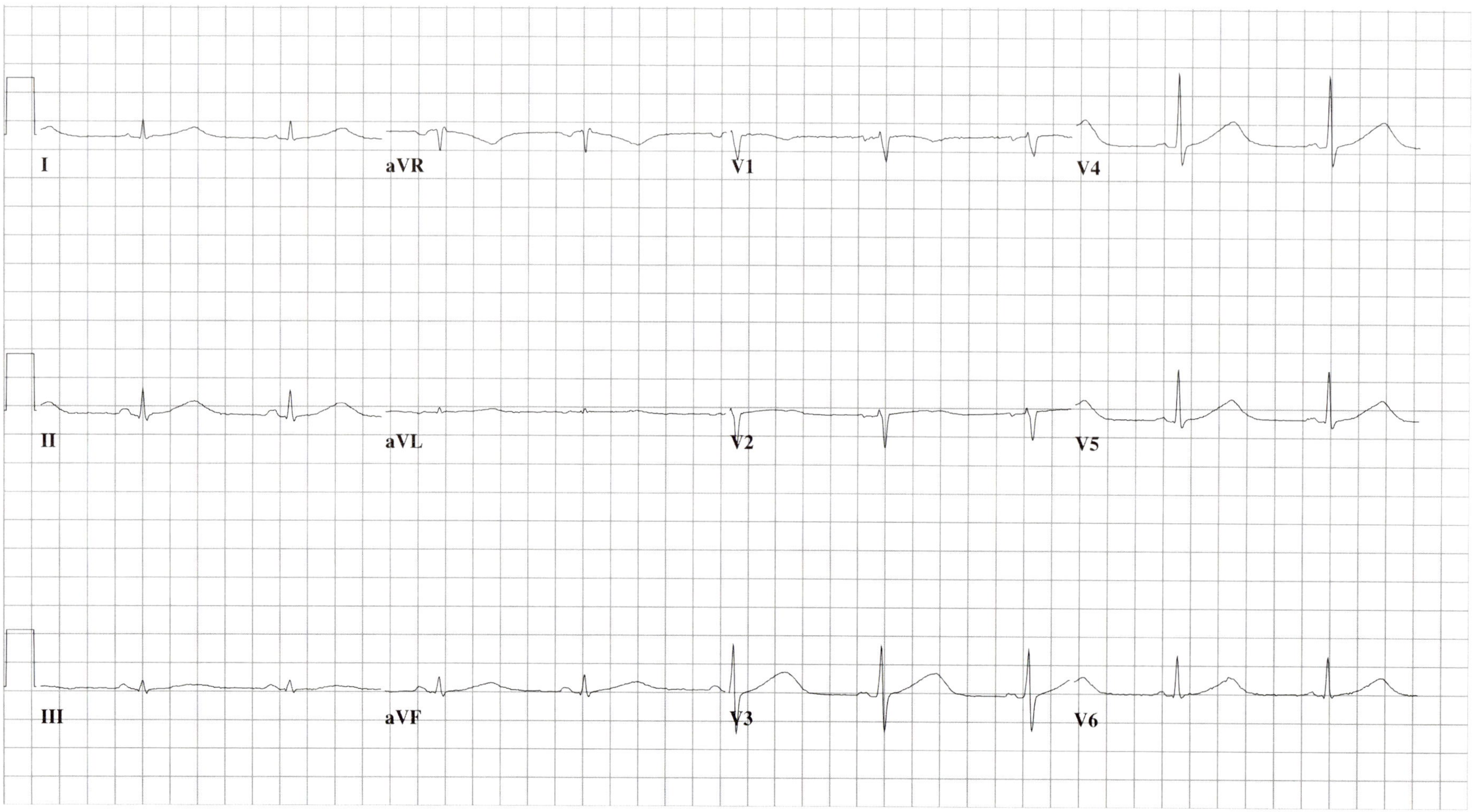

QUESTIONS

83-1. Interpret this ECG: what is the differential diagnosis for this abnormality?

83-2. What is the most likely cause of the abnormality in this patient?

83
P2-4AC
15.0 cm MI 0.9
Gen TIs 1.1
[2d] G78/71 d
FA4/P90
HAR/FS|0
[C] G50/0.80 kHz
FA5/F1/B
TDI
Amplitude (V)
S-T
Interval
Time (s)
3
2.5

ANSWERS

83-1. Interpret this ECG: what is the differential diagnosis for this abnormality?

The rhythm is sinus rhythm. The rate is approximately 50 beats/min. The QRS interval is normal. The QT interval is markedly prolonged to 570 milliseconds. Since the QT interval varies depending on heart rate, the corrected QT interval, or QTc should be calculated using Bazett's formula, which corrects the measured QT for heart rate. This formula is not as accurate at bradycardic and tachycardic heart rates, however.

Normal QT interval is less than 430 milliseconds in men and less than 450 milliseconds in women. The QT interval is considered prolonged when it is greater than 450 milliseconds in men and 470 milliseconds in women. Between 430 to 450 milliseconds and 450 to 470 milliseconds in men and women respectively, the QT is considered borderline prolonged. The QTc in this tracing is prolonged to 550 milliseconds. The differential diagnosis for prolonged QT interval includes electrolyte abnormalities such as hypokalemia and hypocalcemia, medication side effect, and congenital long QT syndrome (LQTS). There are multiple medications that can cause the QT interval to become prolonged including antibiotics, psychotropic medications, and antiarrhythmic medications.

83-2. What is the most likely cause of the abnormality in this patient?

Given that this patient has a family history of sudden cardiac death and has not received any medication, it is likely that she has a congenital LQTS. LQTS is caused by mutations in genes encoding cardiac ion channels. At least 12 different genes have been identified that result in a LQTS phenotype. The mutations in the ion channels result in abnormal repolarization manifested by a prolonged QT interval. Patients are predisposed to polymorphic ventricular tachycardia and sudden cardiac death.

Case #84. A 55-year-old presents with chest pain, dyspnea, and hypotension.

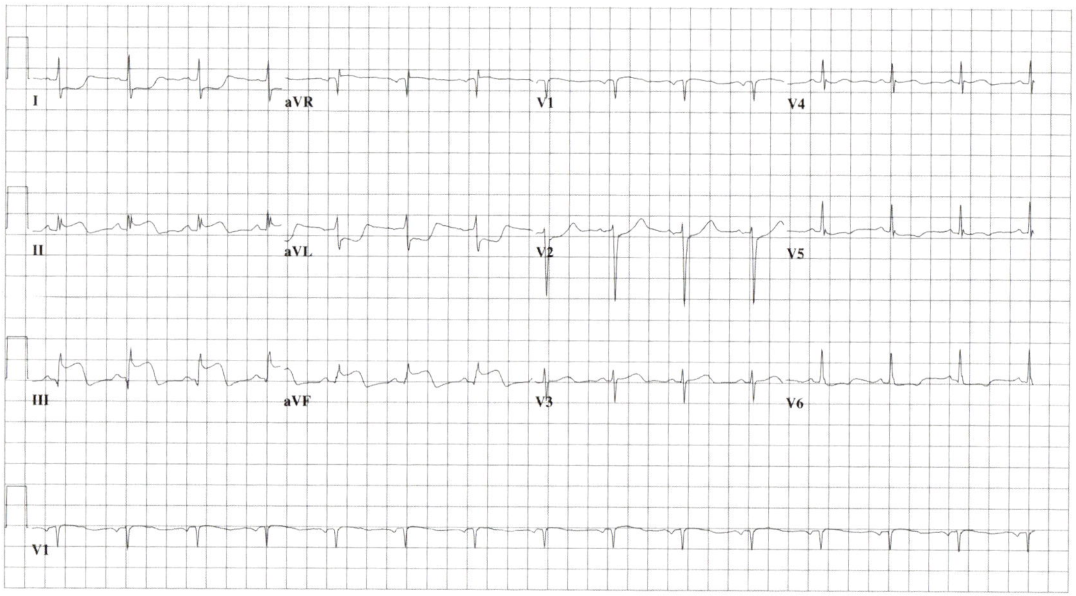

Right-sided leads:

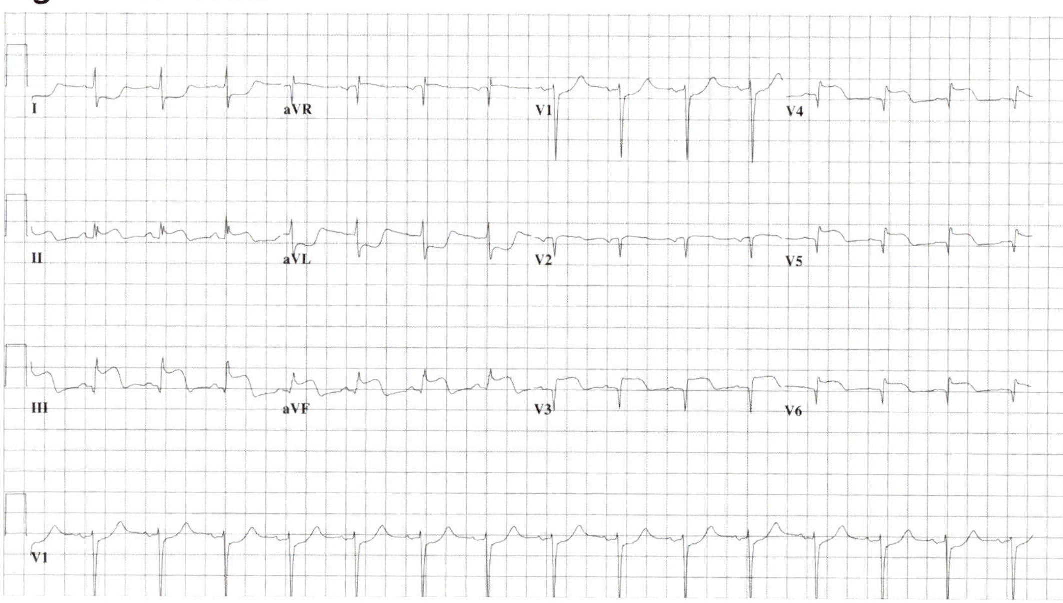

QUESTIONS

84-1. What abnormalities are present?

84-2. How do you diagnose and manage right ventricular myocardial infarction?

83
P2-4AC
15.0 cm MI 0.9
Gen Tls 1.1
[2d] G78/71 d
FA4/P90
[C] G50/0.80 kHz
FA5/F1/B
TDI
S-T
interval
3
2.5

ANSWERS

84-1. What abnormalities are present?

The first tracing demonstrates sinus rhythm. The QRS axis and PR, QRS, and QT intervals are normal. There are no pathologic Q waves. There is ST-segment elevation in leads II, III, and aVF corresponding to the inferior wall of the left ventricle with reciprocal ST-segment depression in leads aVL and I. The fact that there is more ST-segment elevation in lead III compared to lead II coupled with significant ST-segment depression in aVL suggests occlusion of the right coronary artery. In the setting of inferior myocardial infarction due to suspected right coronary occlusion, there is concern for concomitant infarction of the right ventricle.

84-2. How do you diagnose and manage right ventricular myocardial infarction?

Right ventricular myocardial infarction occurs when the right coronary artery is occluded proximally. Ischemia leads to right ventricular failure, which impairs left-sided filling and thus left ventricular preload. With decreased left ventricular preload, cardiac output also decreases. RV infarction should be suspected clinically if a patient has inferior infarction with the triad of hypotension, jugular venous distention, and clear lungs. There are several potential electrocardiographic clues to right ventricular infarction. If greater than 1 mm of ST-segment elevation is present in lead V1 coupled with ST elevation in II, III, and aVF, RV infarction should be suspected. This is not observed in this tracing. Alternately, a right-sided ECG can be performed by leaving the V1 and V2 leads as they are on the chest, and placing the V3 through V6 leads in their mirror-opposite positions on the right side of the chest. The V2 lead becomes V1R, V1 lead becomes V2R, and V3R through V6R are positioned likewise. Greater than 1 mm of ST elevation in lead V4R supports the diagnosis but is neither sensitive nor specific. Treatment should be guided by pulmonary artery catheterization and includes inotropes and judicious volume loading as well as urgent revascularization. Examination of the right-sided ECG in this case reveals 2 mm of ST-segment elevation in V4R, suggesting RV infarction.

Case #85. An asymptomatic 79-year-old man.

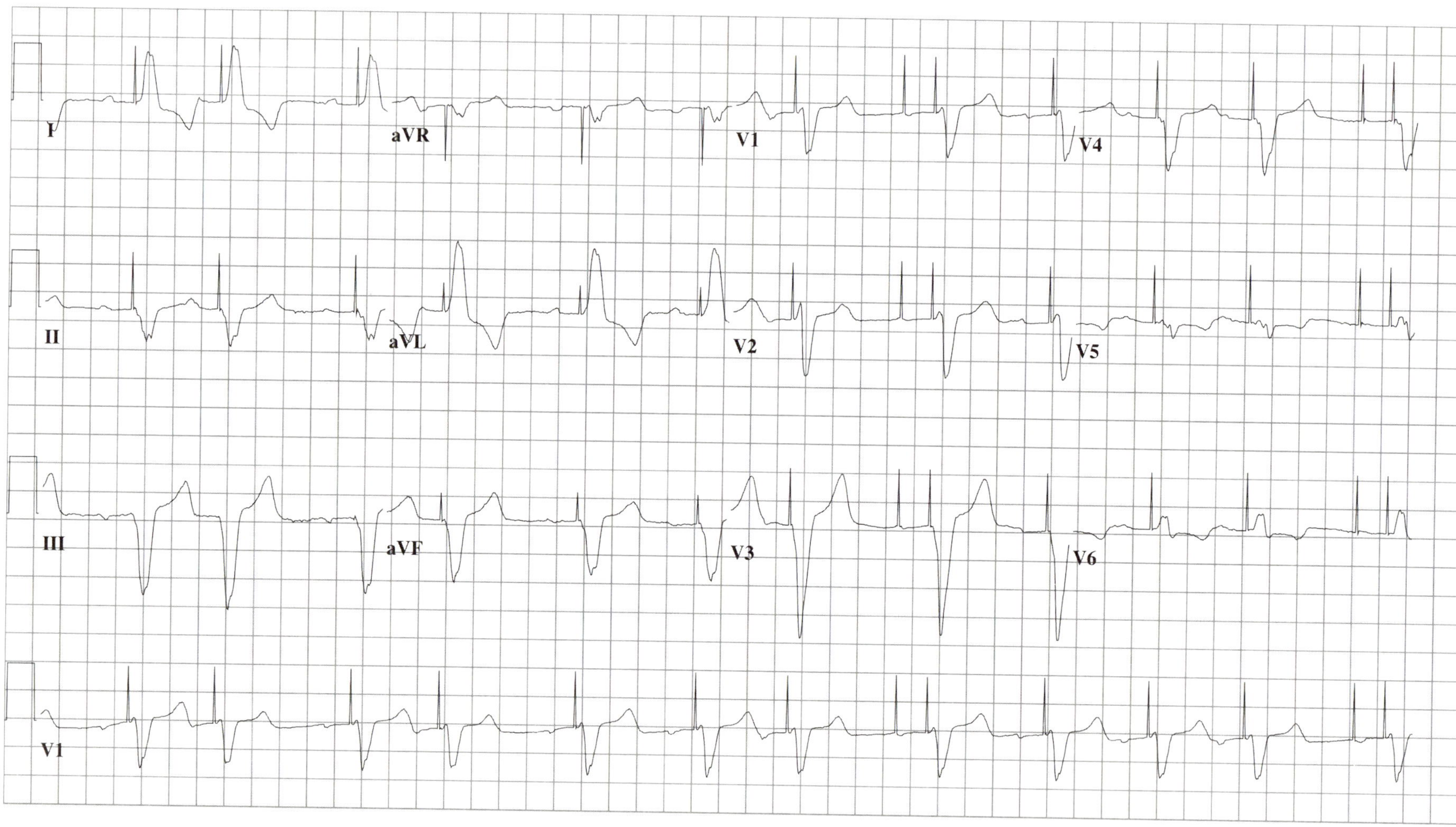

QUESTIONS

85-1. Interpret this ECG: where are the pacemaker leads located?

85-2. What is the set lower rate limit of the pacemaker? What is the set AV delay?

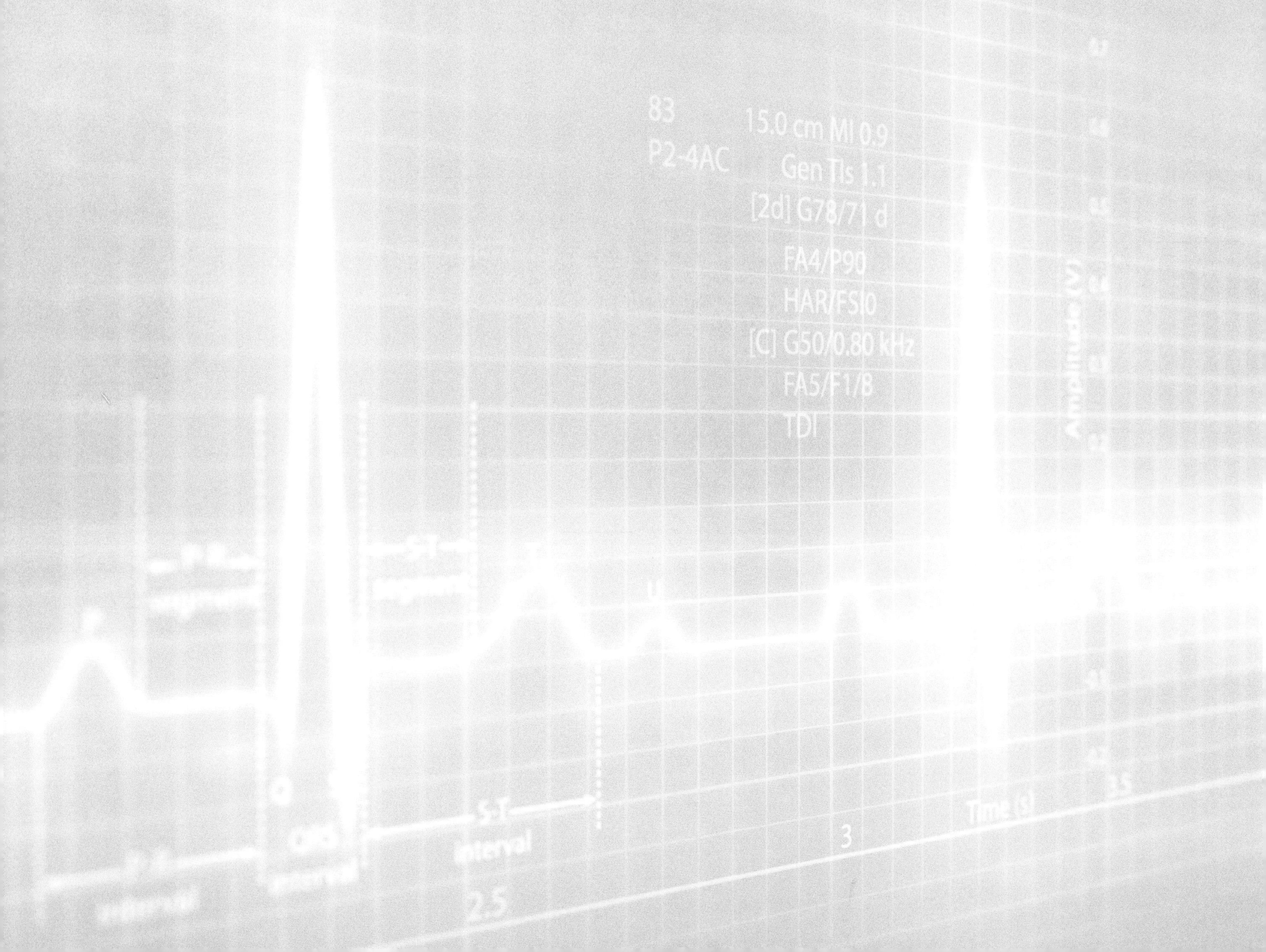
83
P2-4AC
15.0 cm MI 0.9
Gen TIs 1.1
[2d] G78/71 d
FA4/P90
HAR/FSI0
[C] G50/0.80 kHz
FA5/F1/8
TDI
S-T
interval
2.5
3
Time (s)
Amplitude (V)

ANSWERS

85-1. Interpret this ECG: where are the pacemaker leads located?

The rate is 72 beats/min. The atrial rhythm is sinus with both multifocal premature atrial beats and sinus pauses leading to atrial pacing. The figure demonstrates sinus beats, atrial premature beats, and atrial paced beats. None of the atrial activity is conducted to the ventricle, as every QRS is a paced complex. The QRS axis is leftward with left bundle branch morphology, consistent with right ventricular apical pacing. There are secondary ST-segment abnormalities due to the paced ventricular rhythm. Thus, there are pacemaker leads located in both right ventricle and right atrium.

85-2. What is the set lower rate limit of the pacemaker? What is the set AV delay?

Examining the rhythm strip, the pre-pacing interval (the interval measured from the 11th P wave of native atrial activity to the 12th paced P wave, a paced P wave) is 5 big boxes, which equals 1 second. Hence, the lower rate limit is 60 beats/min. A sensed or paced atrial beat will start the timer, and if no atrial activity is sensed in the next second, the pacemaker will deliver a paced P wave. The programmed A-V delay can be assessed by examining the length of time between any P wave and the paced ventricular beat. After sensed or paced atrial activity, a second internal clock starts, now looking for ventricular activity. If no ventricular activity is sensed by the end of this programmed "A-V delay," a ventricular pacing impulse is delivered. In this case, the A-V delay is set to 0.2 seconds.

Sinus P waves are noted with asterisks, and atrial premature beats are noted with carats. There are also atrial paced beats noted. All the QRS complexes are paced beats.

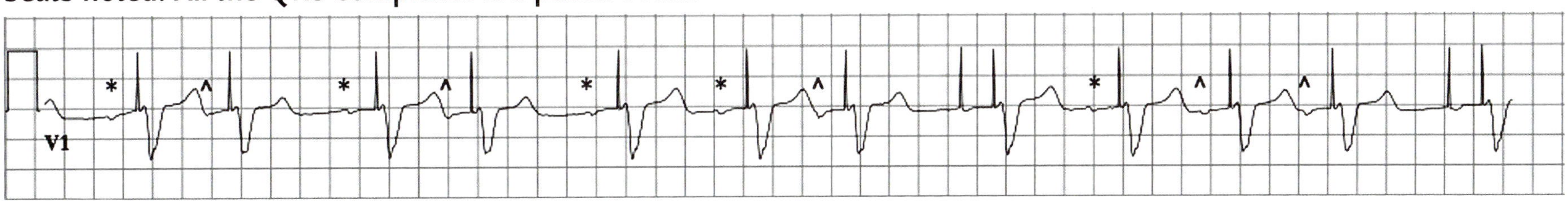

Case #86. A 48-year-old female presents to her physician after experiencing an episode of lightheadedness and palpitations at home. A resting ECG is shown below.

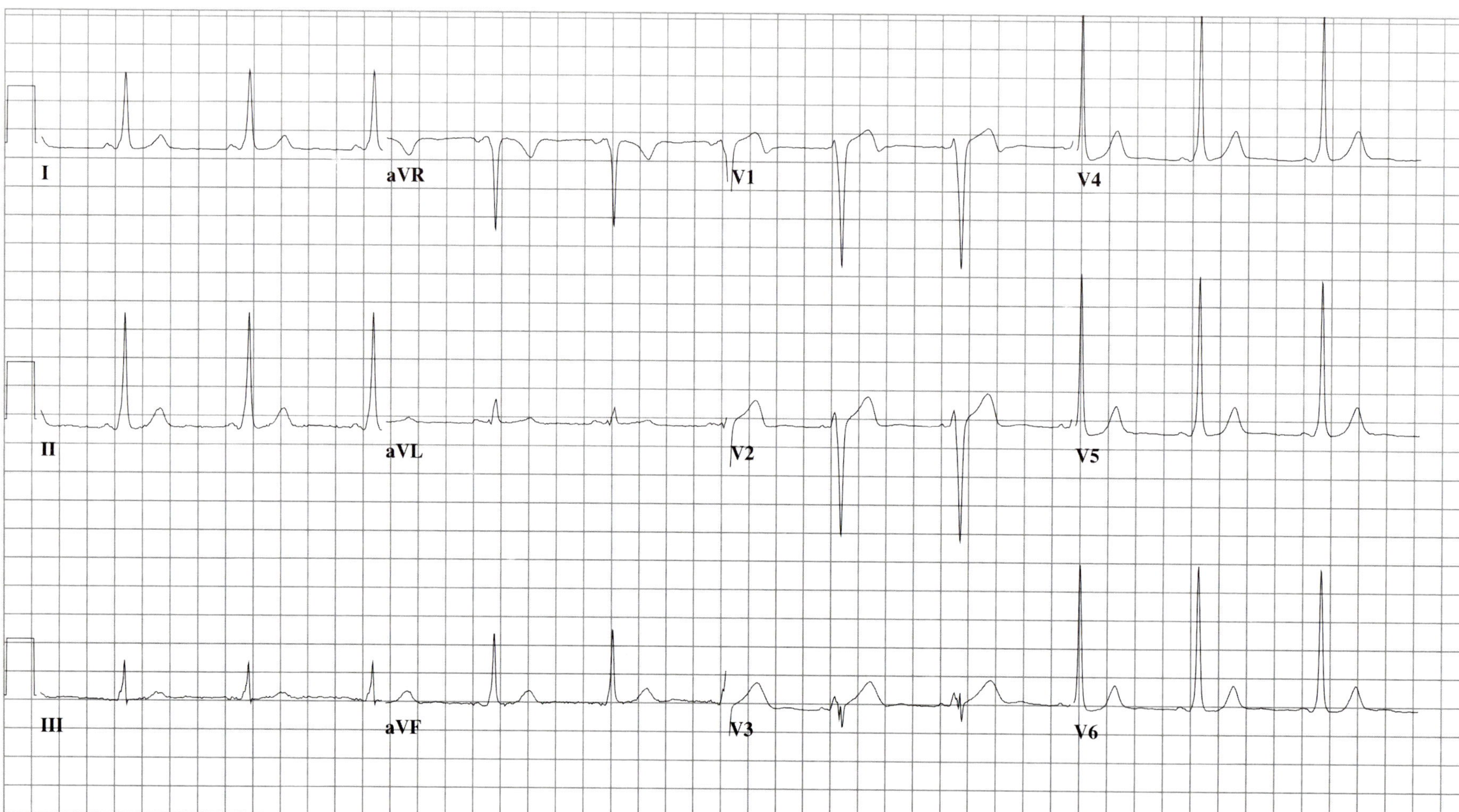

QUESTIONS

86-1. What abnormalities are present on this ECG?

86-2. What arrhythmias would this patient be prone to developing?

83
P2-4AC
15.0 cm MI 0.9
Gen TIs 1.1
[2d] G78/71 d
FA4/P90
HAR/FS|0
[C] G50/0.80 kHz
FA5/F1/8
TDI
Amplitude (V)
S-T
Interval
2.5
3
Time (s)
3.5

ANSWERS

86-1. What abnormalities are present on this ECG?

Sinus rhythm is present at approximately 70 beats/min. The QRS axis is normal. The QRS interval is broad, particularly in leads I and II, with a slurred initial upstroke. The PR interval is short, less than 120 milliseconds. There are no ST-segment and T-wave abnormalities. The presence of a short PR interval and broad QRS with a slurred upstroke suggests the Wolff-Parkinson-White (WPW) ECG pattern. When a WPW ECG is combined with clinical symptoms suggestive of arrhythmia, the WPW syndrome is diagnosed. The short PR interval and slurred upstroke of the QRS are caused by an accessory pathway that provides direct electrical connection between the atria and the ventricles leading to ventricular preexcitation and acting as a substrate for arrhythmia.

86-2. What arrhythmias would this patient be prone to developing?

The accessory pathway present in WPW syndrome provides a path for impulses to travel between the atria and the ventricles bypassing the AV node. Some, but not all, accessory pathways allow impulses to travel both "anterograde," from the atrium to the ventricle, and "retrograde," from the ventricle to the atrium. This property provides the substrate for atrioventricular reentrant tachycardia (AVRT).

Orthodromic AVRT is characterized by anterograde conduction through the AV node and retrograde conduction through the accessory pathway. This results in a regular narrow-complex tachycardia with the loss of any delta wave (because the accessory pathway is conducting retrograde rather than anterograde during arrhythmia).

Antidromic AVRT, in contrast, describes anterograde conduction through the accessory pathway and retrograde conduction through the AV node. Because the accessory pathway provides the anterograde AV conduction during this arrhythmia, the specialized conduction tissue of the Bundle of His and Purkinje fibers is bypassed, and resulting arrhythmia manifests as a wide-complex tachycardia on the surface ECG.

Patients with WPW and bypass tracts with short refractory periods are at significant risk if atrial fibrillation (AF) is present. Recall that the AV node manifests decremental conduction, meaning that at higher heart rates, conduction velocity slows. When AF is present, fibrillation waves may have rates as high as 600 beats/min. Because accessory pathways do not have the property of decremental conduction, patients with WPW and AF can manifest extremely rapid ventricular rates, which can degenerate into ventricular fibrillation or cause hemodynamic collapse. Agents that block the AV node including β-blockers, calcium channel blockers, and digoxin are contraindicated when AF and an accessory pathway are present, as slowing conduction through the AV node can lead to very rapid conduction through the accessory pathway.

Case #87. A 27-year-old woman complaining of a racing heart.

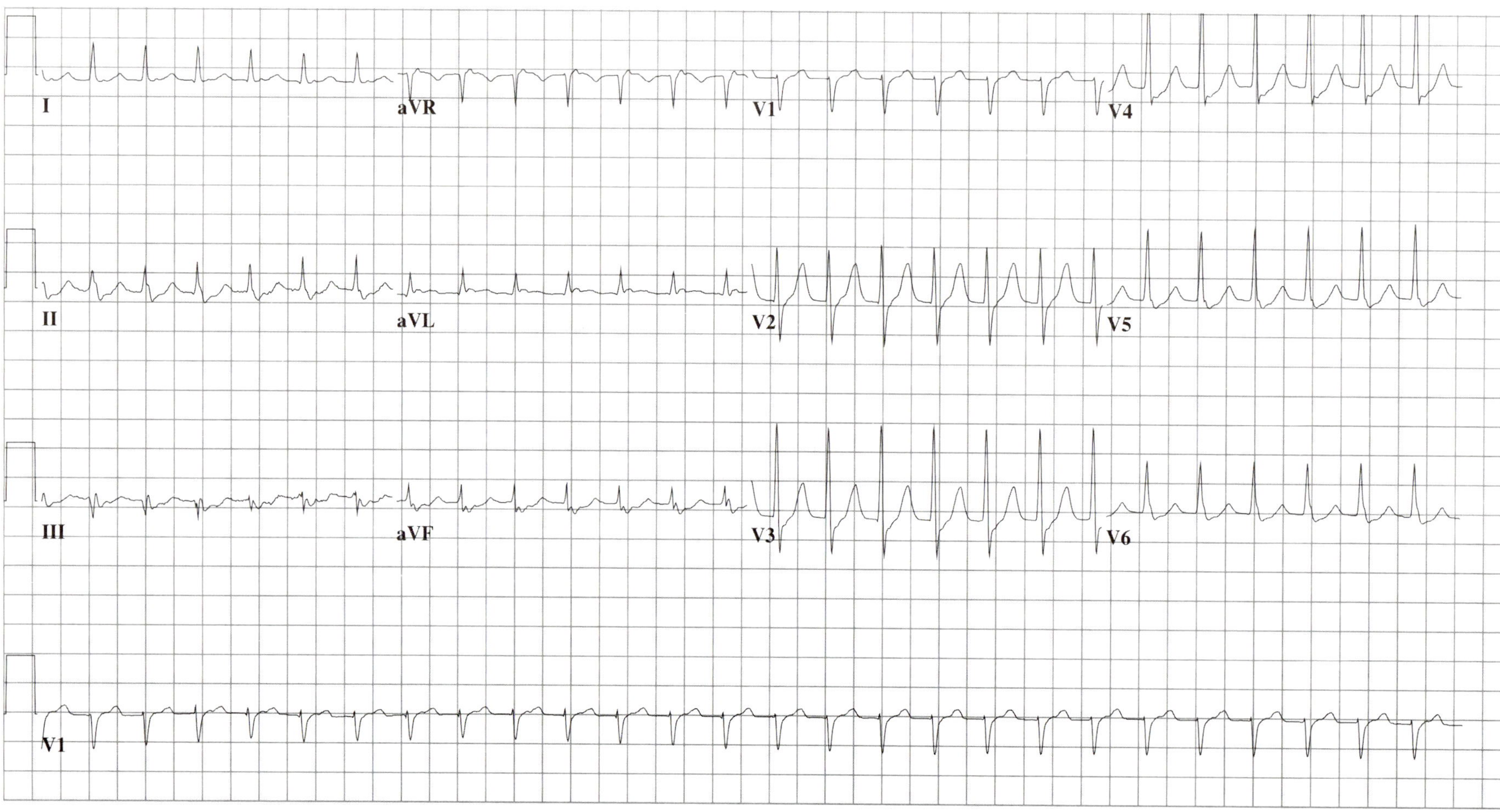

QUESTION

87-1. Interpret this ECG: what is the most likely diagnosis?

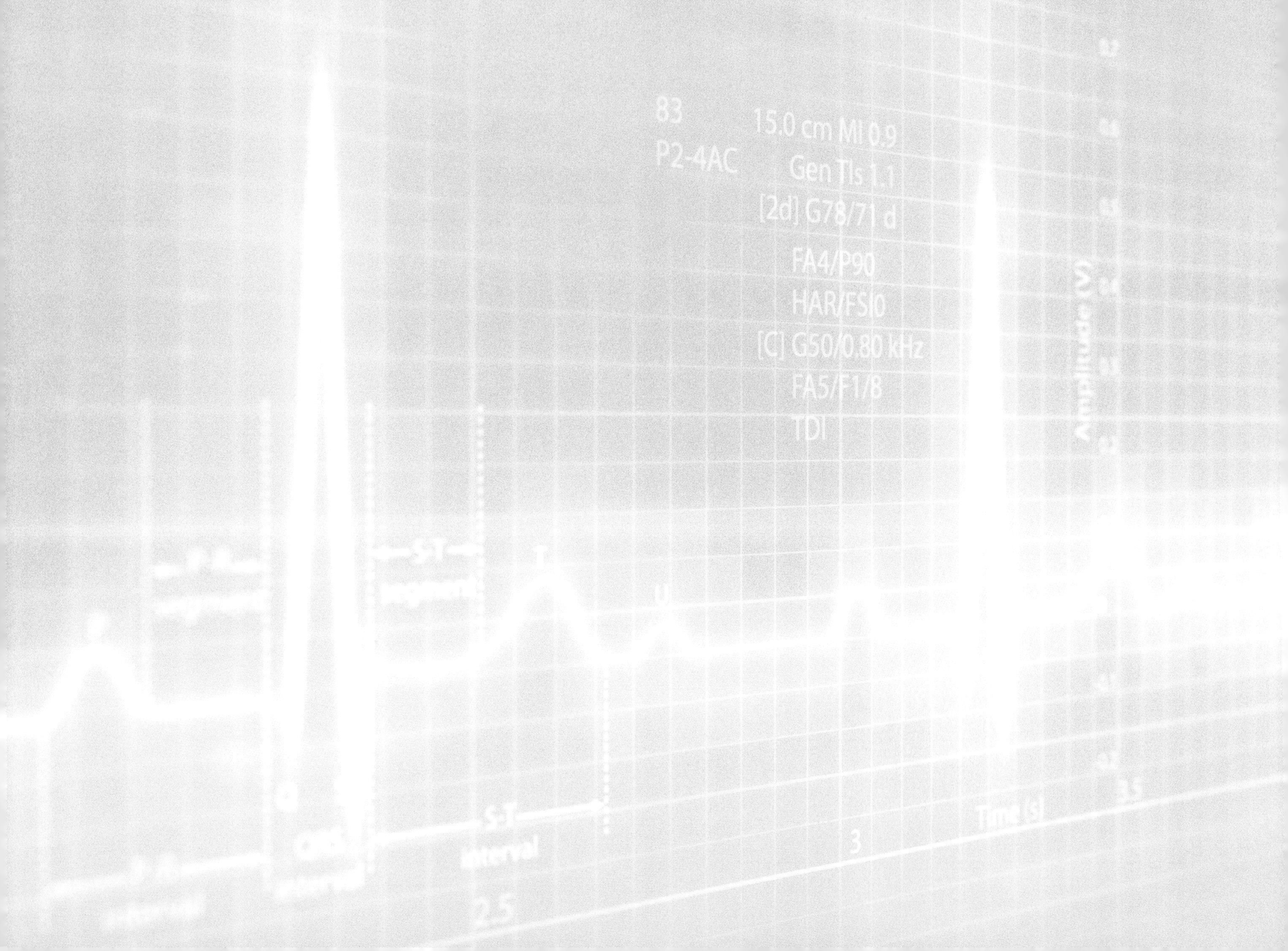
83
P2-4AC
15.0 cm MI 0.9
Gen TIs 1.1
[2d] G78/71 d
FA4/P90
HAR/FS|0
[C] G50/0.80 kHz
FA5/F1/8
TDI
Amplitude (V)
S-T
segment
T
U
S-T
interval
QRS
2.5
3
3.5
Time (s)

ANSWER

87-1. Interpret this ECG: what is the most likely diagnosis?

This tracing reveals a narrow complex tachycardia at a rate of 160 beats/min. Axis and intervals are normal. There is 1 to 2 mm of upsloping ST-segment depression in the inferior, anterior, and lateral leads. When faced with a narrow complex regular tachycardia, the differential includes sinus tachycardia, atrial tachycardia, atrial flutter with constant block, junctional tachycardia, AVRT, and AVNRT. A careful search for P waves, either conducted anterograde or retrograde, can help clarify the diagnosis. Closely examining the terminal part of the QRS complex in lead II, aVF, and V5 reveals a rounded, negative deflection appended to the terminal QRS complex. This is sometimes called a "pseudo S wave" and in this case represents retrograde conduction from the AV node to the atria, suggesting the diagnosis of AVNRT. Other less likely possibilities for this short RP tachycardia include atrial tachycardia with first-degree AV delay, or junctional tachycardia.

Case #88. A 63-year-old gentleman 4 days after cardiac surgery.

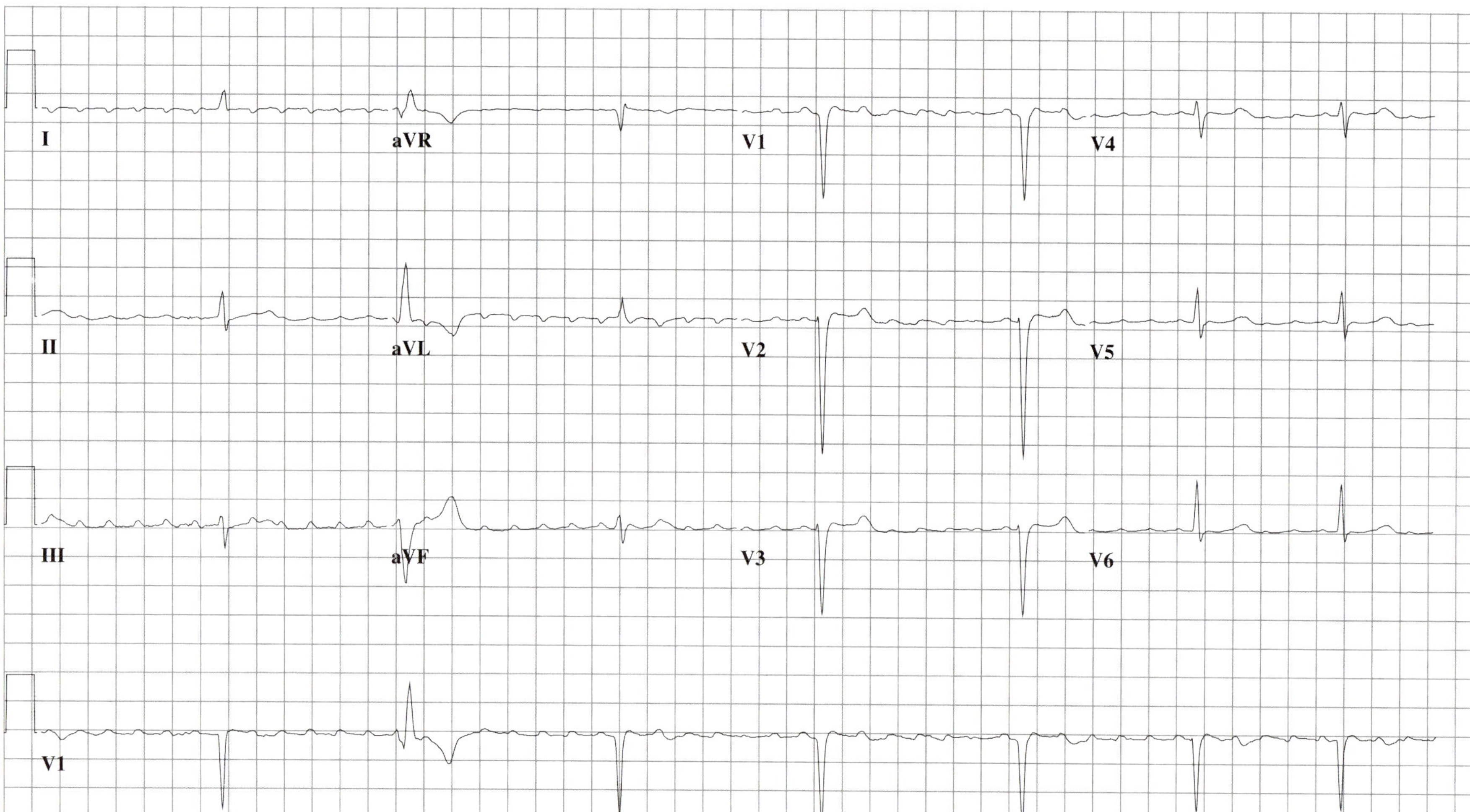

QUESTION

88-1. What is the rhythm?

83
P2-4AC
15.0 cm MI 0.9
Gen Tls 1.1
[2d] G78/71 d
FA4/P90
HAR/FS10
[C] G50/0.80 kHz
FA5/F1/8
TDI
S-T
interval
2.5
3
Time (s)
Amplitude (V)

ANSWER

88-1. What is the rhythm?

The ventricular rate is approximately 42 beats/min. Positively oriented "sawtooth waves" of atrial flutter are visualized best in leads II and III, at a rate of approximately 300 beats/min. There is variable AV conduction manifested as slightly irregular R–R intervals. The second QRS complex of the rhythm strip has right bundle branch block morphology and is either a premature ventricular contraction or a conducted beat with right bundle branch block aberrancy. The QRS axis is normal. There is delayed R-wave progression in the precordial leads. Both tachycardic and bradycardic arrhythmias are common after cardiac surgery.

Case #89. A 53-year-old woman presents with cardiogenic shock after a recent upper respiratory infection. Coronary angiography demonstrates no coronary disease.

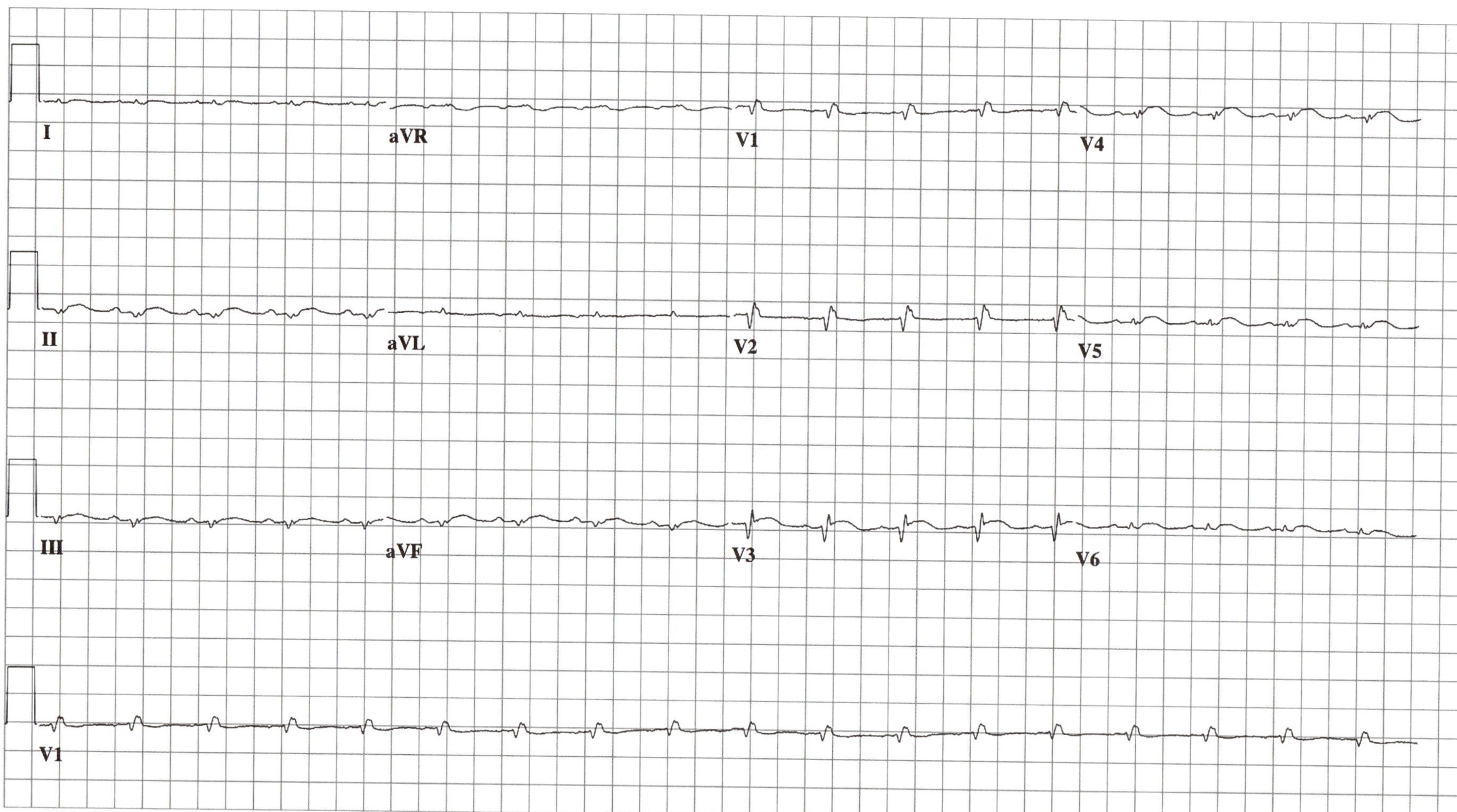

QUESTION

89-1. Interpret this ECG.

83
P2-4AC
15.0 cm MI 0.9
Gen TIs 1.1
[2d] G78/71 d
FA4/P90
HAR/FSI0
[C] G50/0.80 kHz
FA5/F1/8
TDI
S-T
interval
Time (s)
Amplitude (V)
2.5
3
3.5

ANSWER

89-1. Interpret this ECG.

Sinus tachycardia is present, with P waves best seen in lead II. The axis is indeterminate, with striking low voltage throughout the tracing. There is a right bundle branch block pattern present with an RSR′ wave in lead V1. Q waves and ST-segment elevations are present throughout the tracing, most notable in leads V3 through V6 and the inferior leads. Note that, although the magnitude of the ST-segment change is small, relative to the low QRS voltage, this degree of ST-segment change is significant. This patient was suffering from fulminant myocarditis.

Case #90. A 45-year-old patient with nonischemic cardiomyopathy presents with dizziness and lethargy after an increase in his furosemide dose.

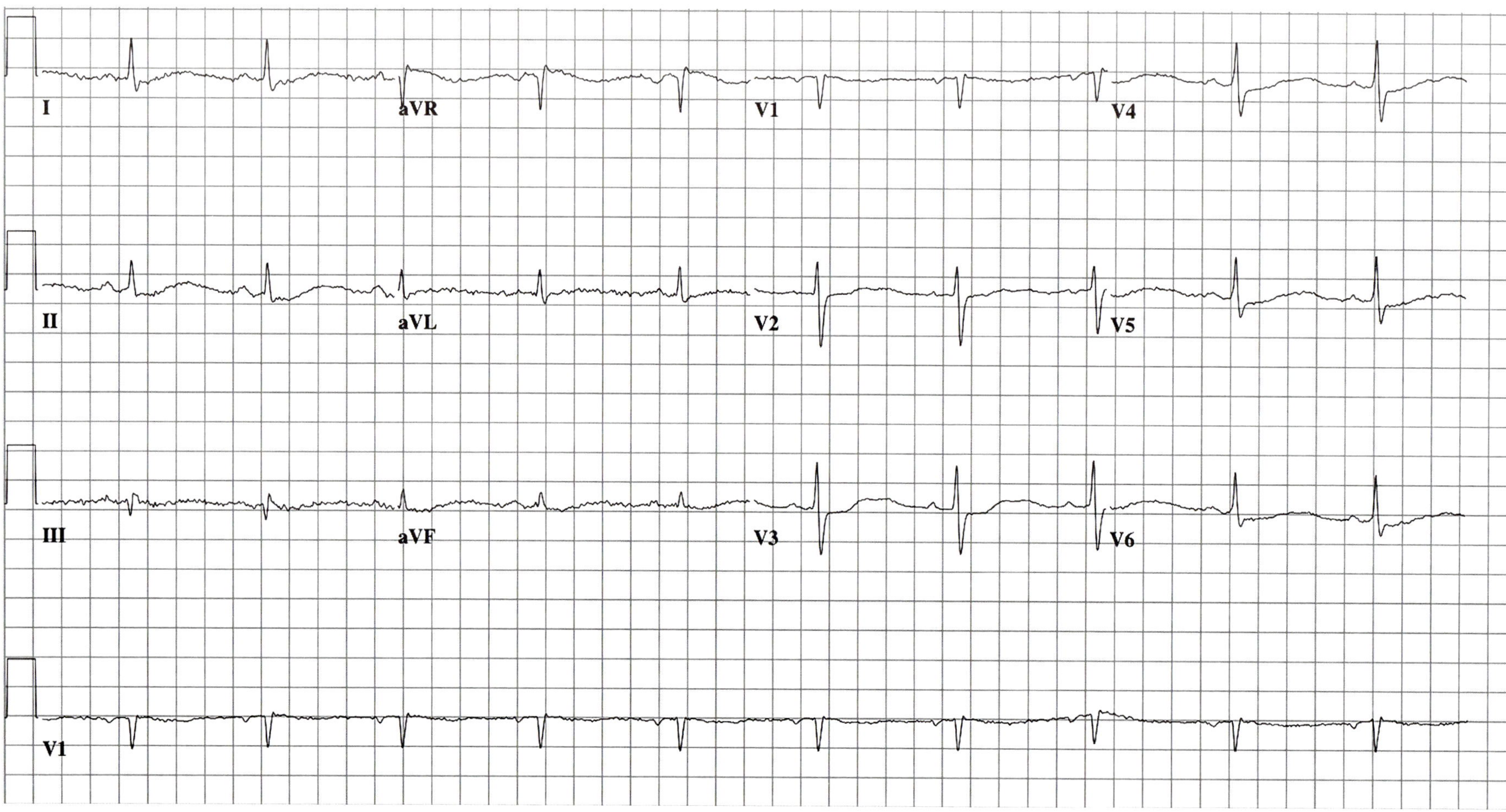

QUESTIONS

90-1. What ECG abnormalities are present?

90-2. What is the most likely diagnosis?

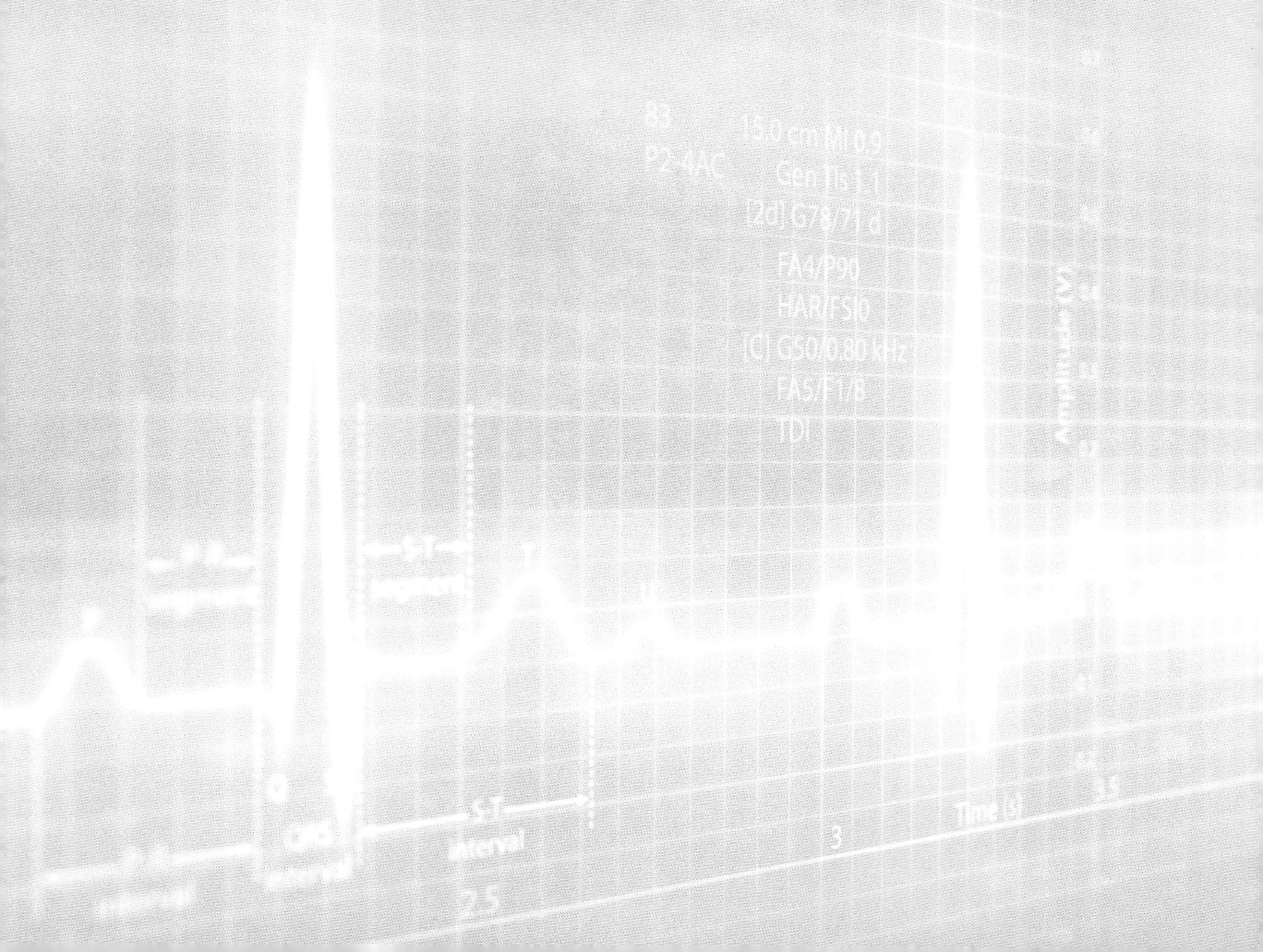
83
P2-4AC
15.0 cm MI 0.9
Gen TIs 1.1
[2d] G78/71 d
FA4/P90
HAR/FS|0
[C] G50/0.80 kHz
FA5/F1/8
TDI
Amplitude (V)
S-T
interval
2.5
3
Time (s)
3.5

ANSWERS

90-1. What ECG abnormalities are present?

There is a fine baseline artifact present in the limb leads. There is sinus rhythm at a rate of 60 beats/min. The QRS axis and the PR interval are normal. There is diffuse flattening of the T waves with a markedly prolonged QT interval. The T waves in leads V2 and V3 have a biphasic or "humped" appearance, suggesting fusion of the T wave with a large U wave, or so-called QT(U) fusion.

90-2. What is the most likely diagnosis?

Diffusely flat T waves with QT-interval prolongation are the ECG manifestations of hypokalemia. The clinical history of a recent escalation of diuretic dosing also suggests hypokalemia. Strict attention to potassium and magnesium homeostasis is essential during adjustment of diuretic dosing in patients with chronic heart failure.

Case #91. An 85-year-old man presents with 45 minutes of severe breathlessness.

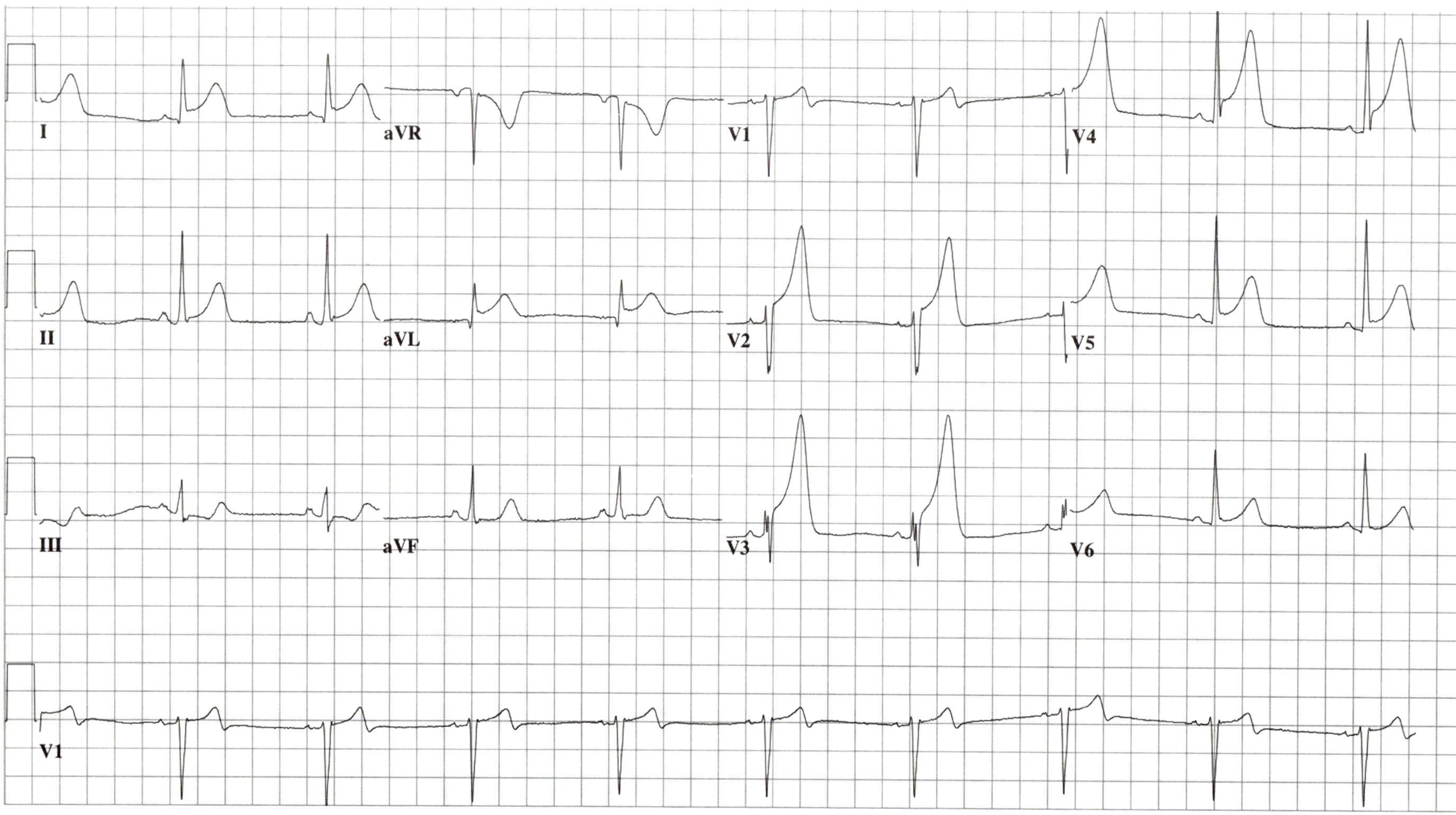

QUESTION

91-1. Interpret this ECG: what is the diagnosis?

83
P2-4AC
15.0 cm MI 0.9
Gen TIs 1.1
[2d] G78/71 d
FA4/P90
HAR/FS|0
[C] G50/0.80 kHz
FA5/F1/8
TDI

ANSWER

91-1. Interpret this ECG: what is the diagnosis?

Sinus bradycardia is present at a rate of 54 beats/min. The axis is normal, and there is no evidence of chamber enlargement. There are tall T waves present in V3 through V5 coupled with ST-segment elevation in leads I and aVL, and V2 through V5 consistent with myocardial injury. The clinical diagnosis is ST-segment elevation myocardial infarction in the anterolateral distribution. Given the hyperacute T waves, upward concavity of the ST segments, and lack of Q waves, this patient is early in the course of their infarction. Recall that, in general, immediately after vessel occlusion, the T waves become tall and hyperacute, followed by ST-segment elevation, Q-wave formation, and finally T-wave inversion. There is significant overlap among patients, however, and ECG findings alone should not be used to determine the chronicity of infarction.

Case #92. A 55-year-old man with a history of atrial fibrillation and pacemaker placement presents for follow-up.

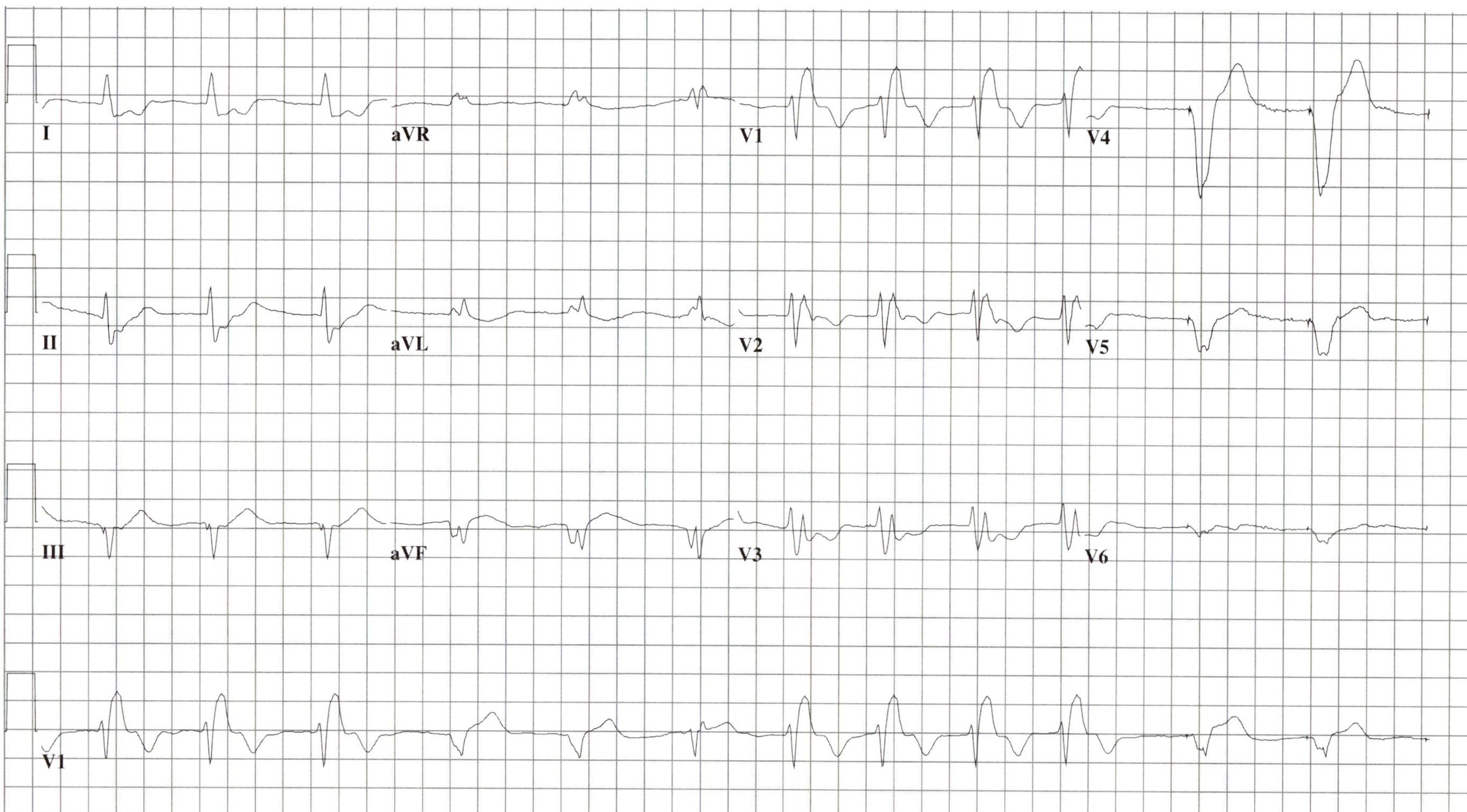

QUESTION

92-1. Interpret this ECG. Explain the different QRS morphologies.

83
P2-4AC
15.0 cm MI 0.9
Gen Tls 1.1
[2d] G78/71 d
FA4/P90
HAR/FSI0
[C] G50/0.80 kHz
FA5/F1/8
TDI
3
2.5

ANSWER

92-1. Interpret this ECG. Explain the different QRS morphologies.

There are 2 distinct rhythms in this tracing. The first 3 beats have a right bundle branch block pattern with an irregular R–R interval and no P waves. The next 2 beats have left bundle branch block morphology, occur at regular intervals, and are preceded by pacemaker impulses. The sixth beat is of indeterminate morphology, appearing similar to a combination of the previous beats. The 7th through 10th beats again are irregularly irregular with right bundle branch block. The final 2 beats are again paced at a regular interval. The rhythm, therefore, is atrial fibrillation. When heart rate becomes slower than the set lower rate limit of the pacemaker (here set at 70 beats/min), demand ventricular pacing occurs, explaining the intermittent paced beats. The left bundle branch block morphology of the paced beats is typical of a pacemaker located in the right ventricle. The sixth beat of the rhythm strip is a "fusion beat" caused by fusion of a concurrent paced impulse and a natively conducted impulse; the morphology appears indeterminate between a paced beat and a natively conducted beat.

Case #93. An 83-year-old female presents to the emergency department after 2 syncopal episodes at home.

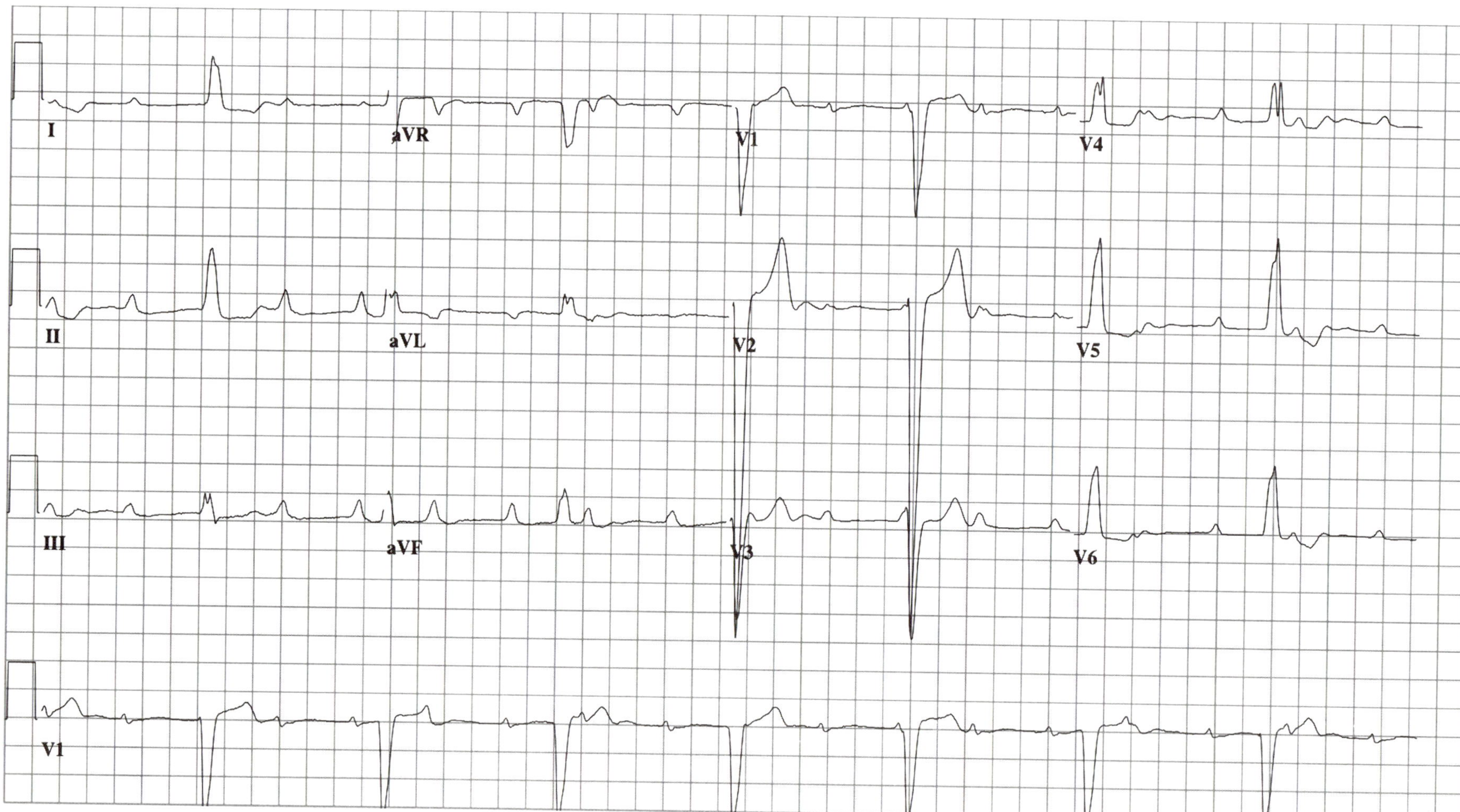

QUESTIONS

93-1. What rhythm is present on this ECG?

93-2. What treatment (if any) is indicated for this patient based on the ECG findings?

83
P2-4AC
15.0 cm MI 0.9
Gen TIs 1.1
[2d] G78/71 d
FA4/P90
[C] G50/0.80 kHz
FA5/F1/8
TDI
Amplitude (V)
S-T
interval
2.5
3
Time (s)
3.5

ANSWERS

93-1. What rhythm is present on this ECG?

The atrial rhythm is sinus at a rate of 100 beats/min. The P waves and QRS complexes do not bear any obvious relationship to each other and atrioventricular dissociation is present, as shown below in the figure. The ventricular rate is approximately 42 beats/min (7 QRS complexes in the 10-second rhythm strip multiplied by 6 yields 42 beats/min). The presence of AV dissociation with an atrial rate faster than ventricular rate is diagnostic of complete heart block. The QRS complex has left bundle branch block morphology and a normal axis.

93-2. What treatment (if any) is indicated for this patient based on the ECG findings?

The patient has symptomatic bradycardia secondary to complete heart block. She should be referred for placement of a permanent pacemaker. Whether a temporary pacemaker is indicated in the interim would depend on the patient's blood pressure, clinical status, and symptoms; if needed, transcutaneous or transvenous pacing could be instituted while awaiting permanent device placement.

P waves, denoted with asterisks, march out independently of the QRS complexes, denoted with arrows. The atrial rate is faster than the ventricular rate. This is diagnostic of complete heart block.

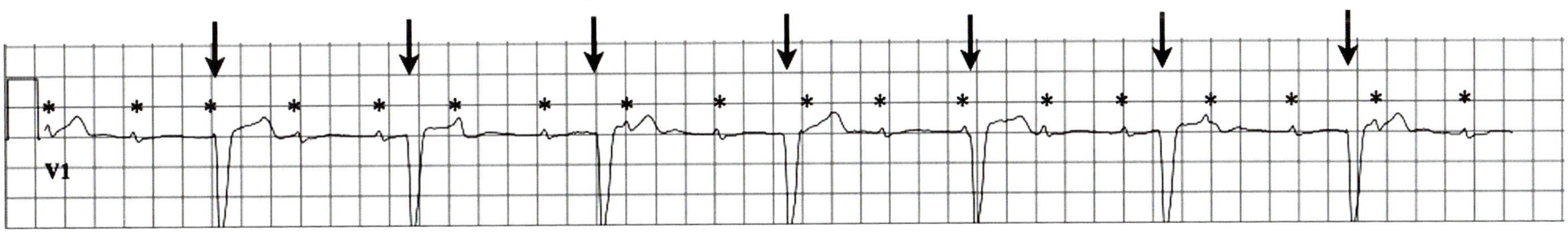

Case #94. An asymptomatic 55-year-old man with a new abnormality on his ECG.

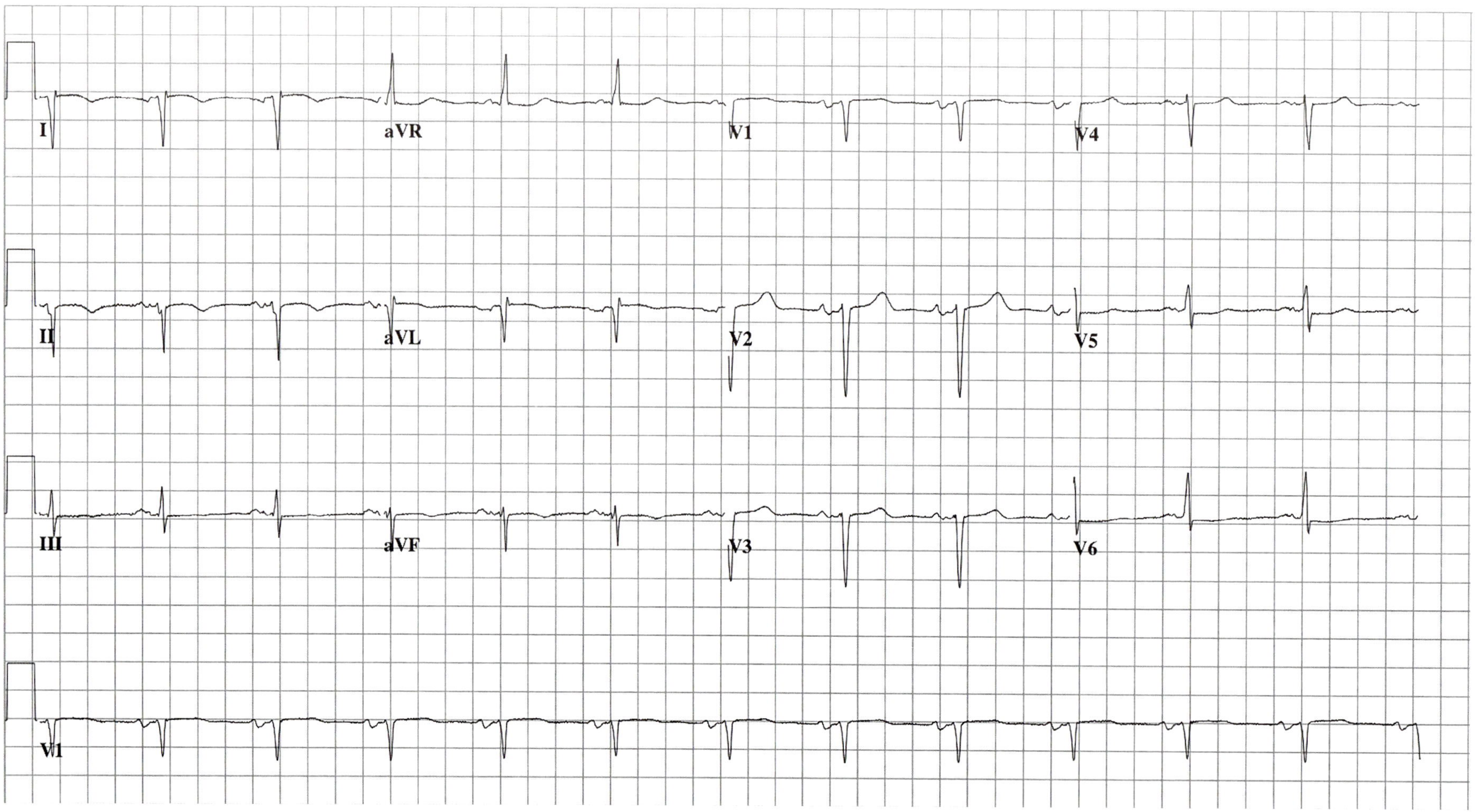

QUESTIONS

94-1. Interpret this ECG.

94-2. What is the abnormality, and how would you correct it?

83
P2-4AC
15.0 cm MI 0.9
Gen TIs 1.1
[2d] G78/71 d
FA4/P90
HAR/FS10
[C] G50/0.80 kHz
FA5/F1/B
TDI
Amplitude (V)
S-T
Interval
2.5
3
Time (s)
3.5

ANSWERS

94-1. Interpret this ECG.

The rate is 75 beats/min. The P waves have an abnormal morphology—biphasic in lead II and inverted in lead I. The axis is extreme rightward at −120 degrees. (The QRS complex is completely negative in lead II, which is oriented at +60 degrees, suggesting that the impulse lies 180 degrees with respect to this lead. Alternately, one can diagnose an extreme rightward axis noting that the QRS complex is downward in lead I and lead aVF placing the axis somewhere in the northwest quadrant.) The differential diagnosis of an extreme axis and negative P wave in lead I includes dextrocardia or right arm-left arm limb lead reversal. In addition to the abnormalities in axis, there are nonspecific T-wave abnormalities present in the precordial leads.

94-2. What is the abnormality, and how would you correct it?

If dextrocardia were present, the heart would be oriented in the right chest and the precordial R-wave progression would therefore be reversed, demonstrating R-wave regression from lead V1 through V6. In contrast, if the limb leads are reversed, the precordial leads are normal in morphology. In this tracing, the negative P wave and extreme axis coupled with R-wave progression in the precordial leads is diagnostic of right arm-left arm limb lead malposition. To "correct" for this on the surface ECG, interpose the tracings in leads aVR and aVL and leads II and III and interpret the negative image of lead I. Lead aVF would be unchanged.

Case #95. A 56-year-old woman presents with cardiac arrest, defibrillated in the field by EMS. Two tracings on arrival to the ED are shown.

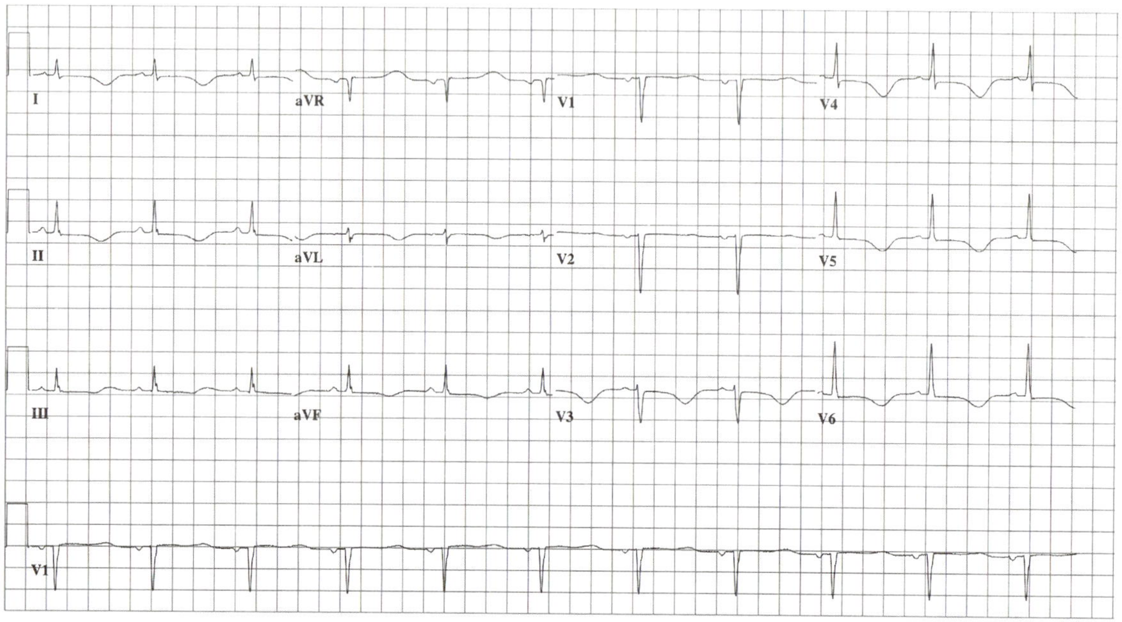

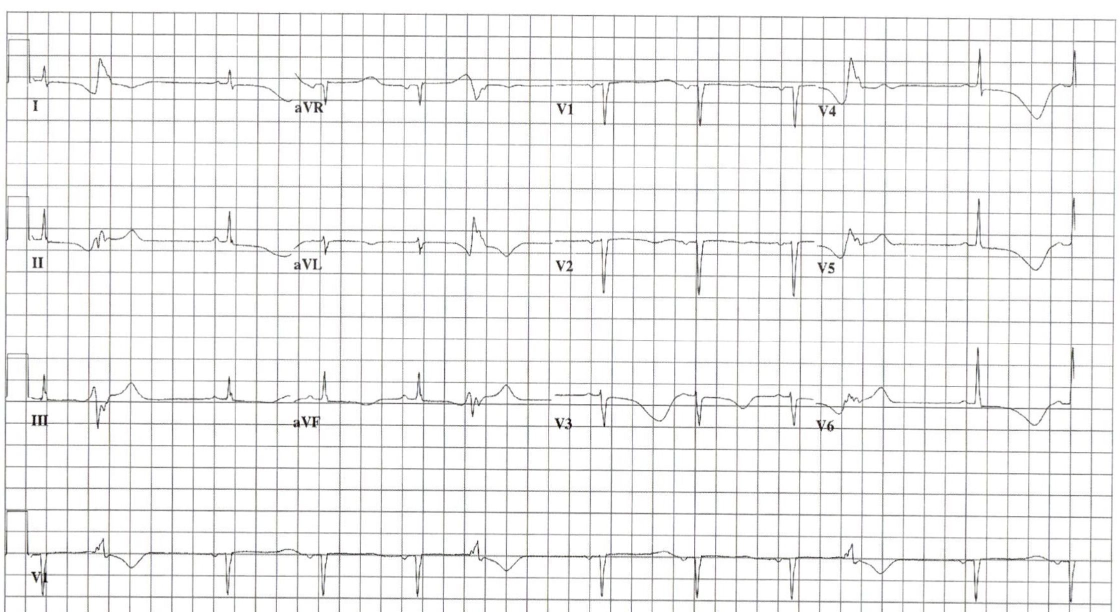

QUESTIONS

95-1. What do the ECGs show?

95-2. Which abnormalities could account for her cardiac arrest?

83
P2-4AC
15.0 cm MI 0.9
Gen TIs 1.1
[2d] G78/71 d
FA4/P90
HAR/FSI0
[C] G50/0.80 kHz
FA5/F1/8
TDI
Amplitude (V)
interval
2.5
3

ANSWERS

95-1. What do the ECGs show?

The rhythm is sinus at a rate of 60 beats/min. Axis is normal. The QT interval is strikingly prolonged to more than 600 milliseconds. The T waves are inverted in the inferior, lateral, and anterior precordial leads. The second tracing reveals premature ventricular beats with compensatory pauses. This finding illustrates the fact that the QT interval depends on the R–R interval: with longer R–R intervals (slower rates as during a compensatory pause), the QT interval also lengthens. In lead V3 of the second tracing, one can see that the beat after a post-PVC pause has a very long and bizarre QT interval compared to the baseline long QT interval of the regular sinus beats. The axis is normal, and there is no chamber enlargement.

95-2. Which abnormalities could account for her cardiac arrest?

The long QT interval is responsible for this patient's arrest, likely giving rise to polymorphic ventricular tachycardia/torsades de pointes. QT-interval prolongation can be congenital or acquired. Congenital causes are inherited mutations in cardiac ion channels, the so-called long QT syndrome. Acquired causes of QT prolongation are common and include medications, electrolyte disturbances, central nervous system diseases, bradycardia, and ischemia.

Case #96. A 59-year-old woman presents to the office complaining of depression and confusion.

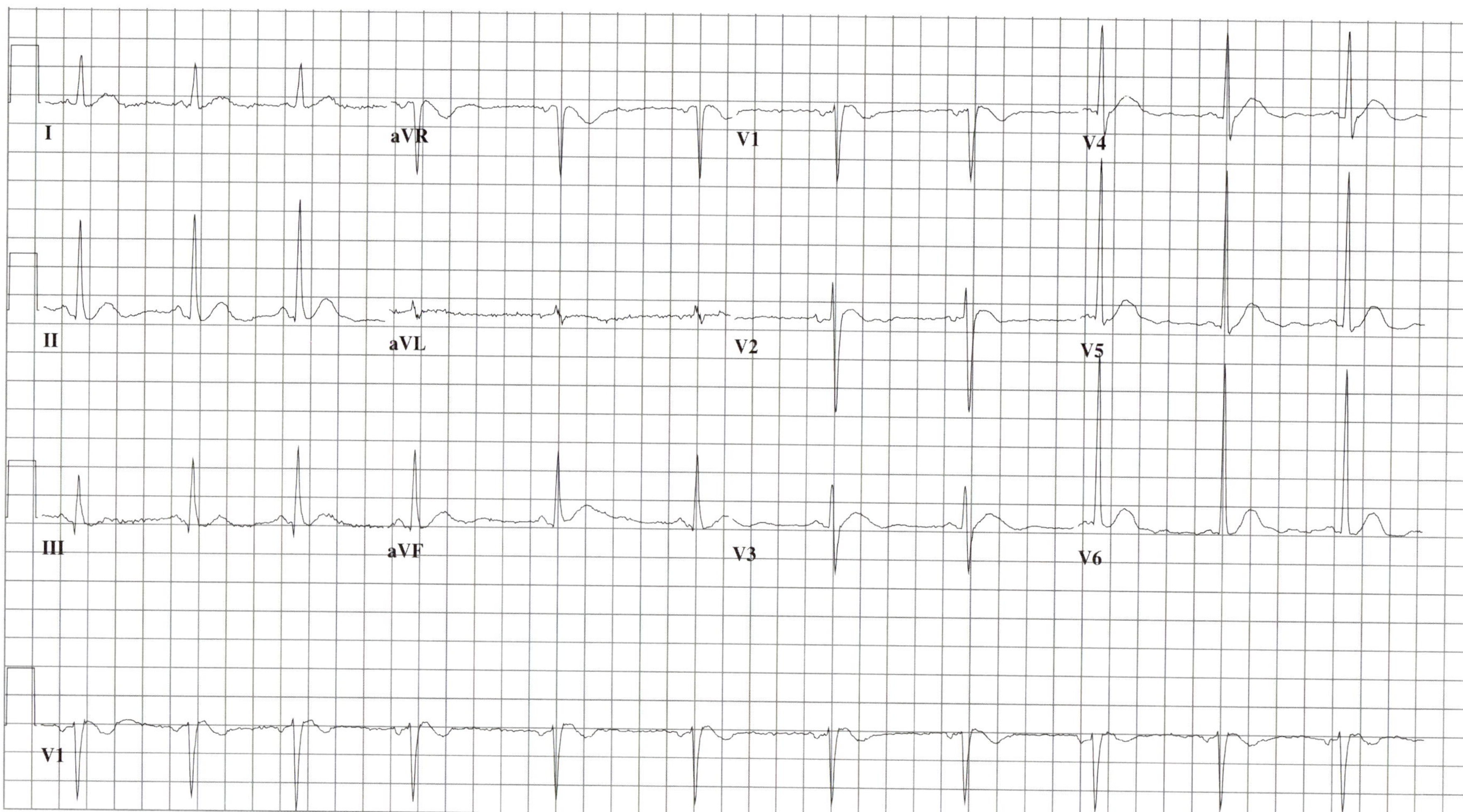

QUESTIONS

96-1. What are the findings?

96-2. What lab test would you order?

83
P2-4AC
15.0 cm MI 0.9
Gen TIs 1.1
[2d] G78/71 d
FA4/P90
HAR/FS10
[C] G50/0.80 kHz
FA5/F1/8
TDI

ANSWERS

96-1. What are the findings?

The rhythm is sinus at a rate of 66 beats/min. The axis is normal. PR and QRS intervals are normal. There is left ventricular hypertrophy diagnosed on the basis of the S wave in lead V1 added to the R wave in V5 greater than 35 mV. The QT interval is abnormal. Most obvious in lead V2, the QT interval is shortened with almost complete loss of the isoelectric ST segment. The T wave "takes off" directly from the J point of the QRS complex.

96-2. What lab test would you order?

A short ST segment with this morphology including loss of the ST segment and the T wave arising directly from the QRS is suggestive of hypercalcemia. Symptoms of hypercalcemia can include bone and abdominal pain, kidney stones, and change in mental status including confusion and depression. Serum calcium level including an ionized fraction should be ordered. Additional helpful studies in the evaluation of patients with hypercalcemia include serum phosphorus and serum parathyroid hormone levels.

Case #97. A 78-year-old man with poorly controlled hypertension presents with worsening dyspnea on exertion.

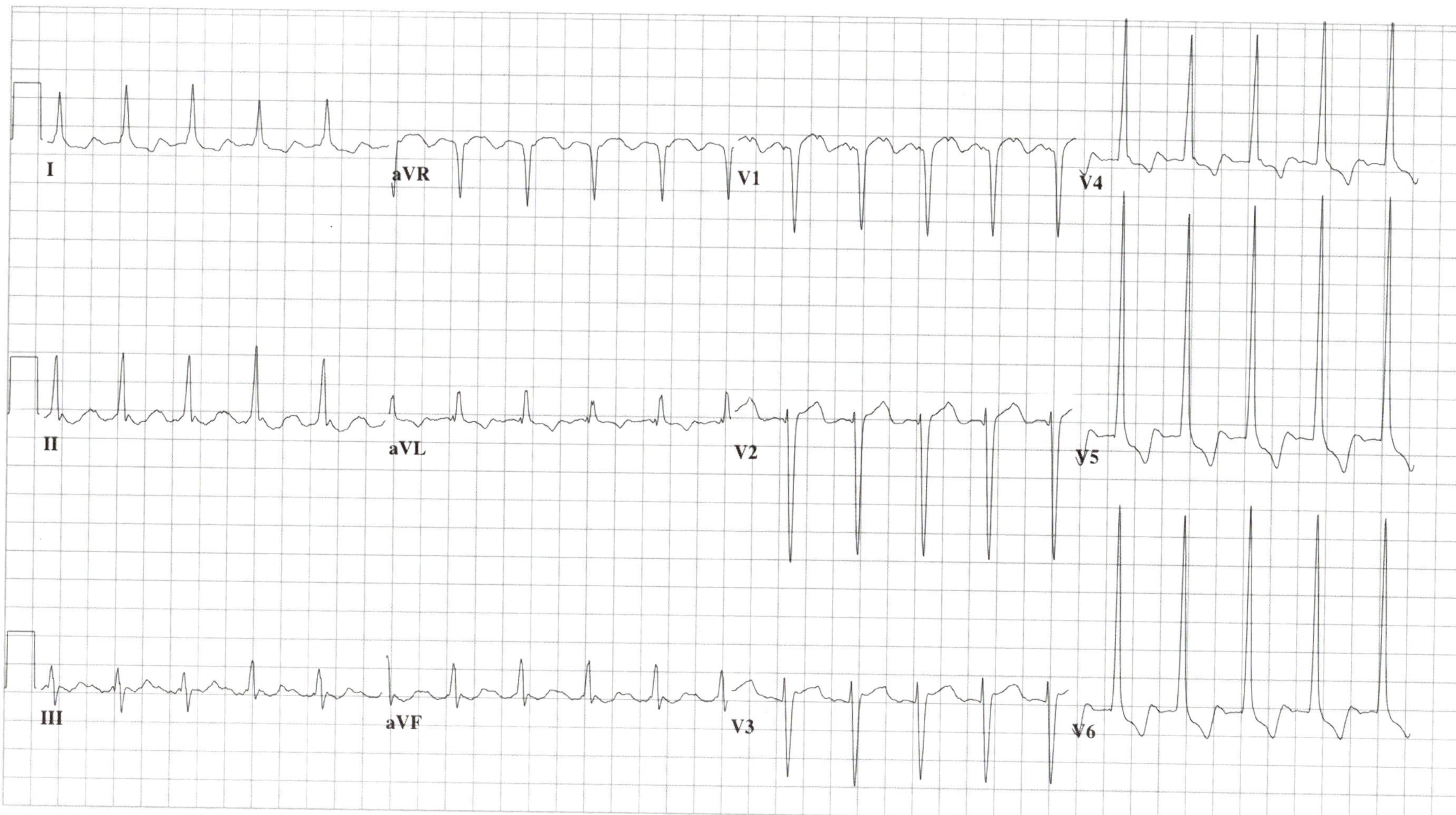

QUESTION

97-1. What abnormalities are present on this ECG?

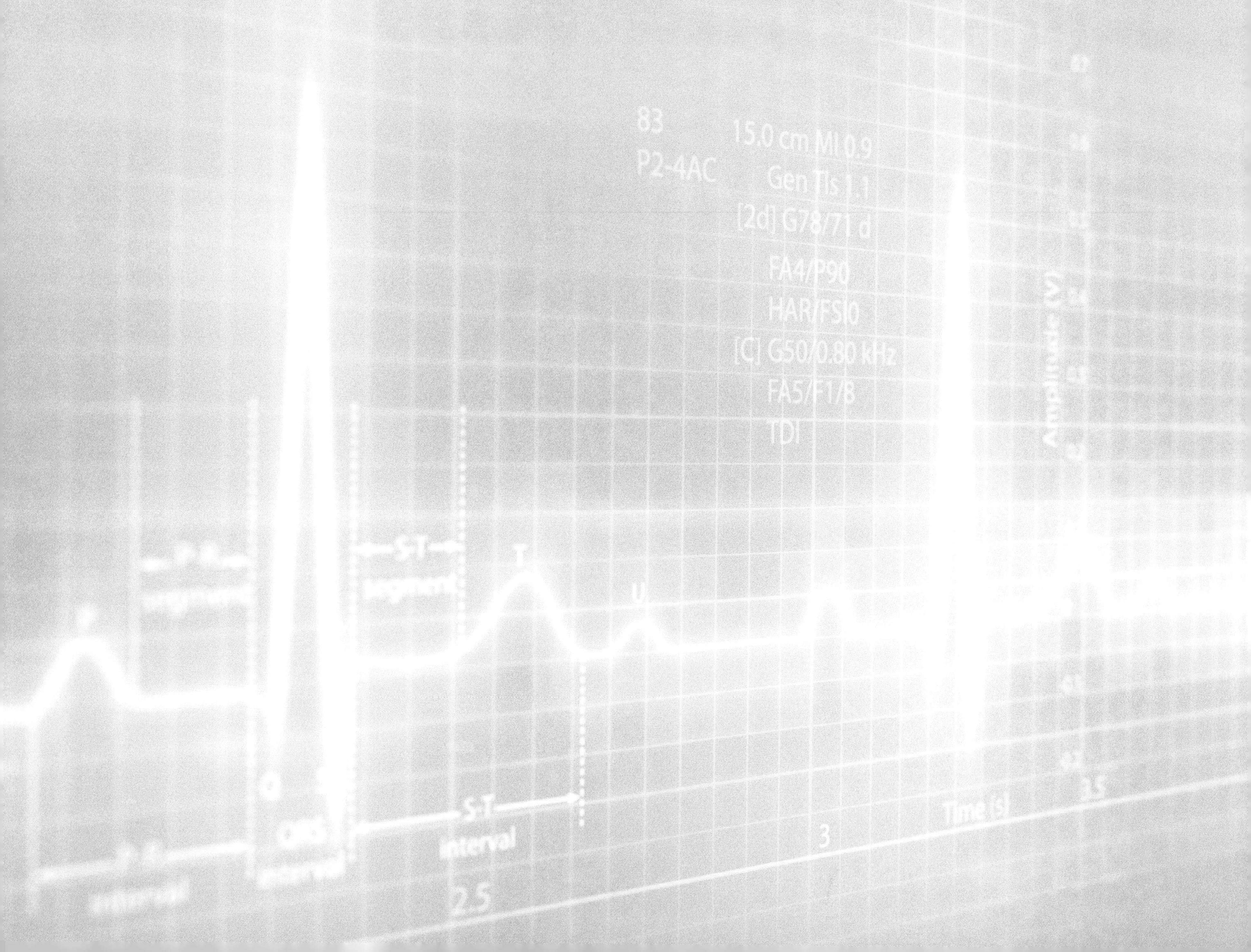
83
P2-4AC
15.0 cm MI 0.9
Gen TIs 1.1
[2d] G78/71 d
FA4/P90
HAR/FSI0
[C] G50/0.80 kHz
FA5/F1/8
TDI
S-T
segment
T
U
S-T
interval
2.5
3
Time (s)
3.5
Amplitude (V)

ANSWER

97-1. What abnormalities are present on this ECG?

This is a rapid, regular, narrow-complex tachycardia at approximately 125 beats/min. Examining lead V1, atrial activity is seen prior to each QRS, and so one might be tempted to diagnose sinus tachycardia. Closer inspection, however, reveals another deflection buried in each T wave, as shown in the figure. These are atrial flutter waves with 2 to 1 AV conduction. The QRS axis appears normal, as does the QRS duration, and there are no pathologic Q waves. There is evidence of left ventricular hypertrophy (the S-wave amplitude in V1 plus R-wave amplitude in V5 or V6 is greater than 35 mV, and the R-wave amplitude in lead aVL is greater than 11 mV). There are downsloping ST-segment depressions and T-wave inversion most evident in leads I, V4, V5, and V6, which may be secondary to the left ventricular hypertrophy or due to subendocardial ischemia in the setting of the tachycardia.

Flutter waves are shown with arrows in lead V1.

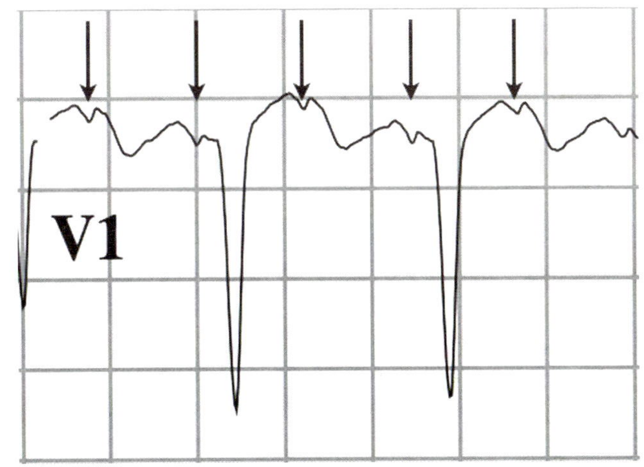

Case #98. A 57-year-old gentleman with nonischemic cardiomyopathy presents with sudden onset of extreme fatigue, malaise, and dizziness.

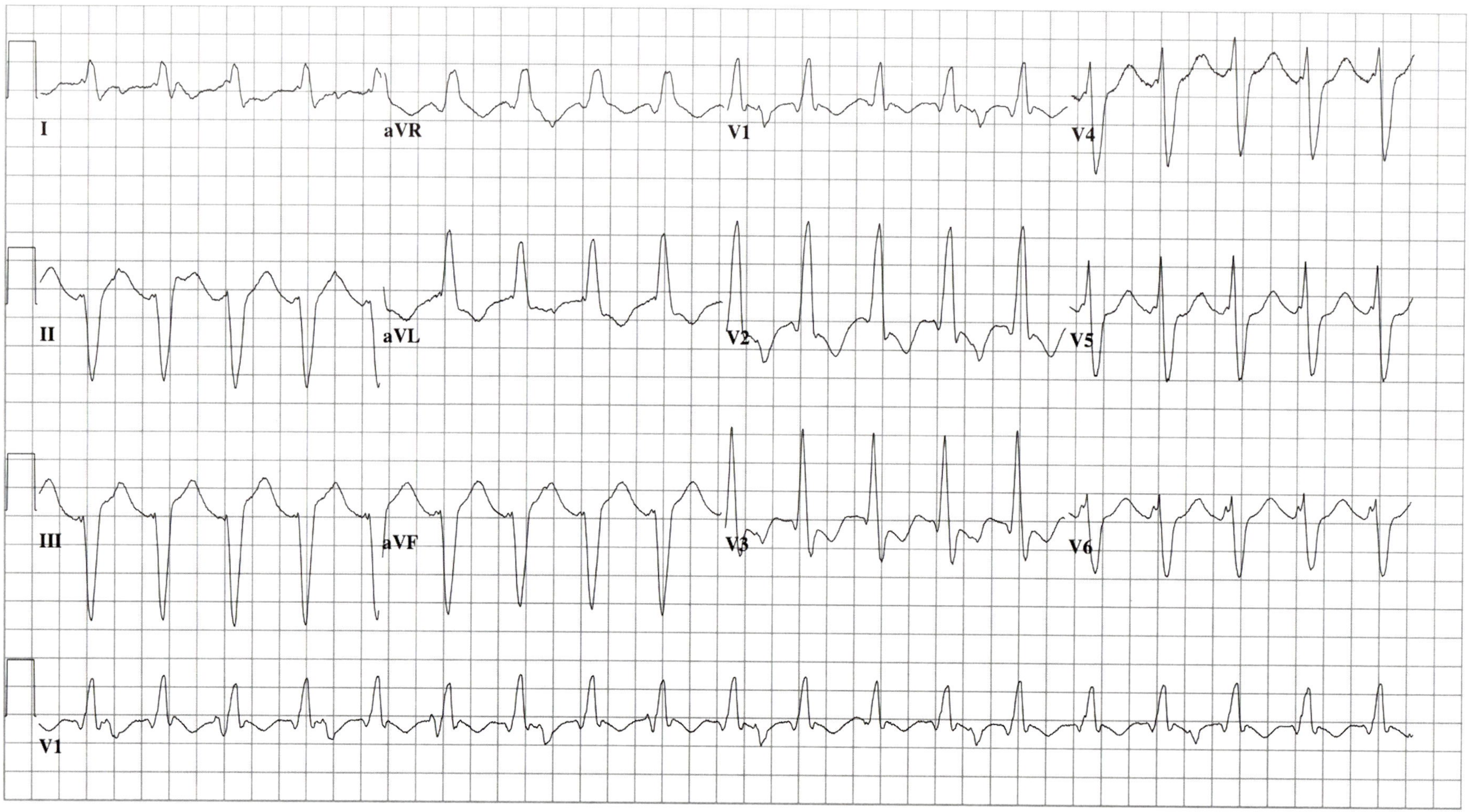

QUESTION

98-1. Interpret this ECG.

83
15.0 cm MI 0.9
P2-4AC
Gen TIs 1.1
[2d] G78/71 d
FA4/P90
HAR/FS0
[C] G50/0.80 kHz
FA5/F1/8
TDI
Amplitude (V)
S-T
interval
Time (s)
2.5
3
3.5

ANSWER

98-1. Interpret this ECG.

The ventricular rate is 110 beats/min. The rhythm is regular. The QRS complex is wide at approximately 150 milliseconds. The differential diagnosis of this wide-complex tachycardia includes supraventricular tachycardia with aberrant conduction versus ventricular tachycardia. There are several sets of published criteria for distinguishing these two possibilities when monomorphic wide-complex tachycardia is present.[1-3] If the QRS complexes across the precordial leads V1 through V6 are all positive (RS complexes) or all negative (QS complexes), "concordance" is present. When present, concordance is suggestive of ventricular tachycardia. This tracing does not demonstrate evidence of concordance in the precordial leads.

Ventricular tachycardias will often demonstrate evidence of atrioventricular dissociation—examining the rhythm strip closely for evidence of P waves without relationship to the QRS can be revealing. In examining the rhythm strip, reproduced here in the figure, p waves can be identified. These p waves are dissociated from the QRS complexes. Note that the p–p interval is approximately 800 milliseconds, whereas the R–R interval is approximately 520 milliseconds. These intervals indicate that the ventricular rate is faster than the atrial rate. It is important to note that atrial and ventricular activity are also dissociated when complete heart block is present; however in that case, the atrial rate would be faster than the ventricular rate.

In sum, this tracing demonstrates ventricular tachycardia with evidence of A-V dissociation; the underlying atrial rhythm is sinus rhythm. The deeply inverted, broad P waves are consistent with left atrial abnormality.

Wide-complex tachycardia with sinus P waves (demonstrating left atrial abnormality) "marching through" diagnostic of ventricular tachycardia.

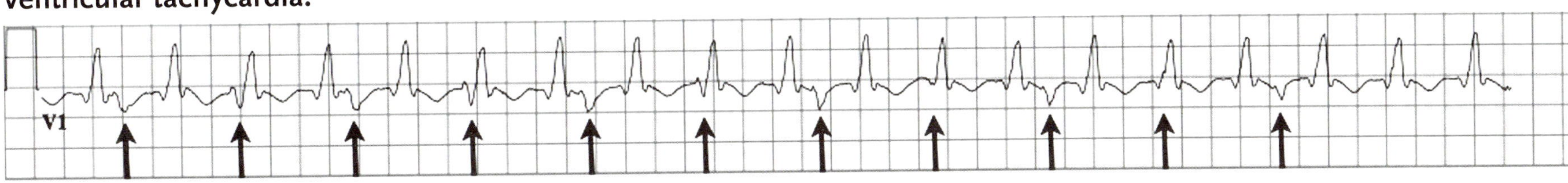

[1]Pava LF, Perafan P, Badiel M, et al. R-wave peak time at DII: a new criterion for differentiating between wide complex QRS tachycardias. *Heart Rhythm* 2010; 7: 922-926.
[2]Vereckei A, Duray G, Szenasi G, et al. Application of a new algorithm in the differential diagnosis of wide QRS complex tachycardia. *Eur Heart J* 2007; 28: 589-600.
[3]Brugada P, Brugada J, Mont L, et al. A new approach to the differential diagnosis of a regular tachycardia with a wide QRS complex. *Circulation* 1991; 83: 1649-1659.

Case #99. A 67-year-old woman presents for follow-up.

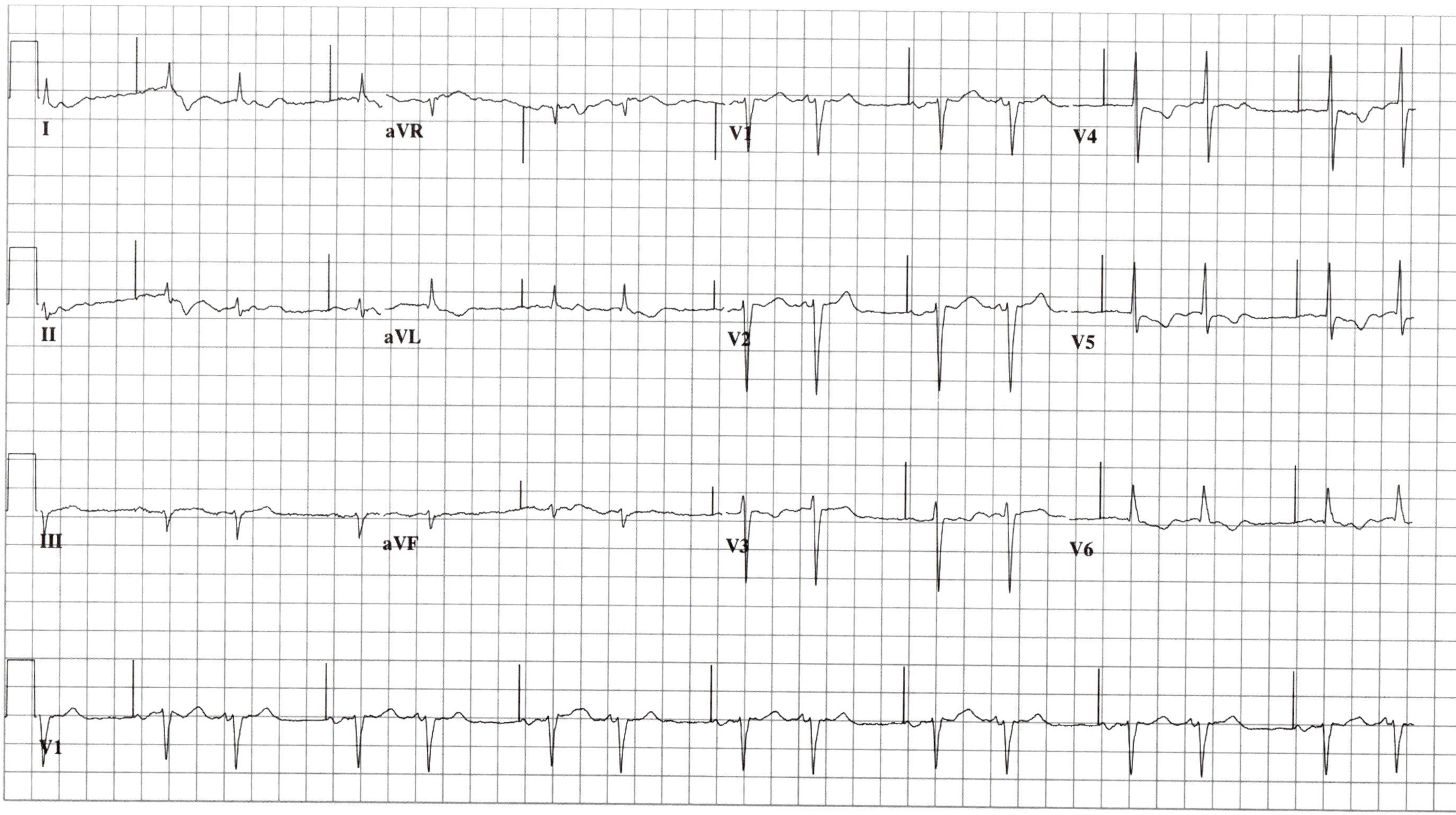

QUESTIONS

99-1. Interpret this ECG: what is the rhythm?

99-2. What is the 3-letter pacemaker code governing the behavior seen on this ECG (assume there is only a single pacemaker lead)? What is the lower rate limit of the pacemaker?

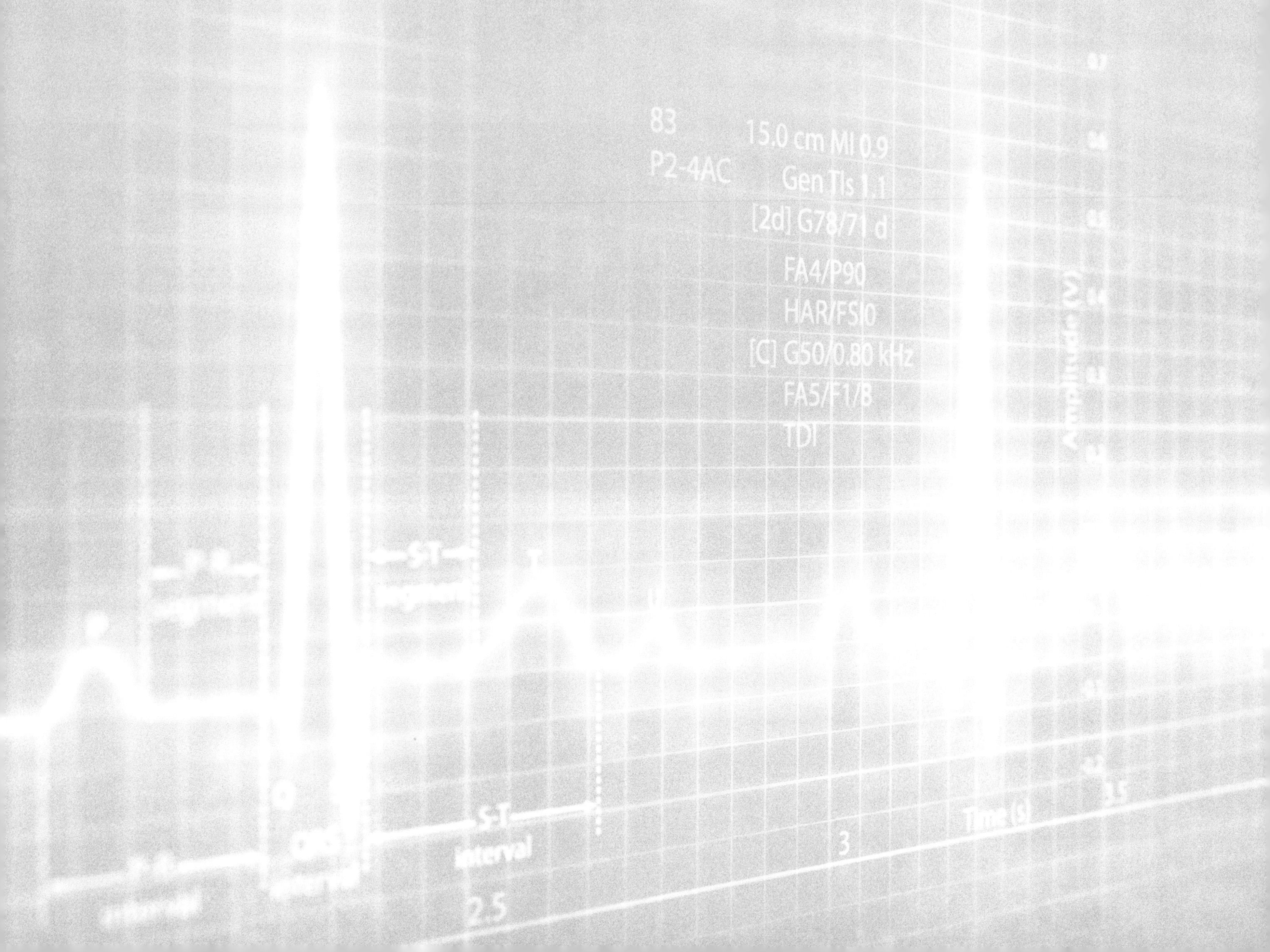
83
P2-4AC
15.0 cm MI 0.9
Gen TIs 1.1
[2d] G78/71 d
FA4/P90
HAR/FS0
[C] G50/0.80 kHz
FA5/F1/B
TDI
S-T
segment
S-T
interval
2.5
3
3.5
Time (s)
Amplitude (V)

ANSWERS

99-1. Interpret this ECG.

The rate is 84 beats/min (there are 14 QRS complexes in the 10-second rhythm strip: $14 \times 6 = 84$). An atrial pacemaker is present with atrial paced beats alternating with an ectopic atrial rhythm with P waves that are negative in the inferior leads and lead I, suggesting a nonsinus mechanism. The figure demonstrates atrial paced beats with asterisks and ectopic atrial beats with carats. There is baseline artifact in the limb leads and low limb-lead voltage. Nonspecific ST-segment and T-wave changes are present in the lateral leads.

99-2. What is the 3-letter pacemaker code governing the behavior seen on this ECG (assume there is only a single pacemaker lead)? What is the lower rate limit of the pacemaker?

A pacemaker lead is present in the atrium because there are spikes before some of the P waves. Pacemakers have a standardized letter code for describing the behavior of the pacemaker.[1] The first letter stands for which chamber is paced. There are three possibilities for the first letter: A for "atrial," V for "ventricular," and D for "dual" or both atrium and ventricle.

The second letter refers to in which chamber the pacemaker has sensing capabilities, and uses the same letters, A, V, or D.

The third letter represents the response to a sensed beat. This letter has three different options, I for "inhibit," T for "trigger," and D for "dual" or both inhibit and trigger. In other words, if the pacemaker is set to I, then it will not fire if there is an intrinsic sensed beat. Conversely, if T is set, the pacemaker will fire if a beat is sensed. If D is set, then it can do both.

In this patient, there are pacemaker spikes only before a P wave; therefore, the chamber paced is the atrium, and the first letter would be A. The chamber sensed is also the atrium, so the second letter would be A. Measuring from the native atrial beat to the next paced beat, as shown in the figure, the time from the native beat to the next paced beat is approximately 0.8 seconds, yielding a lower rate limit of 75 beats/min. One can conceptualize, therefore, that after an atrial paced beat, the pacemaker's clock starts. If no atrial activity is sensed after 0.8 seconds, the pacemaker will fire. If native atrial activity is sensed, the clock resets, and the pacemaker is inhibited.

This behavior can be seen in this tracing and is diagrammed in the figure: as the interval between paced and native atrial beats is less than 0.8 seconds, the pacemaker is appropriately inhibited. Thus, the 3-letter code for this pacemaker is AAI.

---

[1] Kaszala K, Huizar JF, Ellenbogen KA. Contemporary pacemakers: what the primary care physician needs to know. *Mayo Clin Proc* 2008; 83: 1170-1186.

ANSWERS (Cont.)

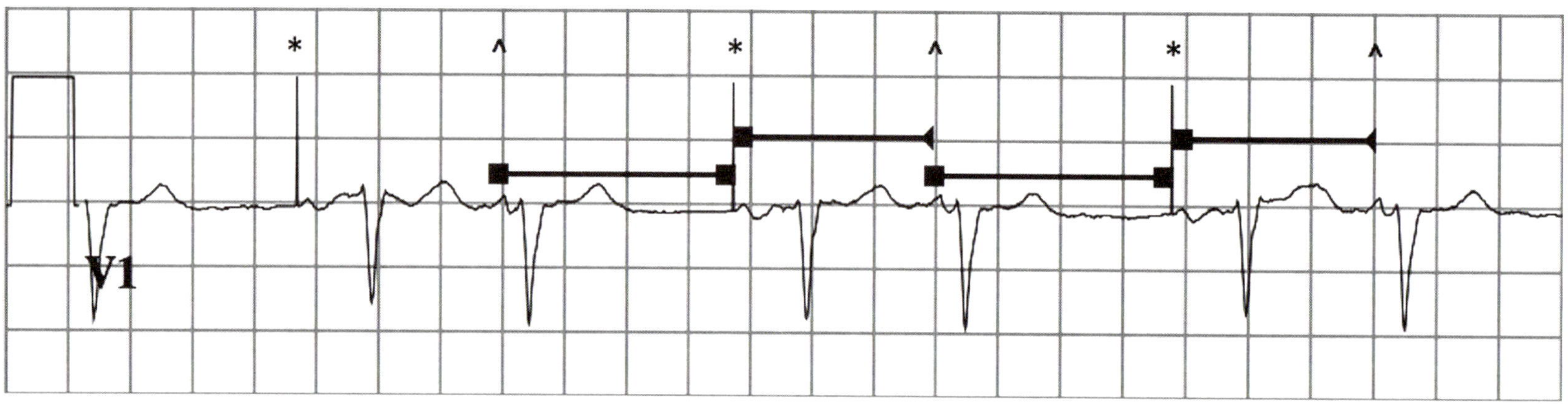

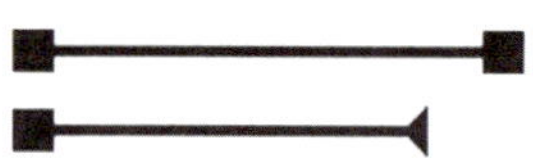

Atrial paced beats are noted with *, alternating with an ectopic atrial rhythm noted with ^. The interval prior to a paced beat, shown here with a line bracketed by boxes, corresponds to the lower rate limit of the pacemaker. The interval between a paced beat and the following native P wave, shown here with a line terminating in a triangle, is less than the interval predicted by the lower rate limit of the pacemaker. Put another way, after a paced beat, the pacemaker clock resets. If the clock runs out without a native impulse being sensed, the pacemaker will fire. If a native beat is sensed prior to the clock running out, the clock will reset.

Case #100. A 70-year-old woman with known right bundle branch block presenting with dyspnea and nausea.

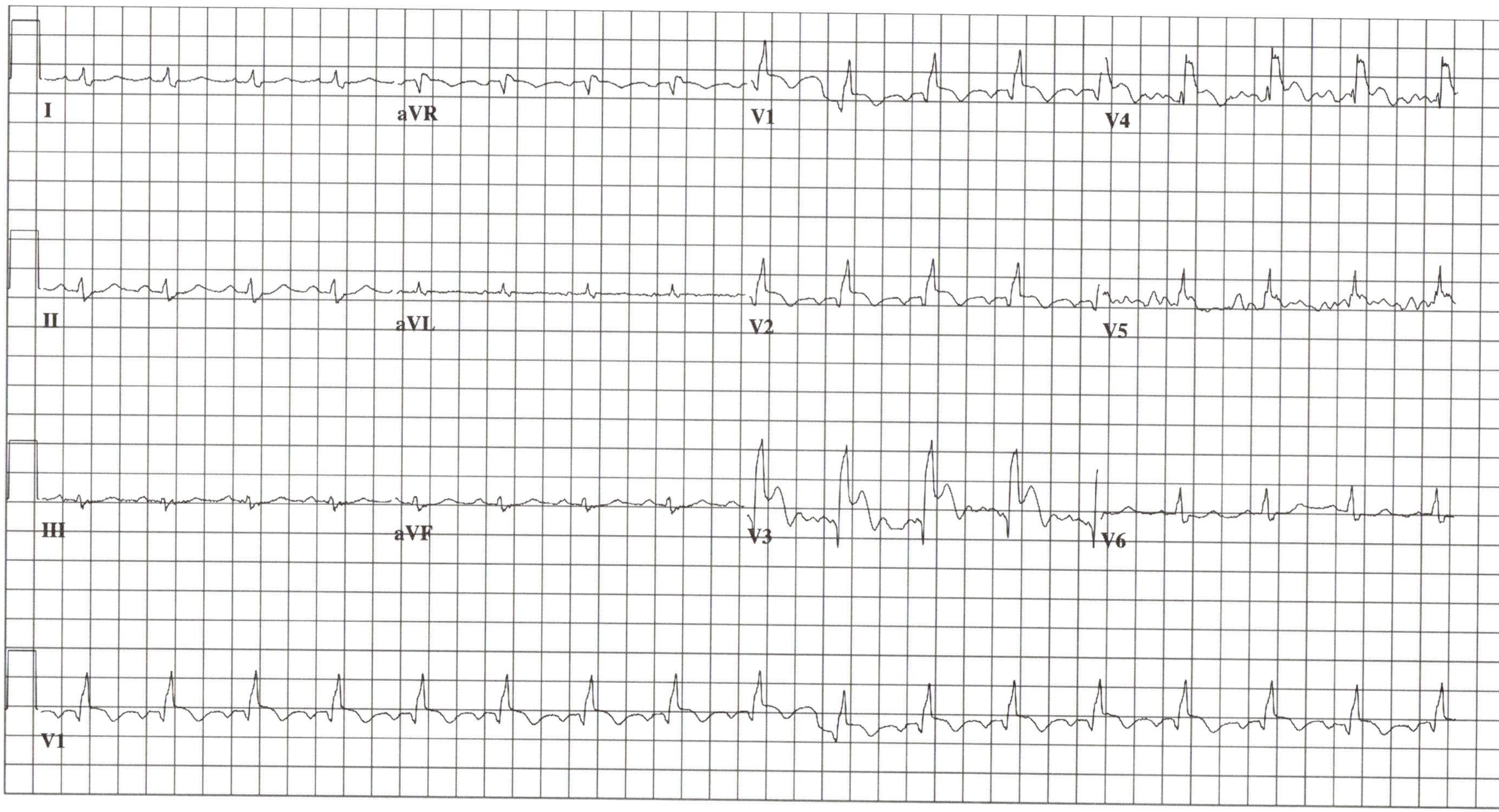

QUESTIONS

100-1. What abnormality is present?

100-2. In which anatomic distribution is this abnormality present?

100-3. What would you do next?

83
P2-4AC
15.0 cm MI 0.9
Gen TIs 1.1
[2d] G78/71 d
FA4/P90
HAR/FS0
[C] G50/0.80 kHz
FA5/F1/8
TDI
S-T
segment
T
U
Amplitude (V)

ANSWERS

100-1. What abnormality is present?

This tracing reveals sinus tachycardia at a rate of 100 beats/min. The axis is normal. Complete right bundle branch block is present, with a qR complex in V1 and broad terminal S wave in V6 and lead I. There are pathologic Q waves in the septal leads of V1 and V2 with ST-segment elevation in leads V1 through V4.

100-2. In which anatomic distribution is this abnormality present?

Recall that in the setting of a typical right bundle branch block, the initial 60 milliseconds of the QRS complex represent LV depolarization, with right ventricular depolarization delayed. This results in an RSR′ complex in V1 and V2 with repolarization abnormalities in these leads including usually T-wave inversion. This is expected when right bundle branch block is present. In this tracing, however, note the pathologic Q waves, ST elevation, and upright T waves in the anteroseptal leads. This is an example of anterior ST elevation myocardial infarction in the setting of preexisting RBBB.

100-3. What would you do next?

This patient requires urgent reperfusion therapy with thrombolytic medications or cardiac catheterization. At angiography, an LAD occlusion was found and successfully treated.

Section III

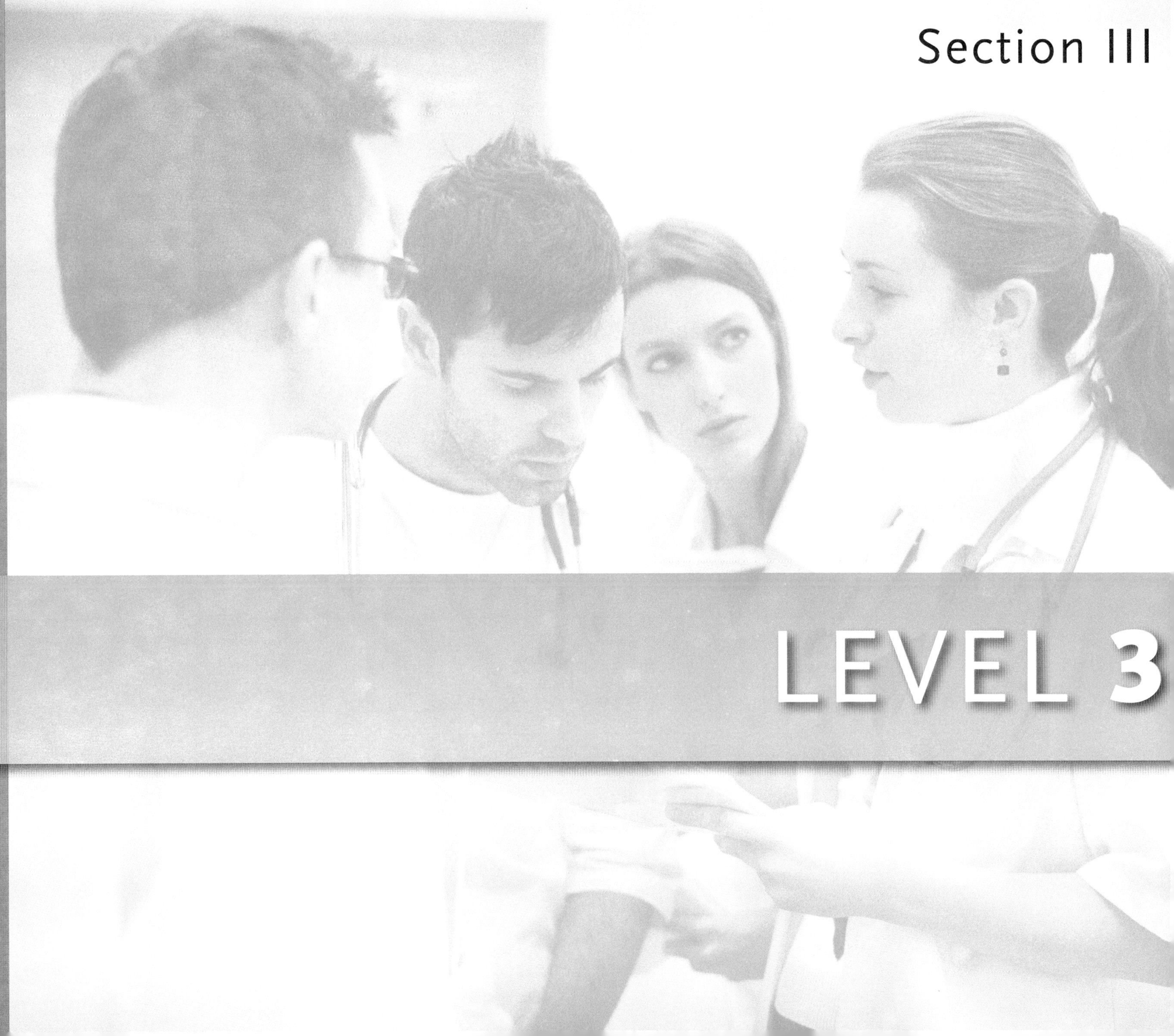

LEVEL 3

Case #101. A 68-year-old male presents with several days of fatigue and palpitations.

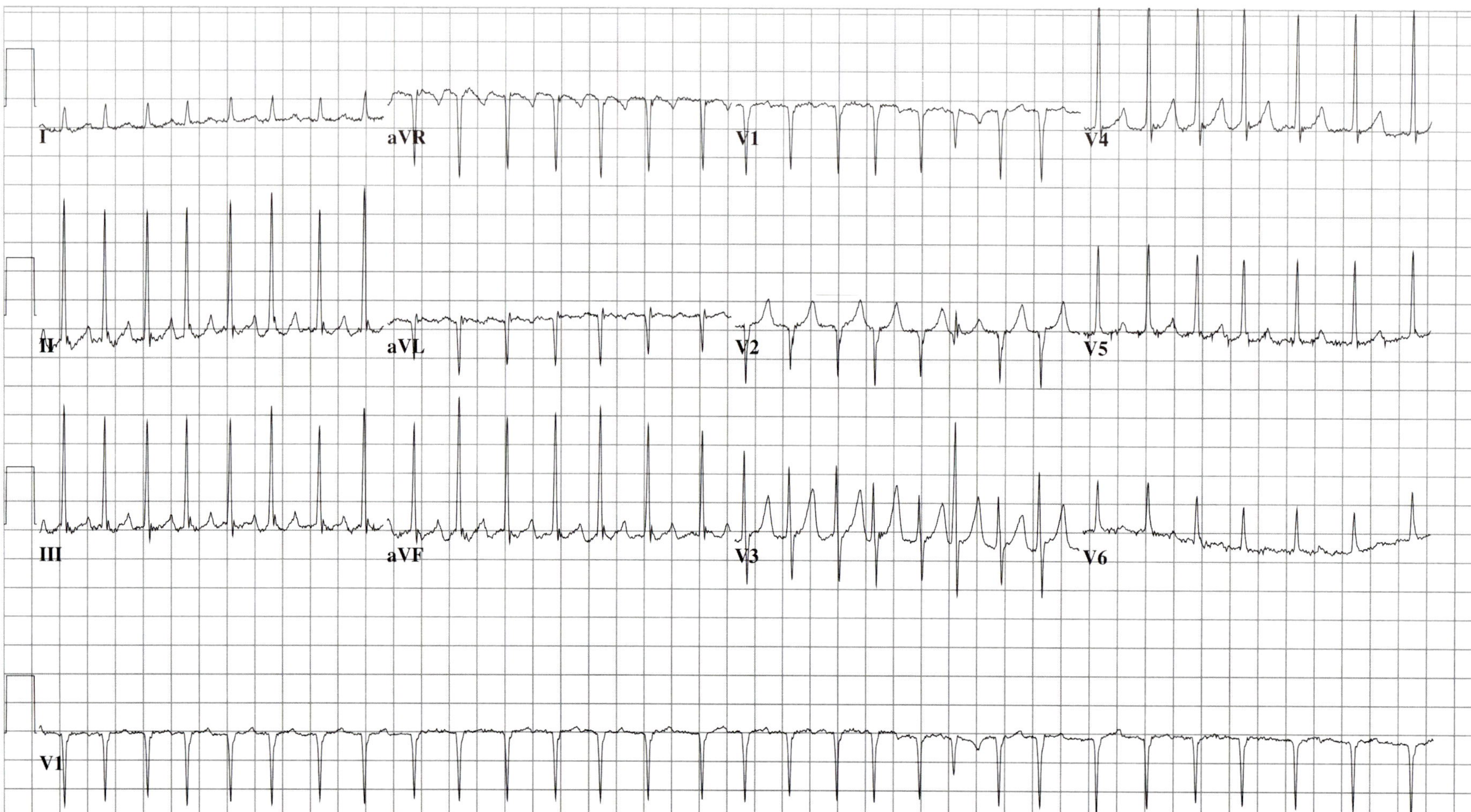

QUESTIONS

101-1. What abnormalities are present on this ECG?

101-2. What are the main clinical consequences of this arrhythmia?

83
P2-4AC
15.0 cm MI 0.9
Gen TIs 1.1
[2d] G78/71 d
FA4/P90
HAR/FSI0
[C] G50/0.80 kHz
FA5/F1/8
TDI
Amplitude (V)
S-T
Interval
2.5
3
3.5
Time (s)

ANSWERS

101-1. What abnormalities are present on this ECG?

This tracing demonstrates a tachycardia with narrow QRS complexes. In this case, the ventricular rate is quite rapid, with the mean rate approximately 180 beats/min. Close inspection reveals that the R–R interval is "irregularly irregular," meaning that the distance between QRS complexes, the R–R interval, is variable without pattern. The differential diagnosis for irregular narrow complex tachycardias includes atrial flutter with variable block, atrial fibrillation (AF), and multifocal atrial tachycardia (MAT). When MAT is present, one can visualize at least 3 distinct, identifiable P-wave morphologies. When AF is present, there is no clear atrial activity on the surface ECG, or there may be small, irregular atrial deflections at a rate of 400 to 600/min. When atrial flutter is present, clear flutter waves are seen with a "sawtooth" morphology. This tracing reveals an irregularly irregular rhythm with no clear atrial activity; therefore, AF is the diagnosis. The remainder of the tracing reveals normal axis, normal intervals, and Q waves in leads V1 and V2.

101-2. What are the main clinical consequences of this arrhythmia?

Atrial fibrillation itself can cause symptoms in some patients including breathlessness, palpitations, and chest pain. In other patients, the arrhythmia can be completely asymptomatic. Sustained rapid heart rates over long periods of time can lead to heart failure and tachycardia-induced cardiomyopathy. When atrial fibrillation is present, atrial contraction is absent, causing atrial stasis and risking left atrial thrombus formation and systemic embolization including stroke.

Case #102. This 46-year-old patient has night sweats, a cough, and an abnormal cardiac contour on chest radiograph.

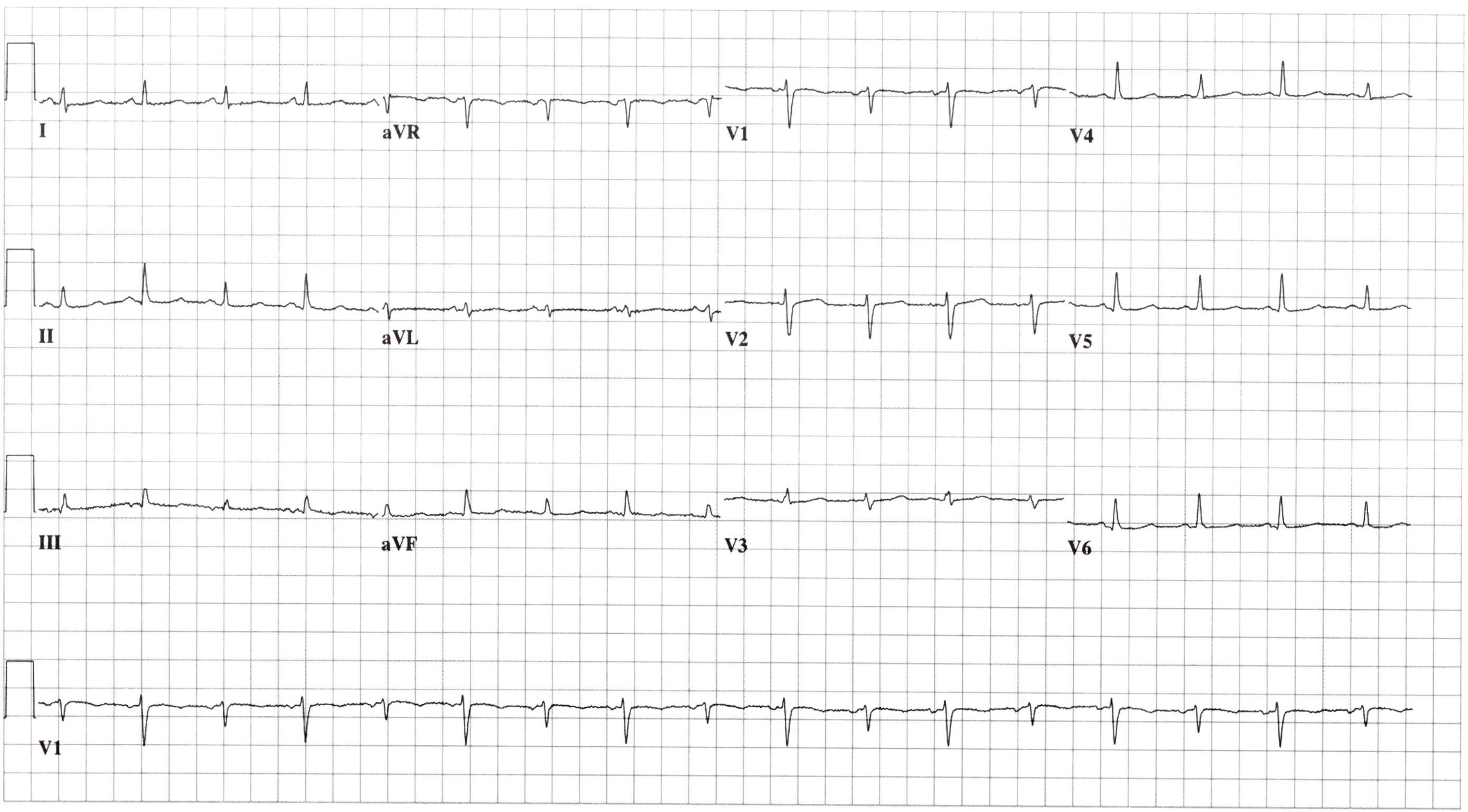

QUESTIONS

102-1. What abnormalities are present on this ECG?

102-2. What further investigation is indicated?

83
P2-4AC
15.0 cm MI 0.9
Gen TIs 1.1
[2d] G78/71 d
FA4/P90
HAR/FS0
[C] G50/0.80 kHz
FA5/F1/8
TDI
Amplitude (V)
S-T
interval
2.5
3
Time (s)

ANSWERS

102-1. What abnormalities are present on this ECG?

This tracing demonstrates sinus tachycardia at 100 beats/min. The axis is physiologic and intervals are normal. The tracing meets criteria for low precordial lead voltage (QRS amplitude <10 mV) and barely misses criteria for low limb lead voltage (QRS amplitude <5 mV). There is beat-to-beat alteration of QRS amplitude, most notable in the rhythm strip and inferior leads. This is called electrical alternans and can be due to abnormalities of conduction or due to the heart swinging to and fro within a large pericardial effusion. Given this patient's history, the likely explanation is the latter. Of note, electrical alternans due to pericardial effusion can occur with every other beat or over several sequential beats depending on the size of the effusion, cardiac size and mass, and heart rate, all of which interact to create a unique period of motion.

102-2. What further investigation is indicated?

An echocardiogram would be indicated to establish the diagnosis of pericardial effusion. Pericardial effusion in general may be due to trauma, aortic dissection, autoimmune disorders, infections including viral, mycobacterial, and bacterial causes, malignancy, medications, radiation therapy, postinfarction or postsurgical, and endocrine or metabolic disorders such as hypothyroidism or uremia. In this patient with night sweats and a cough, tuberculous effusion should be considered. Pericardiocentesis of a tuberculous effusion yields a lymphocytic fluid. Pericardial or pleural biopsy may be required to make the diagnosis.

Case #103. A 74-year-old woman presents with dizziness.

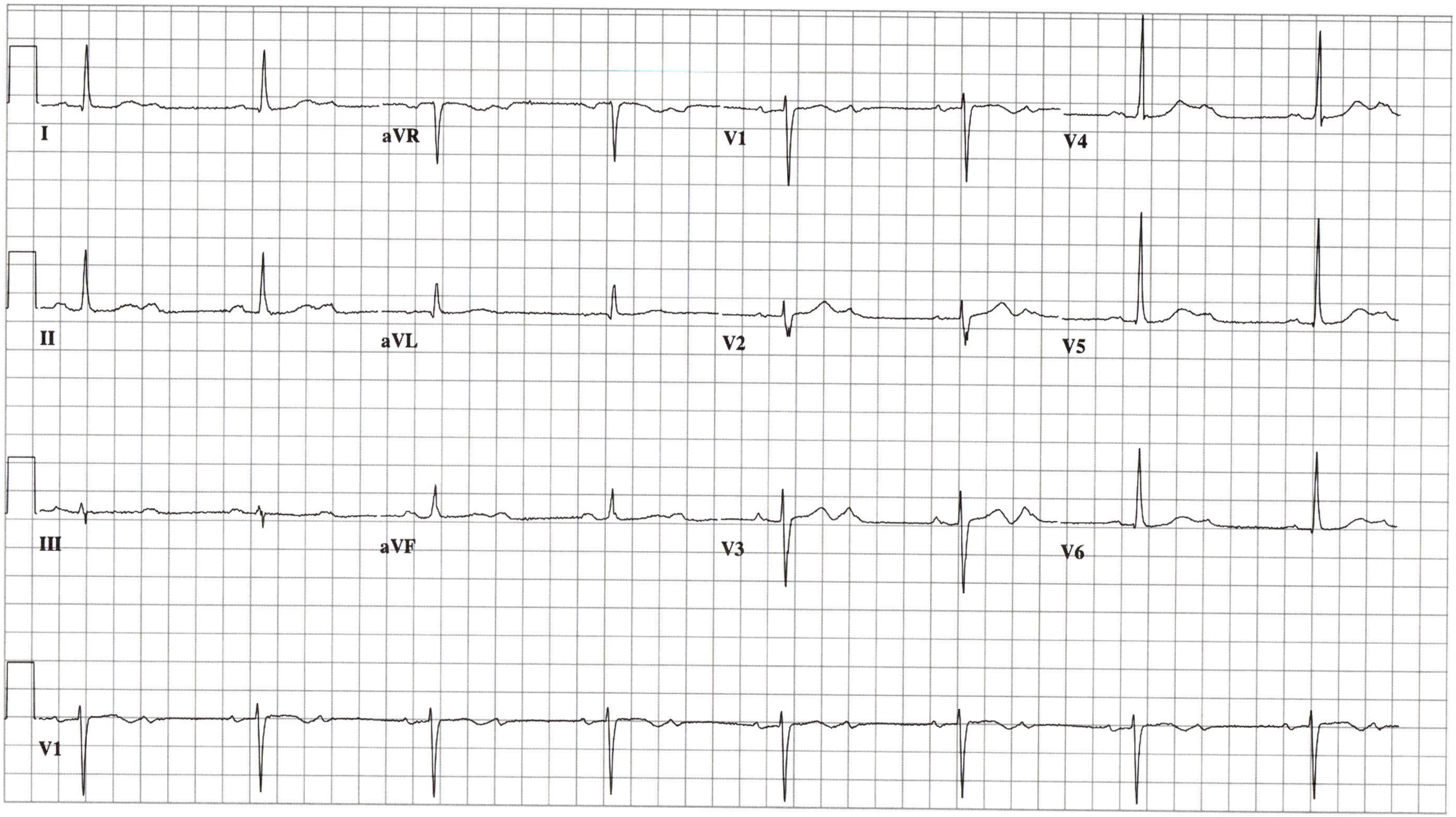

QUESTION

103-1. Interpret this ECG. What abnormalities are present? What accounts for the patient's dizziness?

83
P2-4AC
15.0 cm MI 0.9
Gen TIs 1.1
[2d] G78/71 d
FA4/P90
HAR/FSI0
[C] G50/0.80 kHz
FA5/F1/8
TDI
S-T
interval
2.5
3
Time (s)
3.5
Amplitude (V)

ANSWER

103-1. Interpret this ECG. What abnormalities are present? What accounts for the patient's dizziness?

This tracing demonstrates a regular, narrow complex bradycardia at 46 beats/min. There is a P wave preceding each QRS complex with a PR interval of approximately 200 milliseconds. Following each QRS complex, there is a P wave that is not conducted. The rhythm, therefore, is 2:1 AV block. It is not possible to say definitively whether this block represents Mobitz I or Mobitz II AV block because we would need a second QRS complex and a third P wave to assess if there was PR interval lengthening prior to the nonconducted P wave. The remainder of the tracing has a normal QRS axis and intervals, no atrial or ventricular chamber abnormality/enlargement, and no significant ST-T wave changes. Dizziness is most likely secondary to ventricular bradycardia.

Case #104. A 56-year-old patient with end-stage renal disease is found obtunded after missing several dialysis treatments.

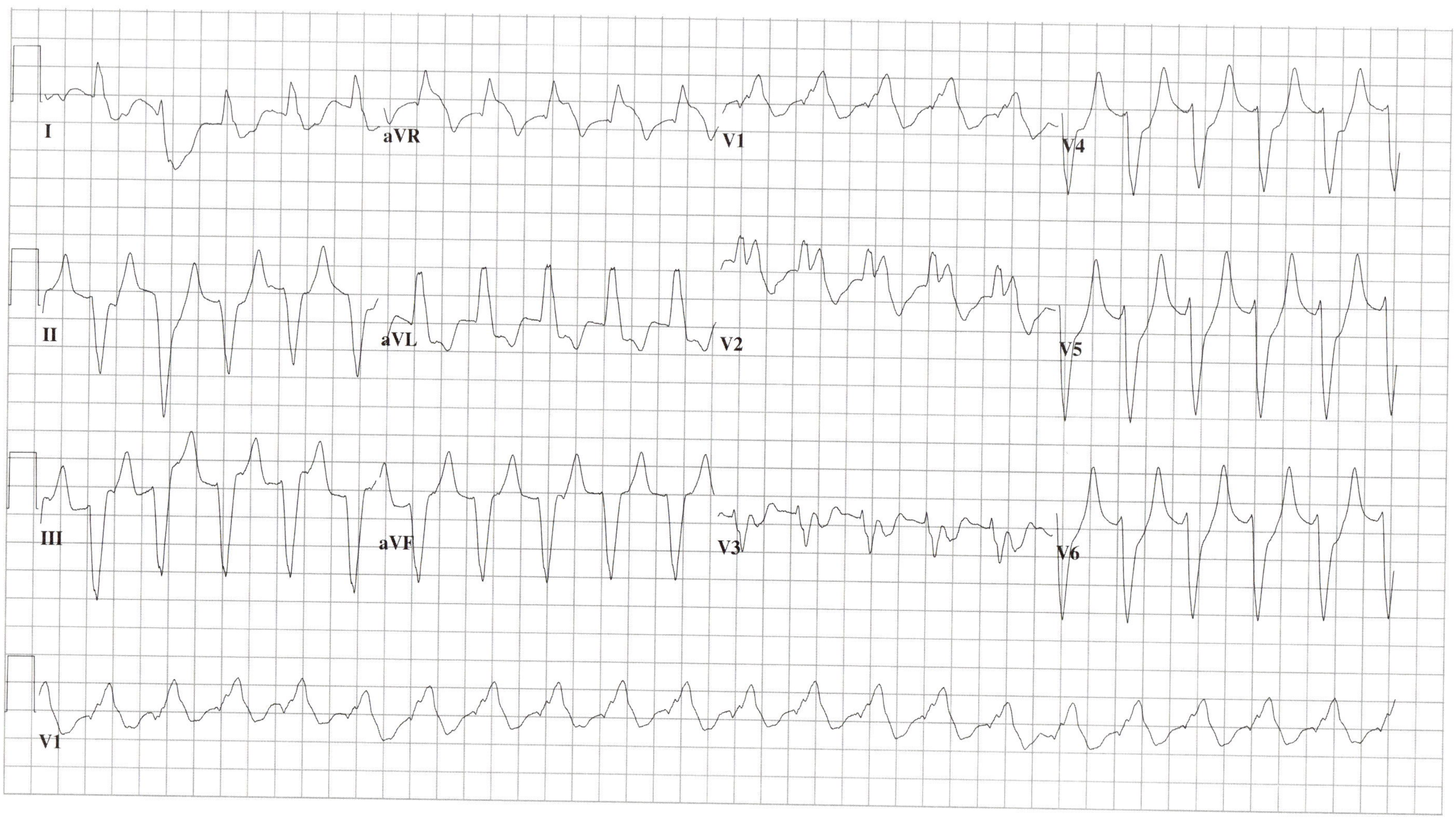

QUESTIONS

104-1. Describe this tracing.

104-2. What is the approach to management of the responsible electrolyte dyscrasia?

83
15.0 cm MI 0.9
P2-4AC
Gen Tls 1.1
[2d] G78/71 d
FA4/P90
HAR/FSI0
[C] G50/0.80 kHz
FA5/F1/B
TDI
3
2.5
Time (s)

ANSWERS

104-1. Describe this tracing.

This ECG shows a regular, monomorphic wide-complex rhythm at a rate of approximately 125 beats/min. There is marked left-axis deviation, even allowing for the baseline artifact present in lead I. Poor R-wave progression, QRS widening, corrected QT-interval prolongation and tall, peaked, pointed T waves are noted. These findings of peaked T waves and QRS widening are consistent with severe hyperkalemia. The electrocardiographic manifestations of hyperkalemia progress in an orderly fashion, starting with tall, peaked T waves, followed by PR-interval prolongation and loss of P-wave amplitude, QRS widening, and finally a sine wave like appearance to the ECG. The level of serum potassium at which ECG changes occur is variable and depends on both chronicity of hyperkalemia and rate of change of potassium.

104-2. What is the approach to management of the responsible electrolyte dyscrasia?

The first priority in therapy of hyperkalemia causing ECG changes is administration of intravenous calcium to stabilize the cardiac membrane potential. This intervention will often cause abrupt narrowing of the QRS complex. Emphasis is then placed on lowering serum levels of potassium. This may be accomplished by driving extracellular potassium into cells or removing potassium from the body. Therapies used to drive potassium into cells include manipulation of insulin receptors (via administration of dextrose and insulin), β-adrenergic receptors (via administration of a β-adrenergic agonist, such as albuterol), and systemic acid–base status (via administration of sodium bicarbonate). Options for removing potassium from the body include enhancement of gut wasting (via administration of the binding resin sodium polystyrene) or renal wasting (via administration of fluids or loop diuretic). Where other measures fail to lower serum potassium with sufficient haste, renal replacement therapy may be instituted with hemodialysis or continuous venovenous hemofiltration.

Case #105. A 75-year-old woman presents with breathlessness, nausea, and left arm pain. Her history is notable for left bundle branch block and dyslipidemia.

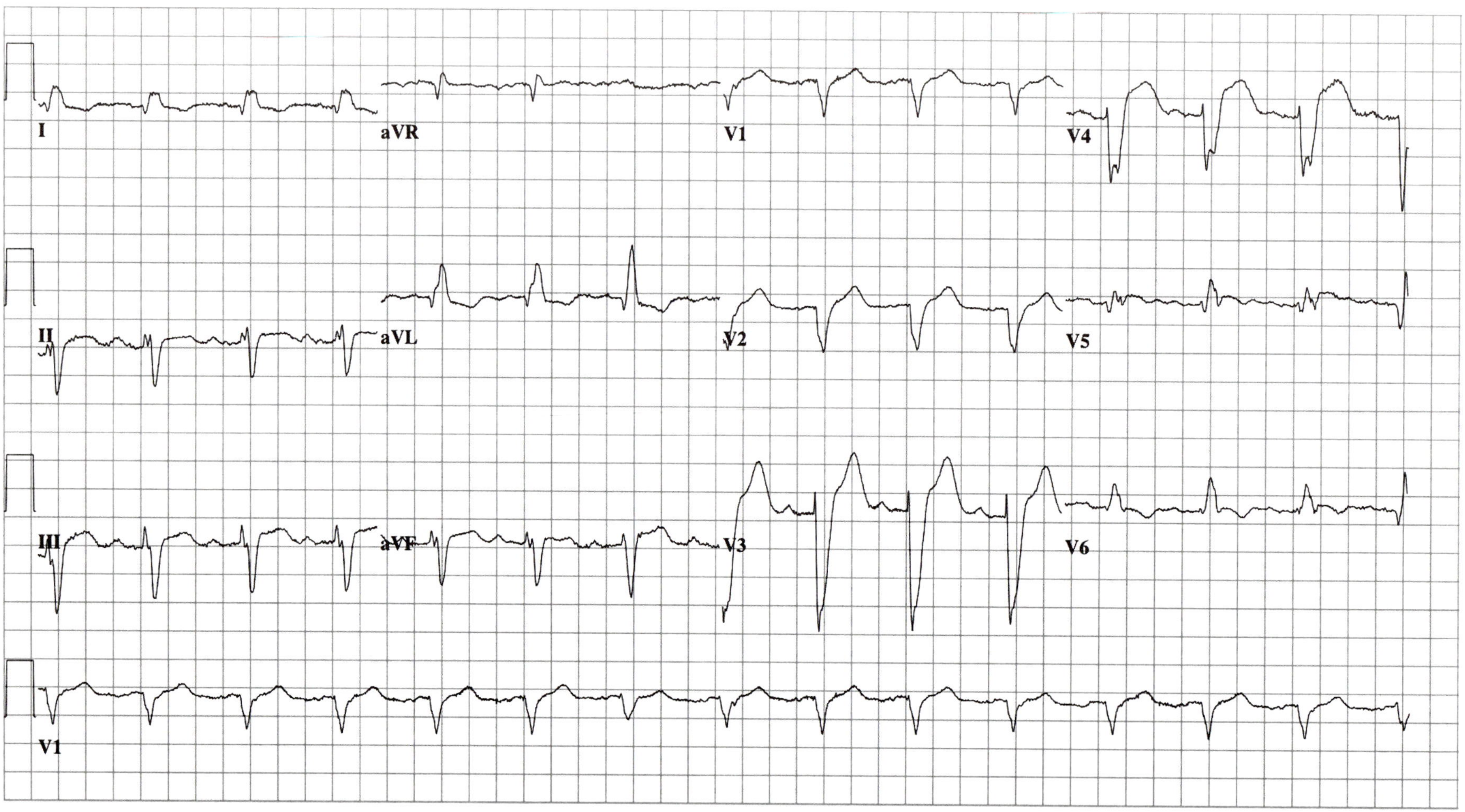

QUESTION

105-1. Interpret this ECG: what findings concern you?

83
P2-4AC
15.0 cm MI 0.9
Gen TIs 1.1
[2d] G78/71 d
FA4/P90
HAR/FS10
[C] G50/0.80 kHz
FA5/F1/B
TDI

ANSWER

105-1. Interpret this ECG: what findings concern you?

Sinus rhythm is present at a rate of 85 beats/min. The axis is leftward. The PR interval is prolonged, consistent with first-degree AV block. The QRS interval is prolonged to greater than 120 milliseconds with a broad notched R wave in I and V6 and rS complexes in the anteroseptal leads consistent with left bundle branch block. The P wave is broader than 120 milliseconds in lead II consistent with left atrial abnormality. Now, assess for ischemia: recall that the presence of left bundle branch block decreases the sensitivity for myocardial infarction, but the diagnosis of MI can still be made. With an uncomplicated left bundle branch block, the ST segment and T wave should be oriented opposite the major deflection of the QRS, that is, if the QRS complex is predominantly positive, the ST segment and T wave should be inverted. Assessing this tracing, the ST segments and T waves are oriented as expected in the inferior leads. Leads I and aVL demonstrate small Q waves. Examination of leads V5 and V6 reveals 1 mm of ST-segment elevation concordant with the major deflection of the QRS complex. These findings are concerning for myocardial injury and infarction.

Sgarbossa et al have enumerated a scoring system for diagnosis of myocardial ischemia in the presence of left bundle branch block:[1]

- The presence of ST-segment elevation ≥1 mm concordant with a predominantly positive QRS complex in at least 1 lead is assigned 5 points.
- The presence of ST-segment depression ≥1 mm in leads V1, V2, or V3 is assigned 3 points.
- The presence of ST-segment elevation ≥5 mm discordant in the opposite direction from a predominantly negative QRS complex is assigned 1 point.
- A score of 3 points or higher has 90% specificity for acute myocardial infarction; however, the sensitivity is only 20%.

[1]Sgarbossa EB, Pinski SL, Barbagelata A, et al. Electrocardiographic diagnosis of evolving acute myocardial infarction in the presence of left bundle-branch block. *New Engl J Med* 1996; 334: 481-487.

Case #106. An 87-year-old woman presents with multiple episodes of near-syncope while doing housework.

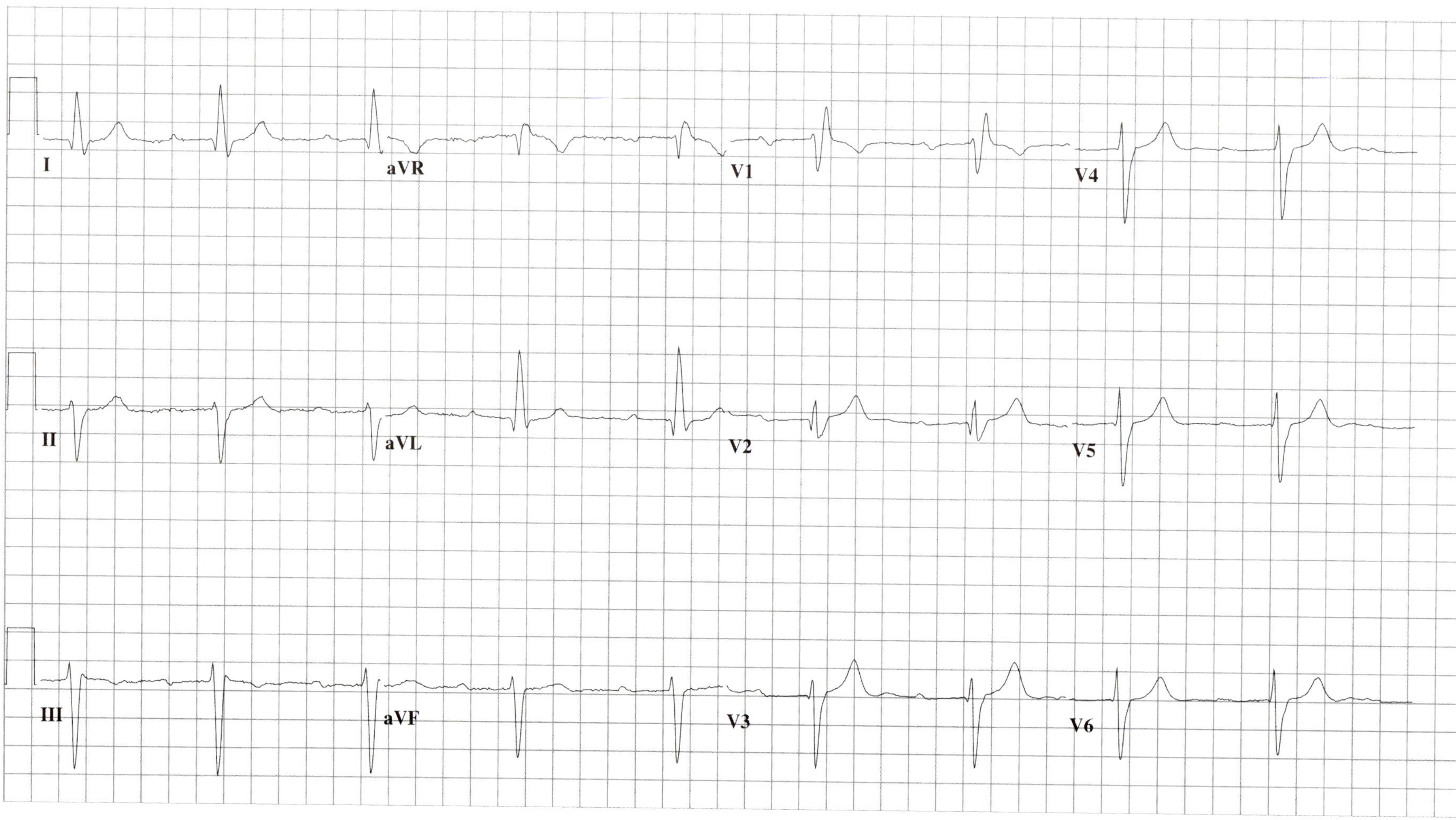

QUESTIONS

106-1. Interpret the ECG: what rhythm is present?

106-2. Which parts of the conduction system are not functioning properly?

106-3. Does this patient need a pacemaker?

83
P2-4AC
15.0 cm MI 0.9
Gen TIs 1.1
[2d] G78/71 d
FA4/P90
HAR/FS|0
[C] G50/0.80 kHz
FA5/F1/8
TDI

ANSWERS

106-1. Interpret the ECG: what rhythm is present?

This ECG demonstrates sinus bradycardia at 54 beats/min. The PR interval is prolonged to 360 milliseconds consistent with AV conduction delay/first-degree AV block. There is left-axis deviation with a frontal plane QRS axis of approximately –60 degrees. The QRS complexes have a small r wave and large S wave in leads II, III, and aVF, and a small q wave and large R wave in leads I and aVL. This morphology coupled with the leftward axis is consistent with left anterior fascicular block. The QRS duration is prolonged at 160 milliseconds. The rSR′ complex in lead V1 and the broad terminal S wave in leads I and V6 is diagnostic of right bundle branch block. There is no evidence of ischemia or prior infarction (the Q waves in leads I, aVL, and V2 are secondary to the left anterior fascicular block), and the QT interval is normal.

106-2. Which parts of the conduction system are not functioning properly?

This patient has evidence of AV conduction delay/first-degree AV block, left anterior fascicular block, and right bundle branch block. The combination of left anterior fascicular block and right bundle branch block is called "bifascicular block." When bifascicular block and AV conduction delay/first-degree AV block are present, the term "trifascicular block" is sometimes used, although this is an imprecise term because the AV conduction delay/first-degree AV block could represent delay at the AV node or below the AV node in the remaining His–Purkinje system. It is not possible to make this determination on a 12-lead ECG.

106-3. Does this patient need a pacemaker?

The presence of symptoms consistent with bradycardia coupled with the significant conduction system disease noted above is a likely indication for pacemaker placement. If the patient's symptoms were not clearly linked to bradycardia and her conduction system disease, an invasive EP study could provide further information.

Case #107. A 37-year-old man with syncope.

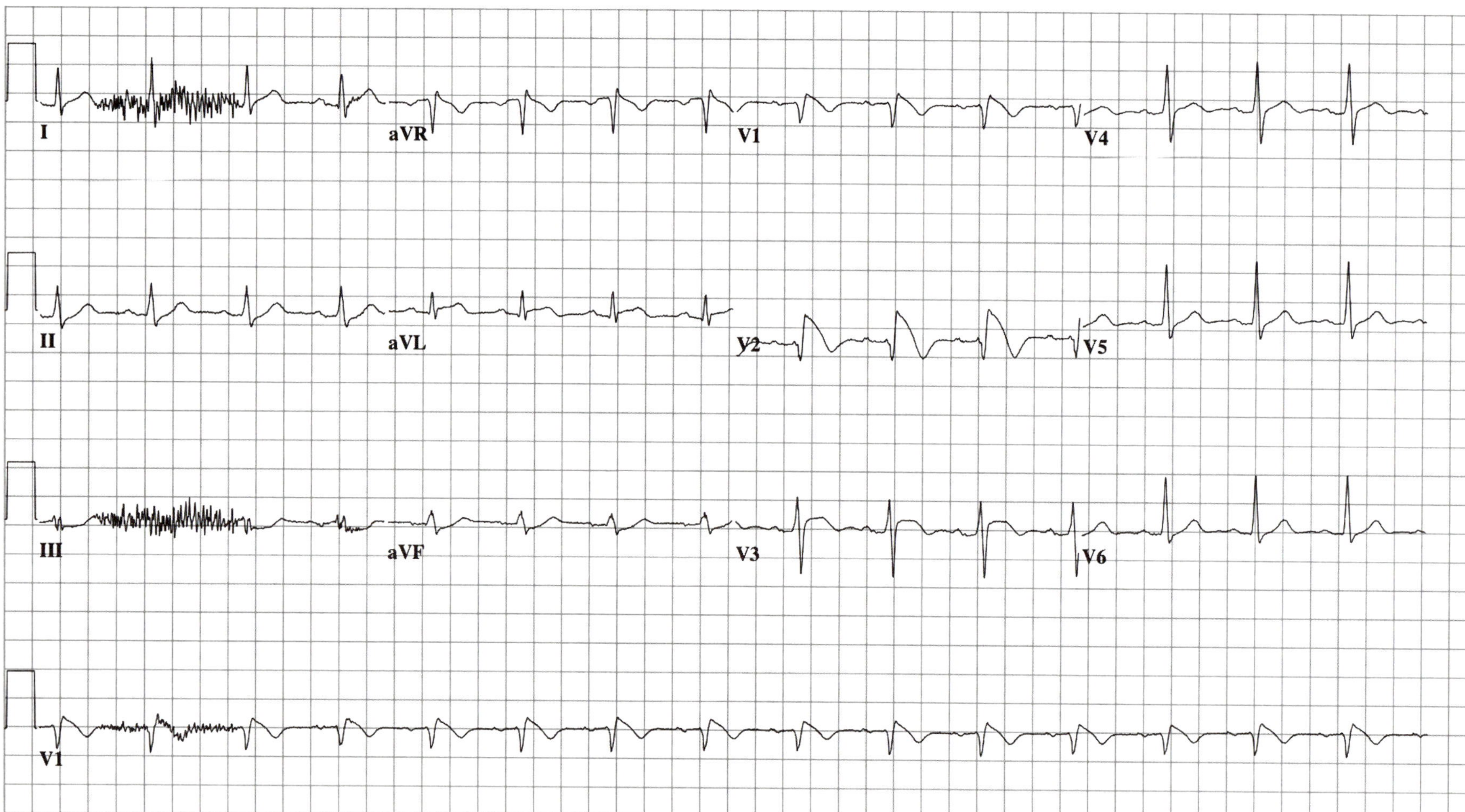

QUESTIONS

107-1. What abnormalities are present on this ECG?

107-2. What is the diagnosis?

83
P2-4AC
15.0 cm MI 0.9
Gen TIs 1.1
[2d] G78/71 d
FA4/P90
HAR/FSI0
[C] G50/0.80 kHz
FA5/F1/B
TDI
3
2.5

ANSWERS

107-1. What abnormalities are present on this ECG?

The rhythm is sinus at approximately 90 beats/min. The axis and intervals are normal, and there is no evidence of chamber enlargement or hypertrophy. Baseline artifact is present in leads I, III, and the initial part of the rhythm strip. ST elevation is present in leads VI and V2 with a downsloping, coved ST segment leading into an inverted T wave.

107-2. What is the diagnosis?

The ST elevation could represent ischemia in the proper clinical context; however, the characteristic morphology demonstrated here is consistent with the Brugada pattern. This specific pattern is a "Brugada type I" pattern, diagnosed if there is greater than 2 mm ST elevation with coved morphology and inverted T waves in greater than 2 precordial leads. If a type I Brugada ECG is seen with one or more of the following criteria, Brugada syndrome is diagnosed: personal history of VT or VF, family history of sudden cardiac death or Brugada ECG, inducible VT, syncope, or nocturnal agonal respirations.[1]

[1]Antzelevich C, Brugada P, Borggrefe M, et al. Brugada syndrome: report of the second consensus conference. *Circulation* 2005; 111: 659-670.

Case #108. A 66-year-old man presents with a complaint of "heart pounding." Two tracings from presentation with the patient's baseline tracing are shown.

Presentation 1:

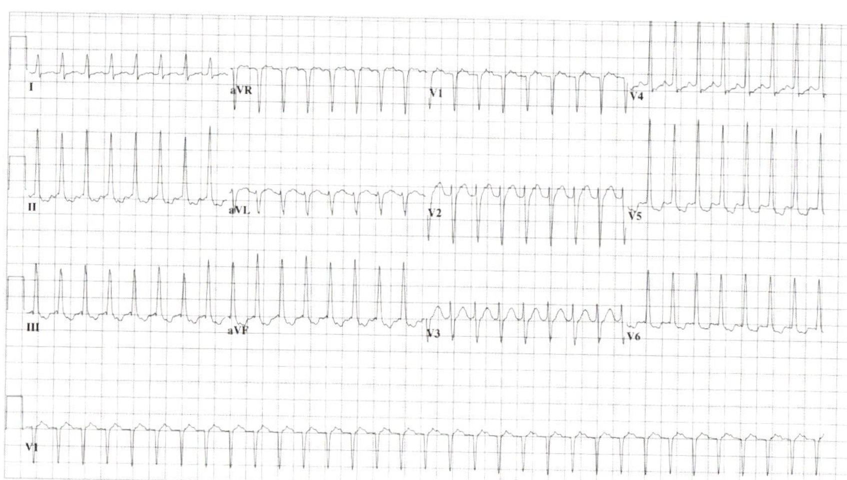

Presentation 2:

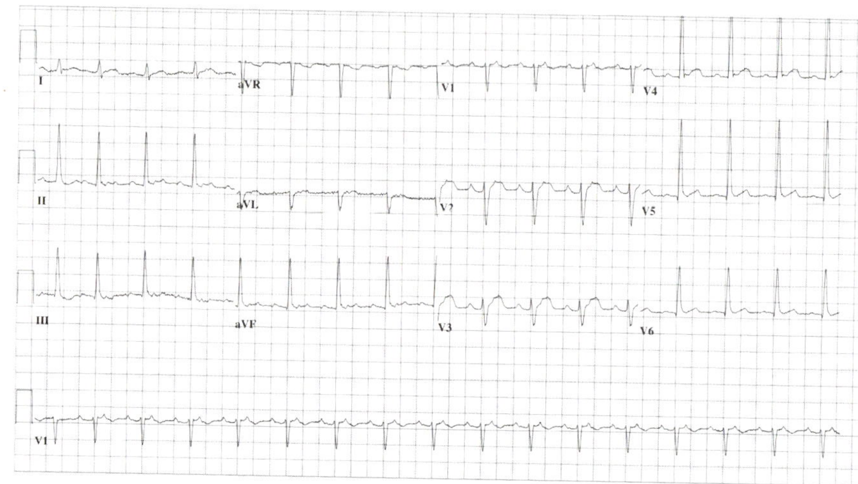

Baseline:

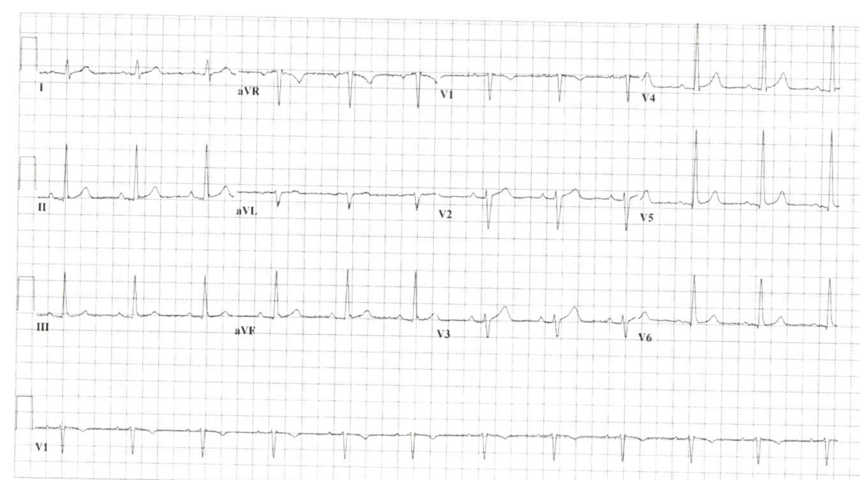

QUESTIONS

108-1. Interpret these ECGs.

108-2. What is the most likely diagnosis for this patient's tachycardia?

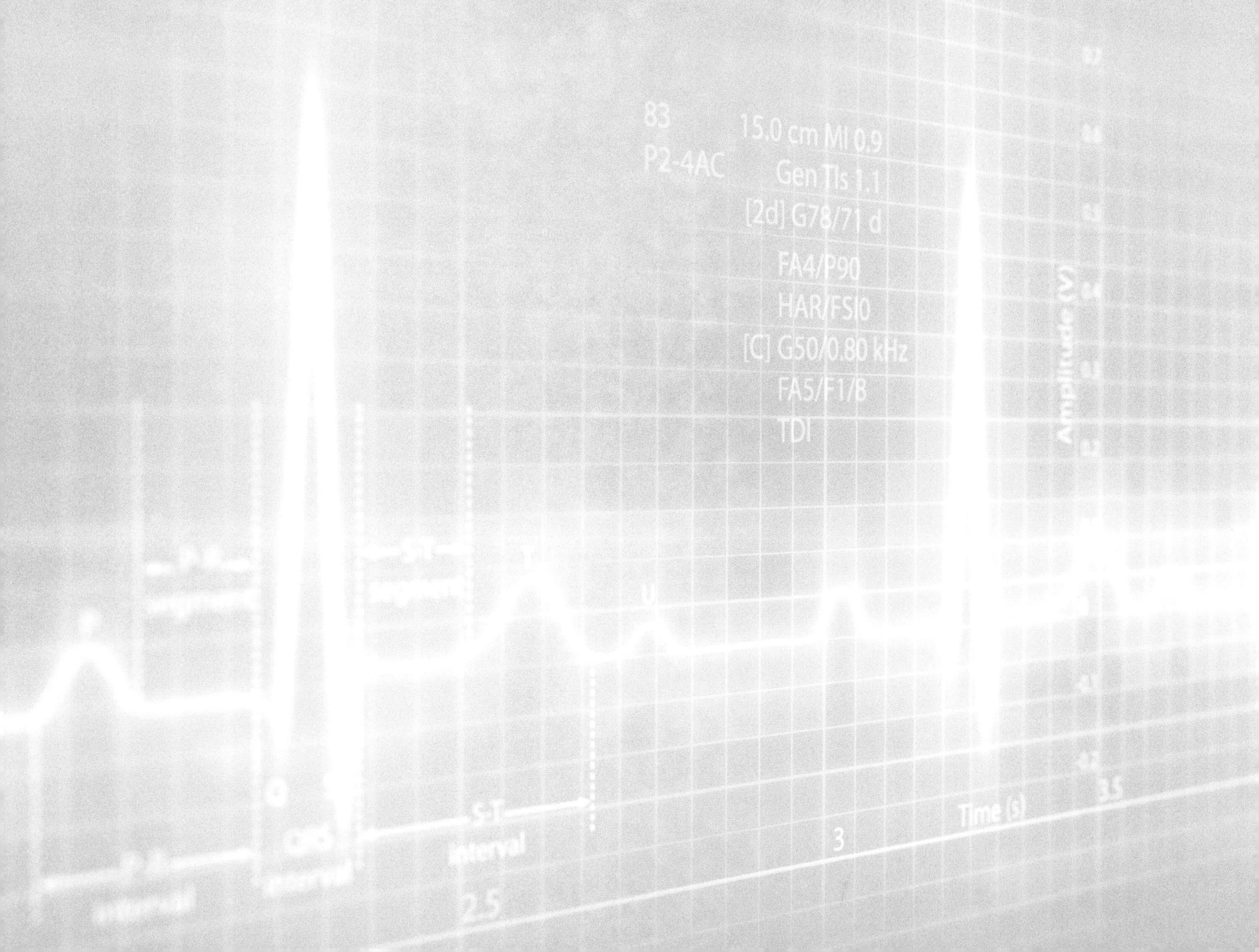
83
P2-4AC
15.0 cm MI 0.9
Gen TIs 1.1
[2d] G78/71 d
FA4/P90
HAR/FSI0
[C] G50/0.80 kHz
FA5/F1/8
TDI
Amplitude (V)
S-T
interval
Time (s)
2.5
3
3.5

ANSWERS

108-1. Interpret these ECGs.

The first tracing demonstrates a rapid, narrow complex tachycardia at a rate of approximately 200 beats/min. The R–R interval is regular. The differential would include sinus tachycardia, atrial flutter, orthodromic AVNRT, AVRT, and atrial tachycardia. There is evidence of atrial activity in lead V1 just following each QRS complex; however, it is impossible to determine from this tracing whether conduction is antegrade or retrograde. Thus, the rhythm is best categorized as a "supraventricular tachycardia." Valsalva maneuvers or adenosine could create transient A-V block and clarify the diagnosis: if flutter waves or atrial activity is unmasked, then atrial tachycardia or atrial flutter could be diagnosed. If the rhythm terminates, AVNRT or AVRT could be diagnosed. The QRS axis is normal. There are downsloping ST-segment depressions in V5 and V6 that likely reflect subendocardial ischemia at this rapid heart rate.

The second tracing reveals that the ventricular rate has slowed by half to 100 beats/min. Every other atrial impulse now conducts to the ventricle, and it is clear that there are regular atrial impulses at a rate of approximately 200 beats/min. The atrial activity is upright in the anteroseptal leads and isoelectric in leads I and aVL.

The final tracing is the baseline tracing and is normal overall. The most notable finding is that the sinus P waves appear quite distinct from the P waves seen in the first 3 tracings.

108-2. What is the most likely diagnosis for this patient's tachycardia?

This tachycardia most likely represents an atrial tachycardia, initially with 1-to-1 conduction, then with 2-to-1 block. Both the atrial rate and the abnormal morphology of the P waves are typical for this dysrhythmia.

Case #109. A 35-year-old woman with prior history of malignancy treated with adriamycin presents for follow-up.

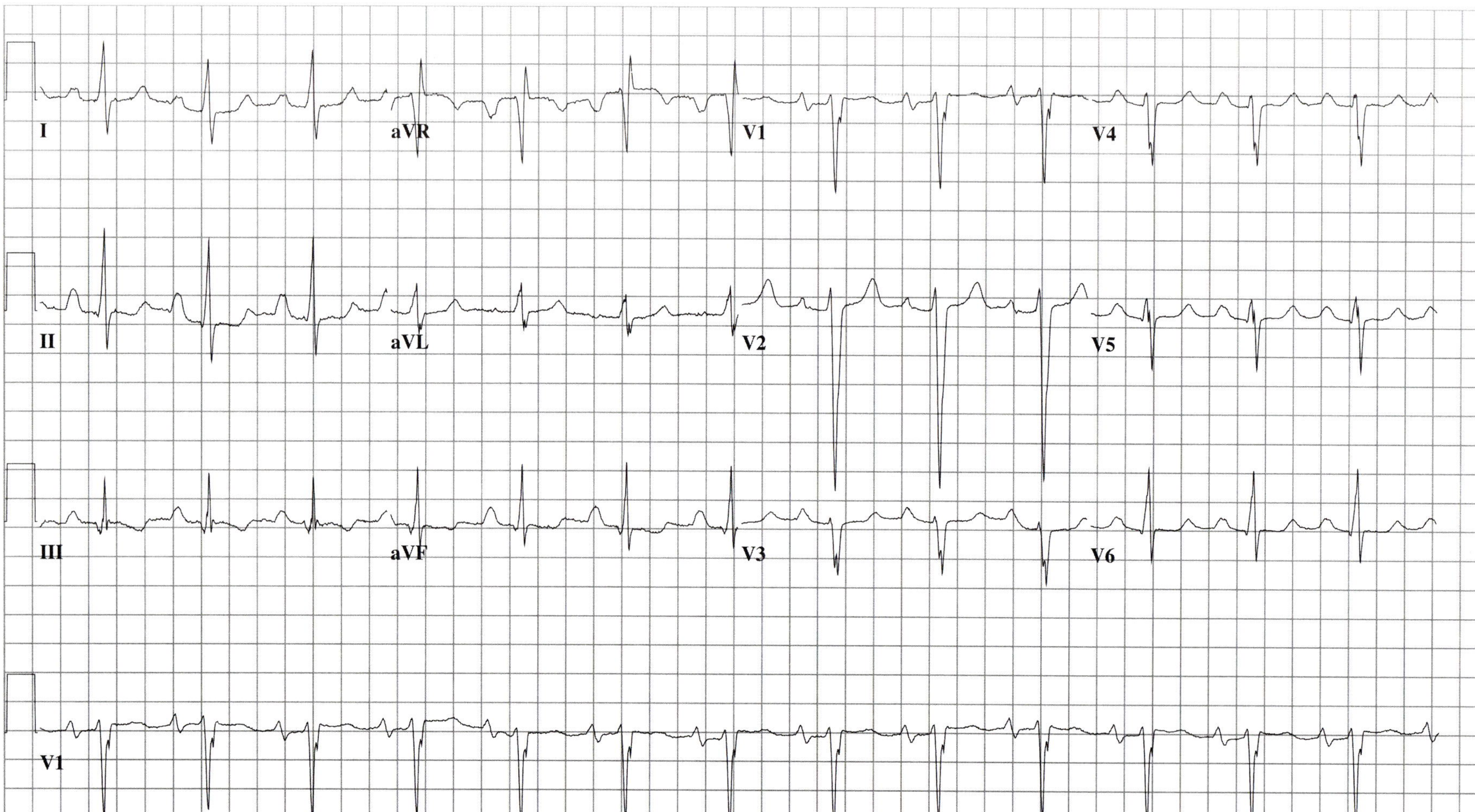

QUESTIONS

109-1. What are the abnormalities?

109-2. What is the differential diagnosis for biatrial abnormality?

83
P2-4AC
15.0 cm MI 0.9
Gen TIs 1.1
[2d] G78/71 d
FA4/P90
HAR/FSI0
[C] G50/0.80 kHz
FA5/F1/8
TDI
Amplitude (V)
S-T
interval
QRS
interval
Time (s)
2.5
3
3.5

ANSWERS

109-1. What are the abnormalities?

This tracing demonstrates normal sinus rhythm at a rate of 80 beats/min. There is a normal axis. The QRS duration is normal, and there is first-degree AV block with prolongation of the PR interval to greater than 200 milliseconds. There is evidence of left atrial abnormality: the P-wave breadth in lead II is greater than 120 milliseconds and there is a biphasic P wave in lead V1 with the negative terminal deflection wider than 40 milliseconds and deeper than 1 mV. There is also evidence of right atrial abnormality by 2 criteria: the P wave in lead II is taller than 2.5 mV, and the P wave in lead V1 is taller than 1.5 mV.

109-2. What is the differential diagnosis for biatrial abnormality?

Some of the classic etiologies of biatrial abnormality include valvular heart disease, intracardiac shunts, dilated cardiomyopathy, and restrictive cardiomyopathies.

Case #110. **A 70-year-old gentleman with ischemic cardiomyopathy treated with implantable cardioverter-defibrillator (ICD) placement presents with several ICD discharges. While a 12-lead ECG is being recorded, this event transpires.**

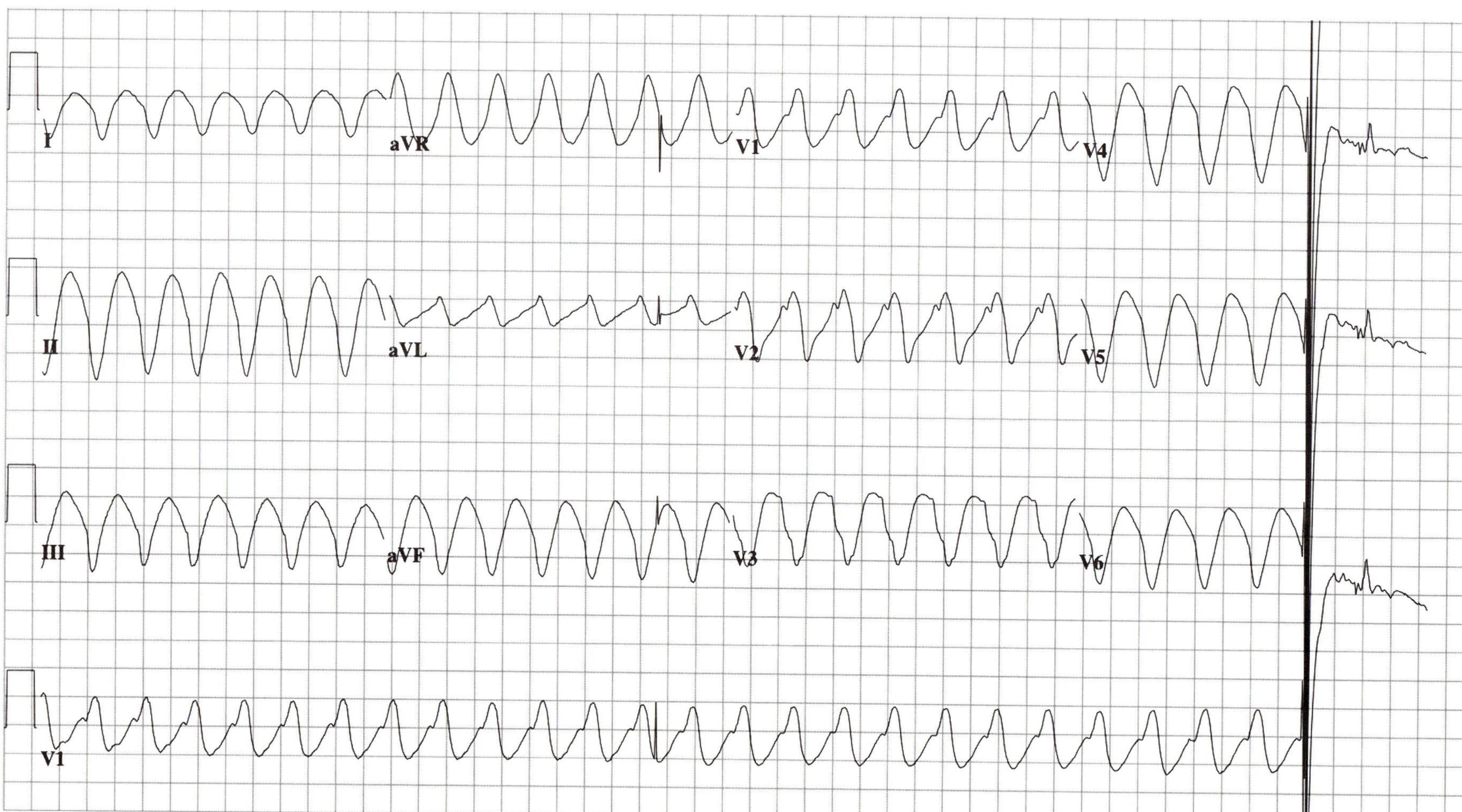

QUESTIONS

110-1. What does the ECG reveal?

110-2. How would you evaluate this patient?

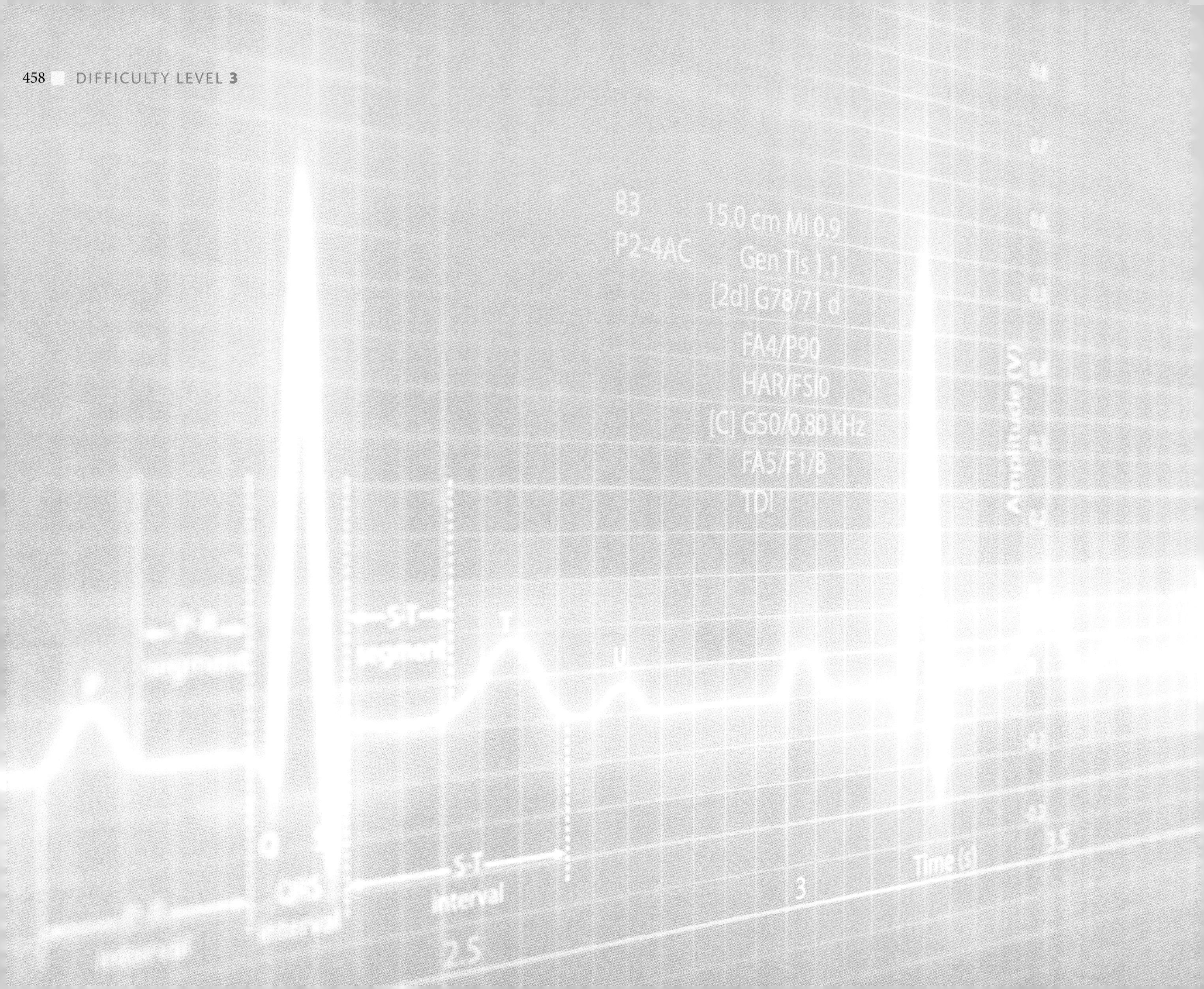
83
15.0 cm MI 0.9
P2-4AC
Gen TIs 1.1
[2d] G78/71 d
FA4/P90
HAR/FS0
[C] G50/0.80 kHz
FA5/F1/8
TDI
Amplitude (V)
S-T
segment
T
U
S-T
interval
2.5
3
Time (s)
3.5

ANSWERS

110-1. What does the ECG reveal?

The majority of the tracing consists of a monomorphic wide-complex tachycardia at a rate of upwards of 160 beats/min. The QRS axis is negative in the inferior leads and lead I and upward in lead aVR—so-called "extreme axis" oriented in the northwest frontal plane quadrant. The differential diagnosis includes ventricular tachycardia versus supraventricular tachycardia with aberrant conduction. This arrhythmia is most consistent with ventricular tachycardia given the extreme axis and history of ischemic cardiomyopathy. Applying the Brugada criteria[1] to distinguish ventricular tachycardia from supraventricular tachycardia:

1. Assess the precordial leads for presence of an R-S complex (see the figure for definitions). In this case, there is an R-S complex in lead V2. If no R-S complex were seen, ventricular tachycardia would be diagnosed.
2. In leads with an R-S complex, if the distance from the onset of the R wave to the nadir of the S wave is greater than 100 milliseconds, VT is diagnosed, as in this case. This criterion connotes slowed conduction of the initial ventricular depolarization, as occurs when depolarization is via ventricular muscle rather than the normal His–Purkinje system.

The remainder of the Brugada criteria assess for A-V dissociation and abnormal QRS morphology. Application of the remaining criteria is not needed in this case, given that ventricular tachycardia is diagnosed.

At the end of the tracing, an impulse is seen followed by resumption of a narrow QRS rhythm. This impulse is the discharge from the patient's ICD.

Diagram of R, RS, and QS complexes. The bracket under the RS complex demonstrates the distance of the onset of the R wave to the nadir of the S wave.

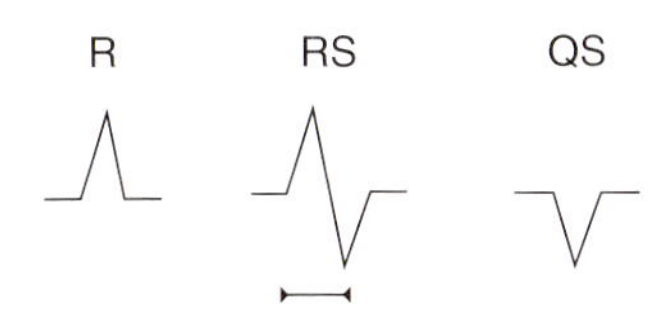

[1] Brugada P, Brugada J, Mont L, et al. A new approach to the differential diagnosis of a regular tachycardia with a wide QRS complex. *Circulation* 1991; 83: 1649-1659.

ANSWERS (Cont.)

110-2. How would you evaluate this patient?

ICD discharges can be appropriate discharges to treat malignant ventricular arrhythmia, as in this case, or inappropriate discharges secondary to the device interpreting a supraventricular tachycardia as ventricular tachycardia and delivering therapy that is not indicated.[2] Interrogation of the ICD can be invaluable in making this distinction.

For this patient's appropriate ICD discharge, any electrolyte abnormalities should be corrected and myocardial ischemia should be treated if present. If both of those reversible factors are assessed and adequately treated, antiarrhythmic therapy or an alteration in ICD programming may be useful in reducing the likelihood of future ICD shocks.

[2]Gehi AK, Mehta D, Gomes JA. Evaluation and management of patients after implantable cardioverter-defibrillator shock. *J Am Med Assoc* 2006; 296: 2839-2347.

Case #111. A 67-year-old man with a heavy tobacco use history admitted to the ICU with respiratory failure.

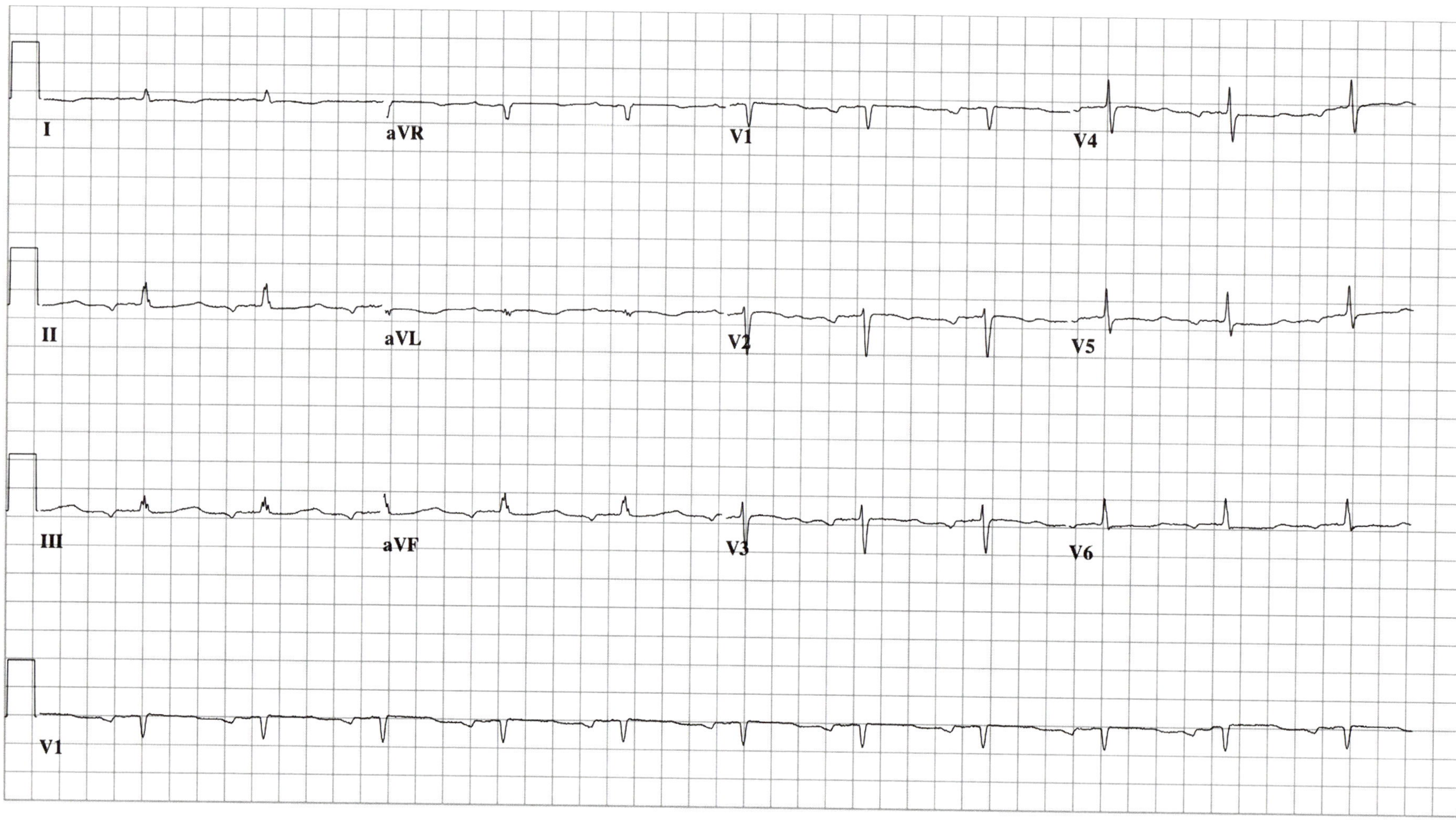

QUESTIONS

111-1. What abnormalities are present on this ECG? What is the rhythm?

111-2. What is the differential diagnosis for the abnormality of voltage?

Case #112. A 54-year-old hospitalized patient.

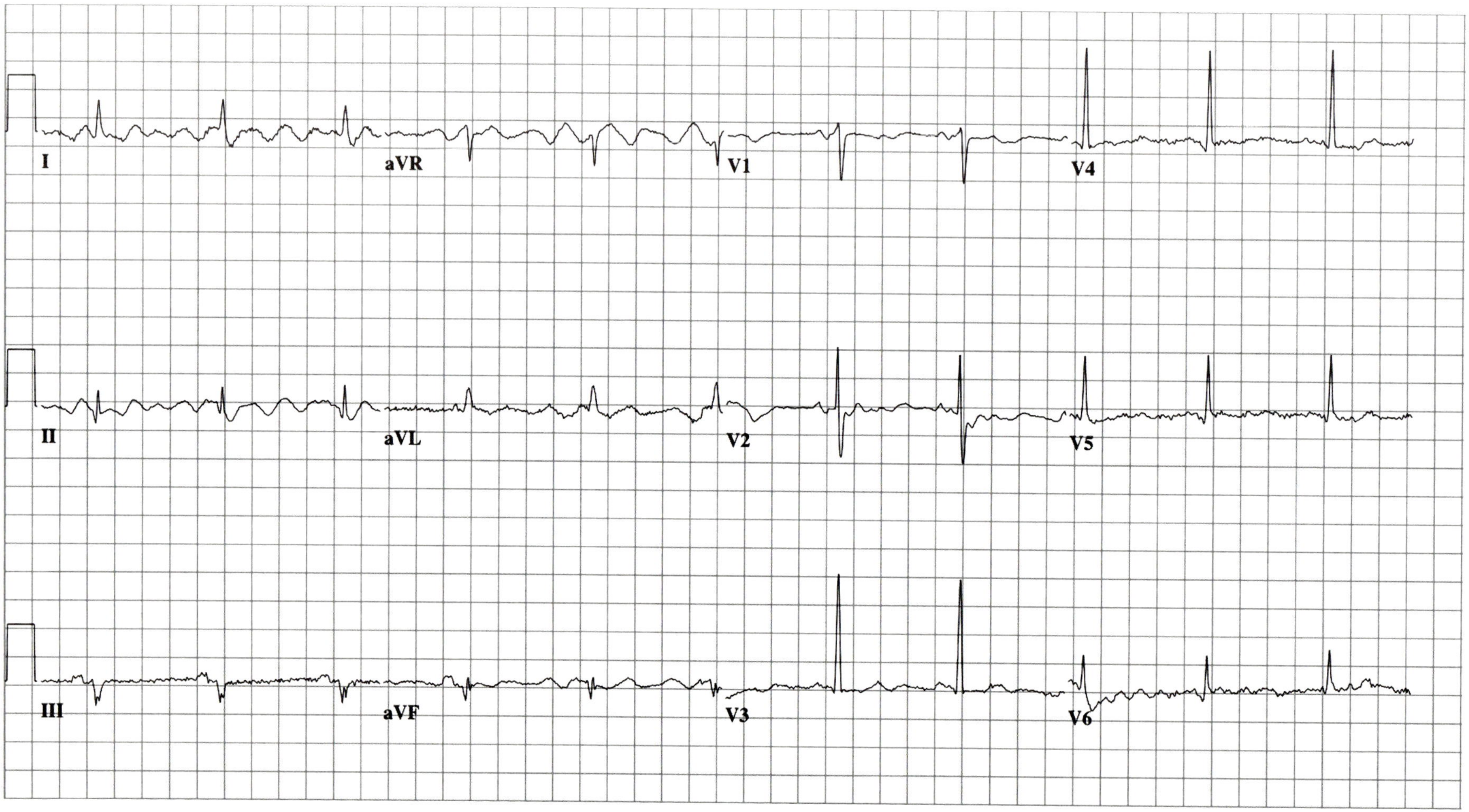

QUESTIONS

112-1. Interpret this ECG.

112-2. What is the differential diagnosis for this finding?

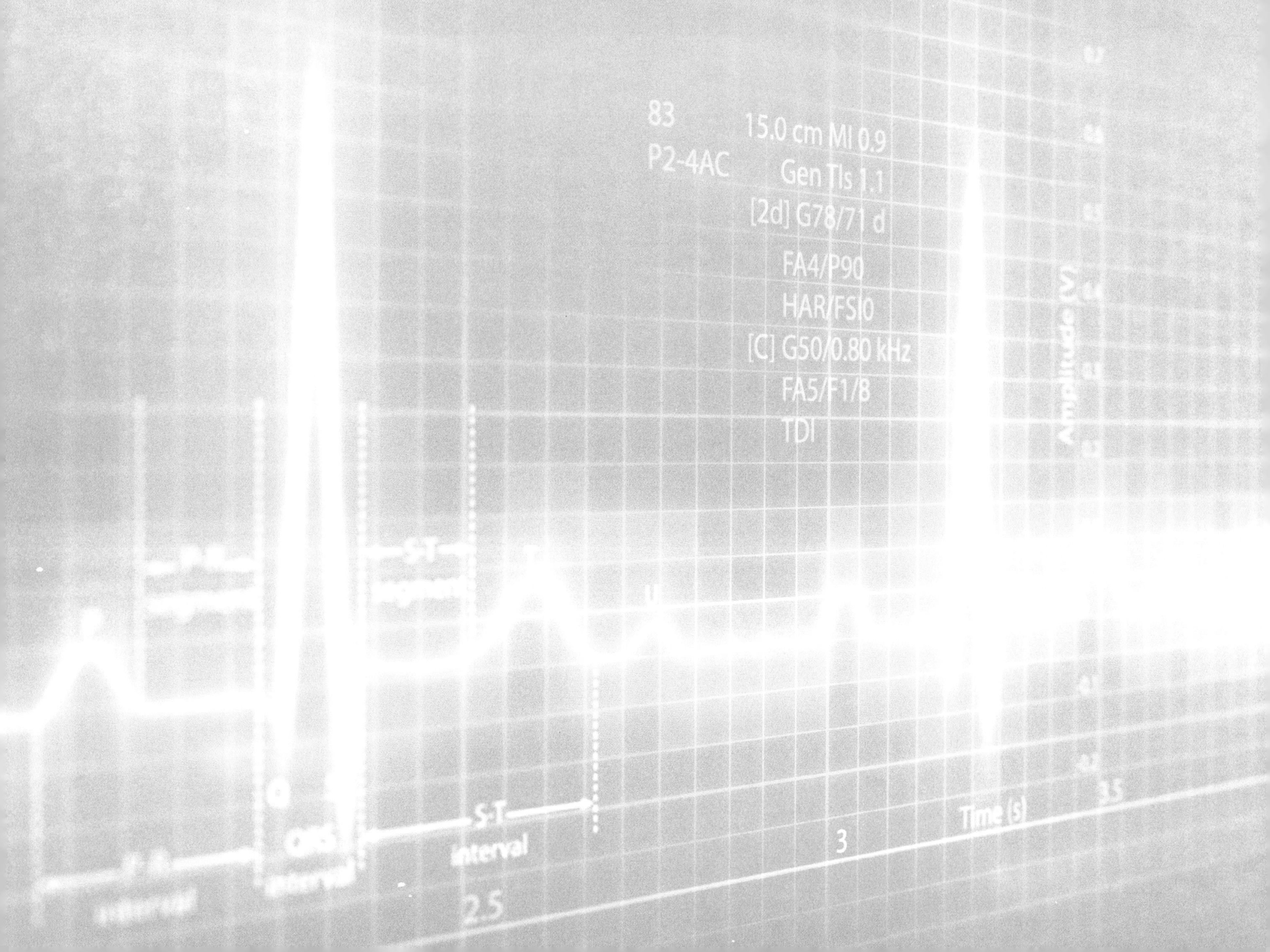
83
P2-4AC
15.0 cm MI 0.9
Gen TIs 1.1
[2d] G78/71 d
FA4/P90
HAR/FSI0
[C] G50/0.80 kHz
FA5/F1/8
TDI
Amplitude (V)
S-T
interval
3
2.5
Time (s)
3.5

ANSWERS

112-1. Interpret this ECG.

On first glance, this tracing demonstrates a coarse irregular rhythm; however, P waves can be visualized clearly in V1 and III, suggesting the coarse "rhythm" is actually baseline artifact. The axis is normal; there is no evidence of chamber enlargement. Nonspecific T-wave abnormalities are also present.

112-2. What is the differential diagnosis for this finding?

Although initially suggesting atrial arrhythmia, the diagnosis of baseline artifact is clear after careful inspection. Recall that leads I, II, and III are created by measuring electrical signals between combinations of the limb leads involving the right and left arms and the left leg. Lead III (created by measuring the electrical signal between the left arm and the left leg) is free of baseline artifact, suggesting by process of exclusion that the right arm is the source of the baseline artifact. A parkinsonian tremor or volitional activity could be the cause of this artifact. Parkinsonian tremors are typically 6 Hz, corresponding to an artifact frequency of approximately 6 cycles/s. The "rate" of this baseline artifact is approximately 5 cycles/s (1 second divided by 200 milliseconds).

Case #113. A 77-year-old gentleman presents with dizziness and dyspnea at rest.

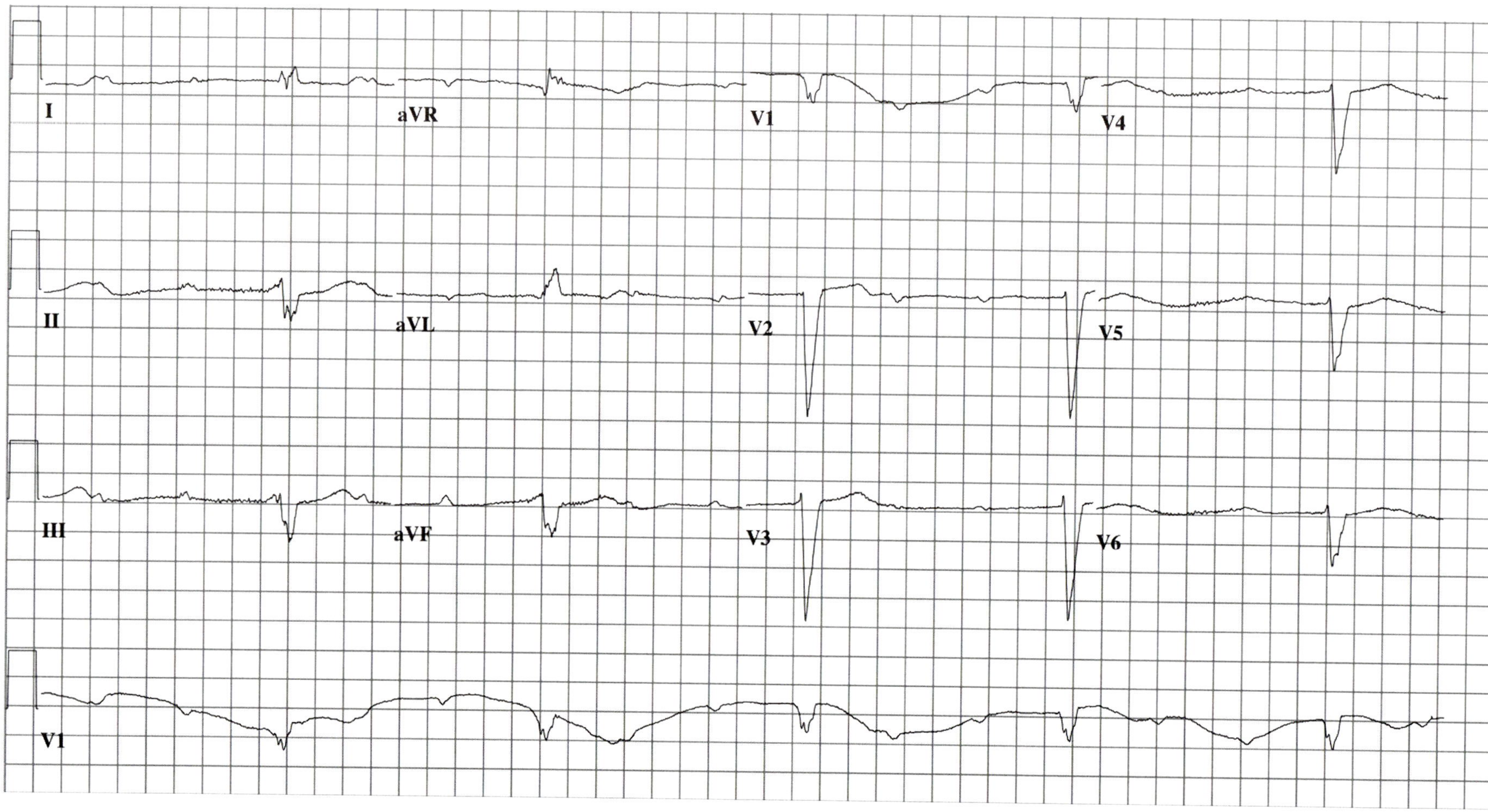

QUESTIONS

113-1. Interpret this ECG: what is the diagnosis?

113-2. Where in the heart does the escape rhythm originate from?

113-3. What would you do next?

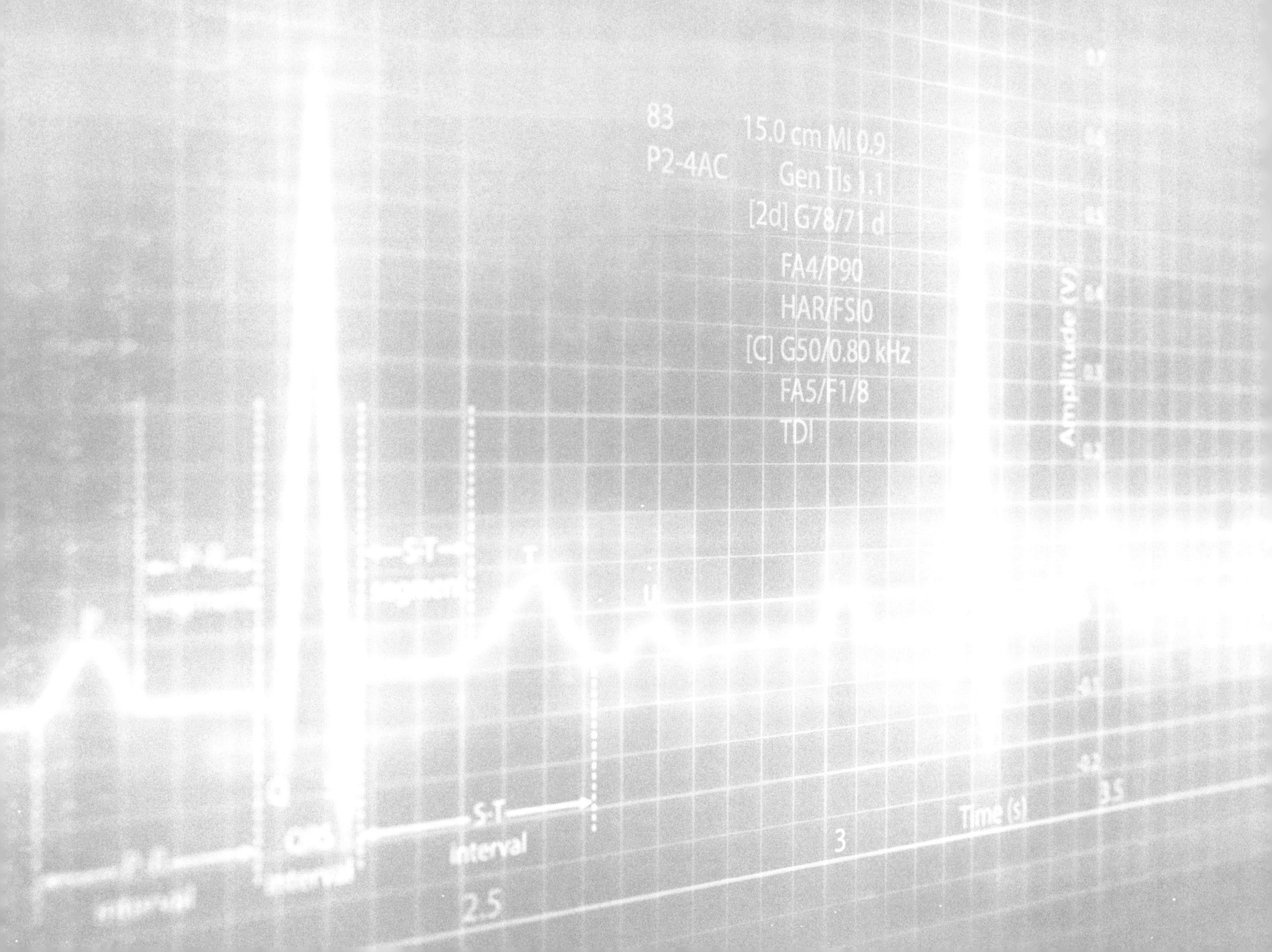
83
P2-4AC
15.0 cm MI 0.9
Gen TIs 1.1
[2d] G78/71 d
FA4/P90
HAR/FSI0
[C] G50/0.80 kHz
FA5/F1/8
TDI
Amplitude (V)
S-T
T
U
S-T
interval
2.5
3
Time (s)
3.5

ANSWERS

113-1. Interpret this ECG: what is the diagnosis?

There are clear P waves evident at a rate of approximately 75 beats/min, best visualized in the rhythm strip despite the prominent baseline artifact. The P waves are upright in lead II and biphasic in lead V1 consistent with a sinus mechanism. The QRS complex is wide (approximately 160 milliseconds) with a morphology that does not meet criteria for either right or left bundle branch block. The ventricular rate is very slow, 30 beats/min. There is no relationship between P waves and QRS complexes and the atrial rate is faster than the ventricular rate. Hence, complete heart block is present.

113-2. Where in the heart does the escape rhythm originate from?

The QRS morphology and the ventricular rate are typical of a ventricular escape rhythm. Escape rhythms originating from the AV node are often narrow (unless preexisting conduction system disease is present) and typically have rates between 50 and 60 beats/min. Escape rates tend to become progressively slower as one moves lower in the His–Purkinje system.

113-3. What would you do next?

This patient with complete heart block, severe symptoms, and a wide complex ventricular escape should have a pacemaker implanted. A temporary transvenous pacemaker can be placed at the bedside while permanent pacemaker placement is being arranged.

Case #114. The 77-year-old man from the prior case now status post an intervention.

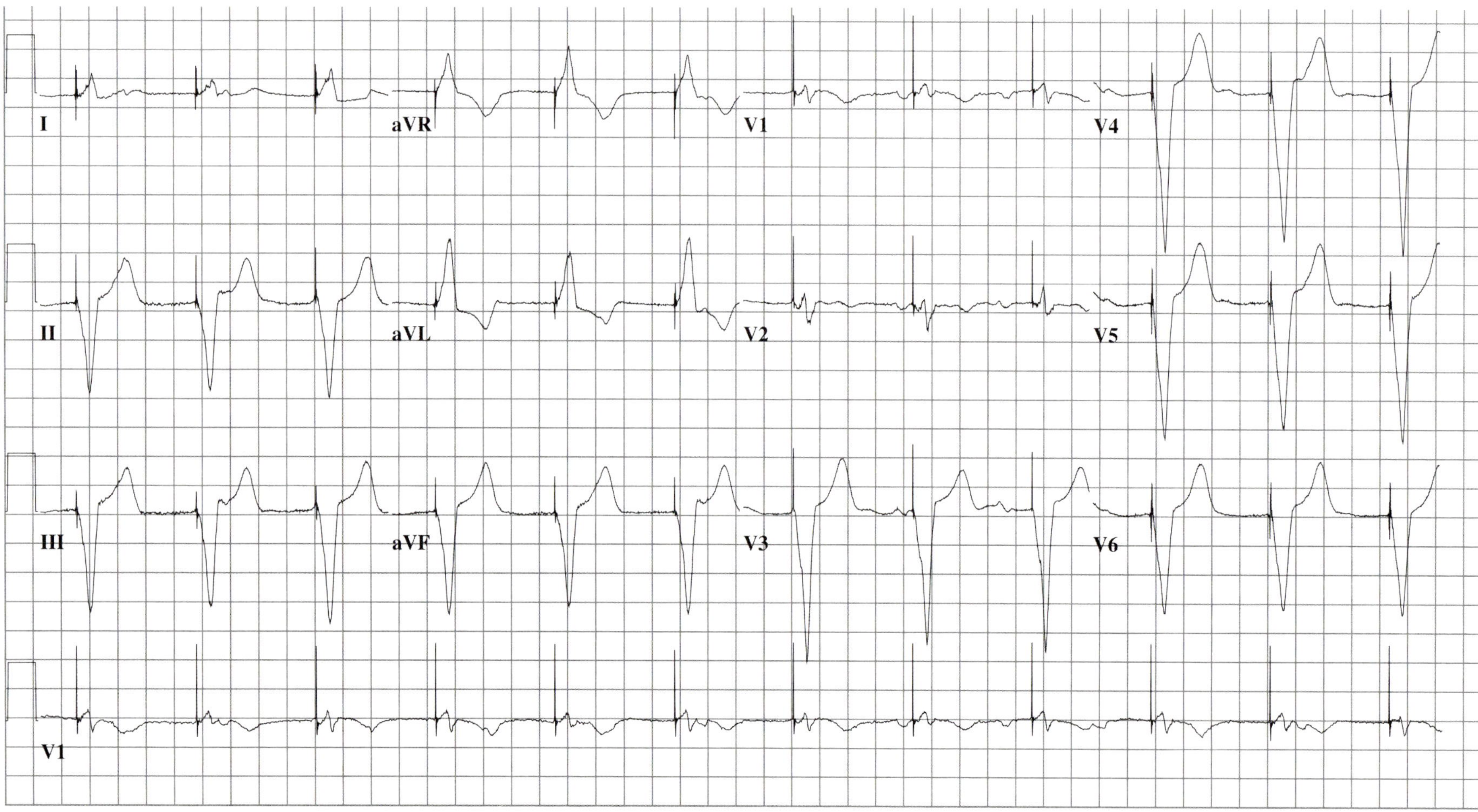

QUESTIONS

114-1. Interpret this ECG.

114-2. Describe the interaction between the atria and ventricles in this tracing.

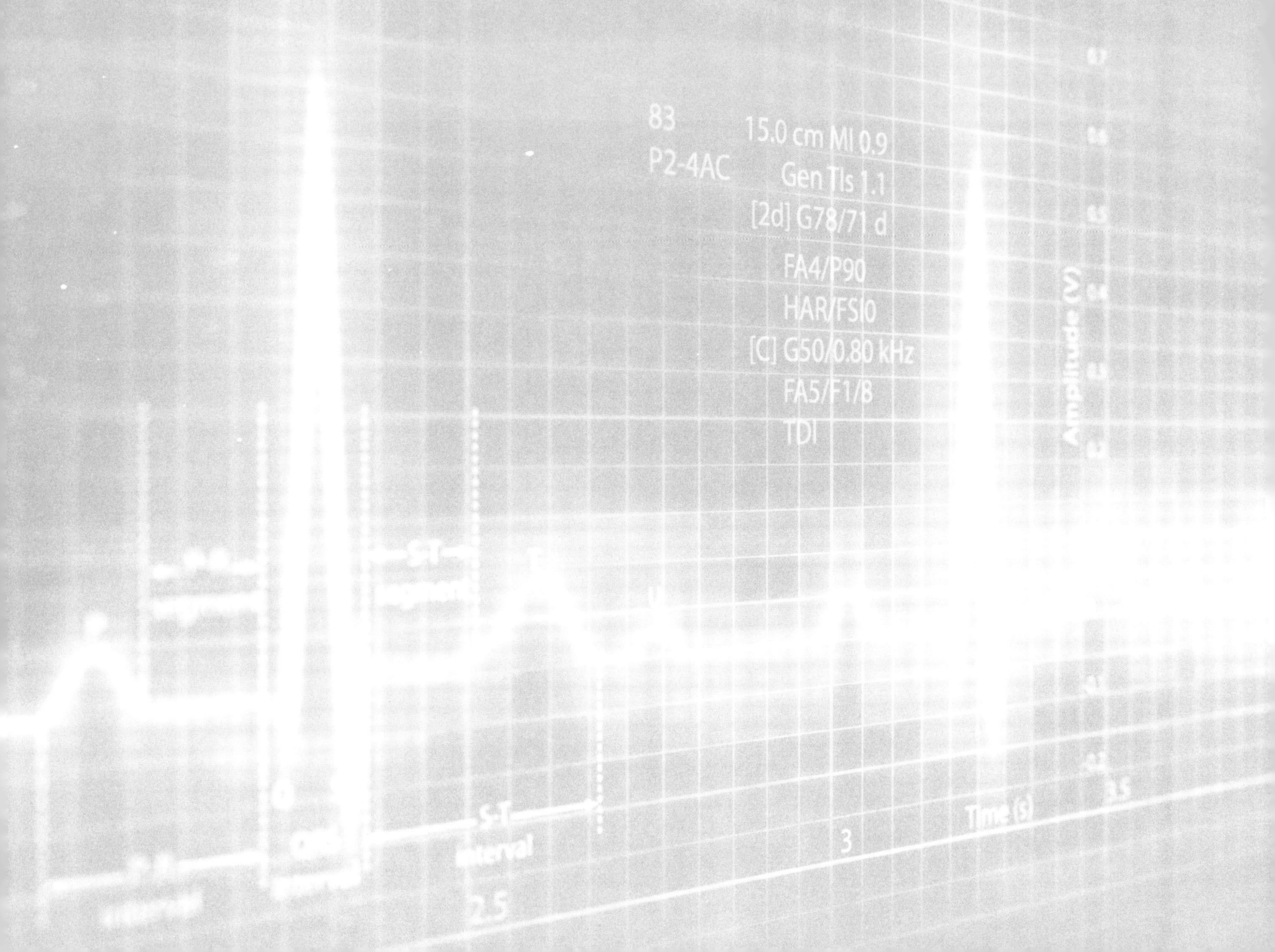
83
P2-4AC
15.0 cm MI 0.9
Gen TIs 1.1
[2d] G78/71 d
FA4/P90
HAR/FSI0
[C] G50/0.80 kHz
FA5/F1/8
TDI
Amplitude (V)
S-T
interval
Time (s)
3
2.5

ANSWERS

114-1. Interpret this ECG.

The ventricular rate is 70 beats/min and regular. The sinus rate is approximately 80 beats/min. By examining the rhythm strip closely, it is apparent that the P waves continue to lack any relationship with the QRS complexes, and therefore complete heart block is still present. The ventricular rhythm, however, is now paced with a leftward axis, wide QRS, and pacemaker impulses clearly evident at the onset of the QRS complexes. The ST segments and T waves point opposite the major deflection of the QRS complex as is expected with ventricular pacing.

114-2. Describe the interaction between the atria and ventricles in this tracing.

As in the prior case, there is no relationship between the atrial and ventricular activity. The ventricular rate has increased now that a pacemaker has been placed, but the atrial impulses still march through totally independent of the ventricular impulses. This would be expected given that pacemaker placement does not "fix" the conduction system disease that caused complete heart block. Temporary transvenous pacemakers placed at the bedside are single-lead devices placed in the right ventricle, but permanent pacemakers often use leads in both the right atrium and the right ventricle. AV synchrony could be restored by placing a permanent pacemaker with right atrial and right ventricular leads and pacing both chambers sequentially.

Case #115. A 78-year-old man with chest pressure and dyspnea requiring inotropic therapy.

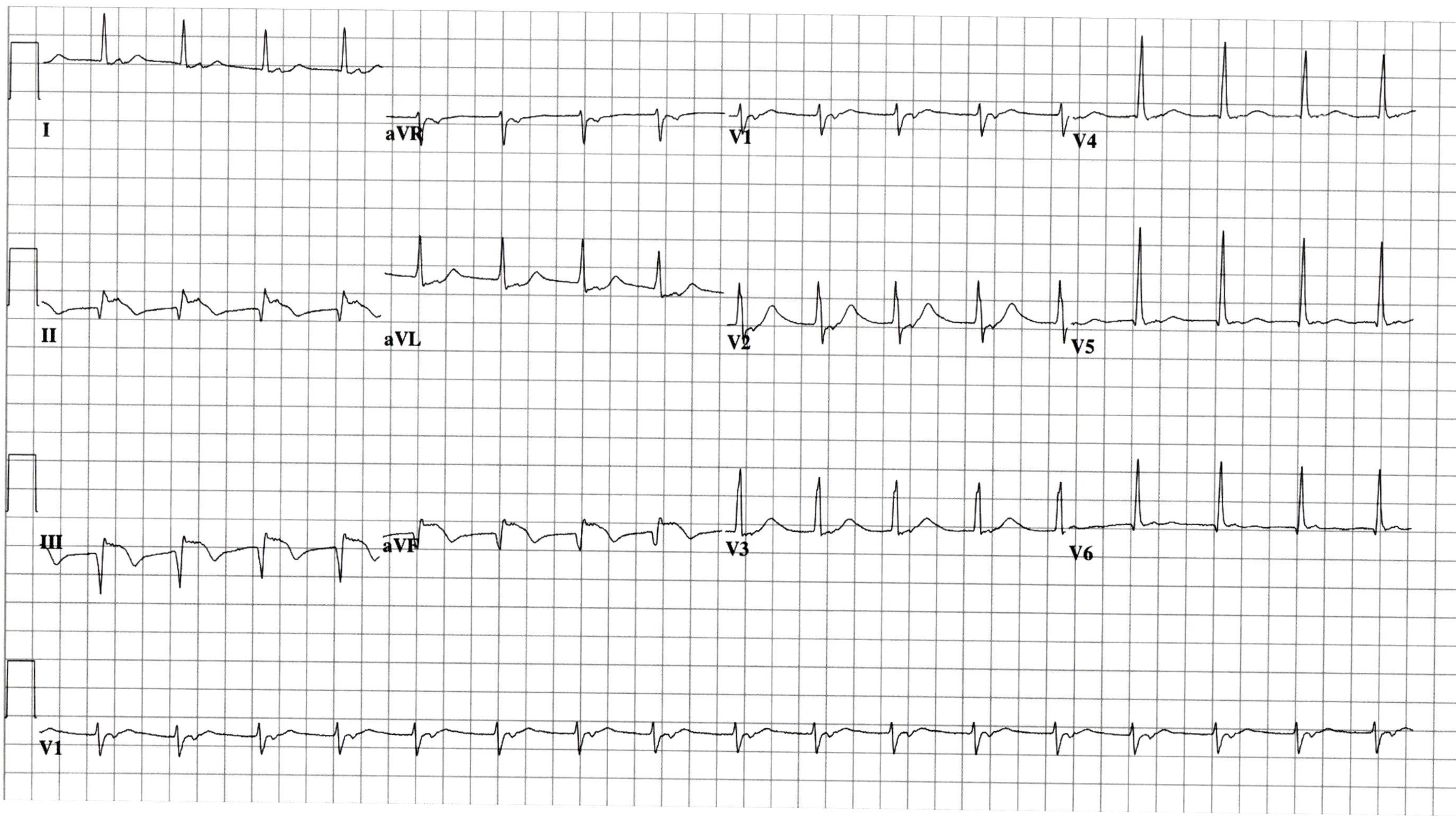

QUESTIONS

115-1. What is the rhythm?

115-2. What other abnormality is present?

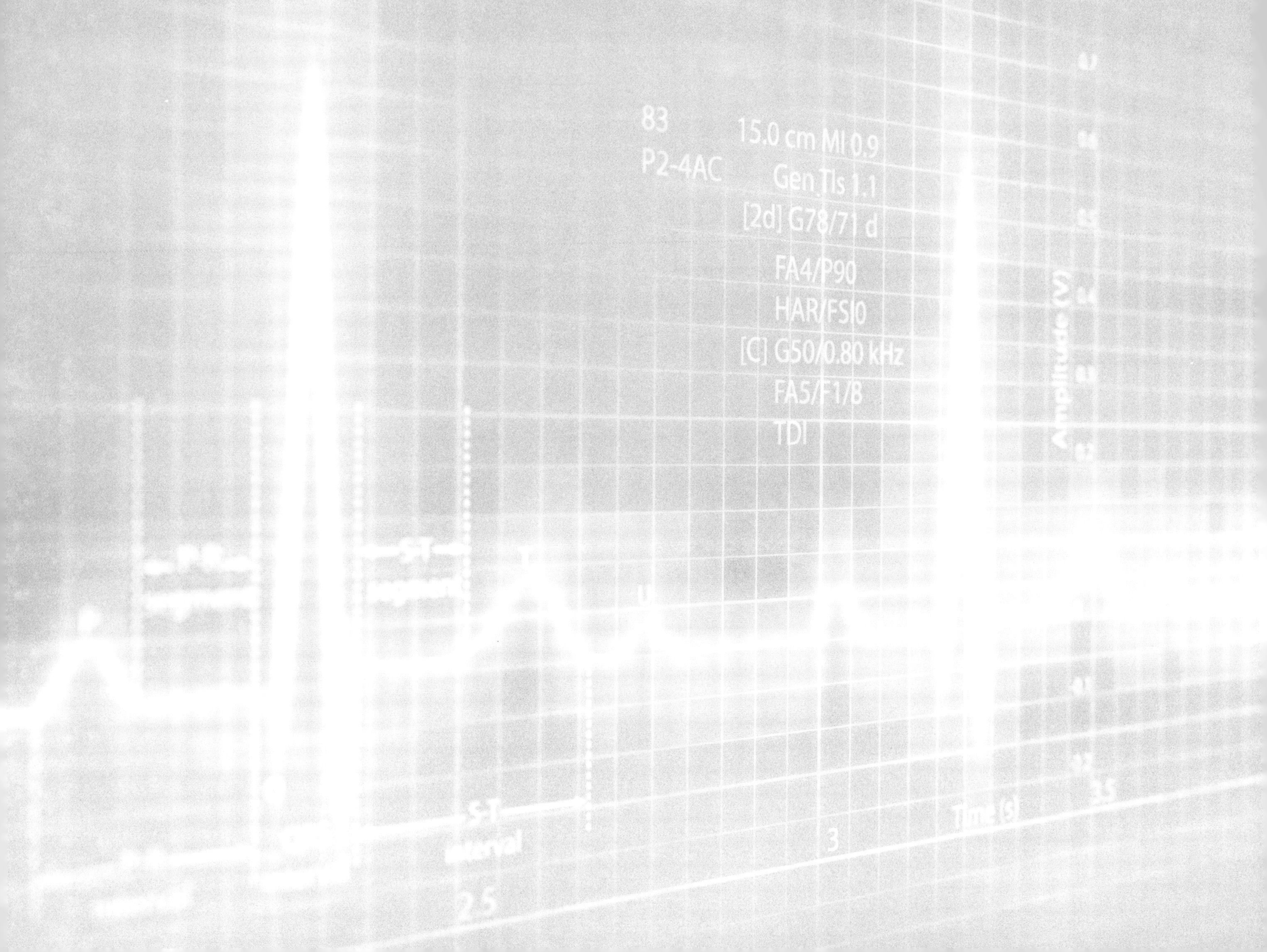
83
P2-4AC
15.0 cm MI 0.9
Gen TIs 1.1
[2d] G78/71 d
FA4/P90
HAR/FS|0
[C] G50/0.80 kHz
FA5/F1/8
TDI
Amplitude (V)
S-T
interval
Time (s)
2.5
3

ANSWERS

115-1. What is the rhythm?

There is a tachycardic, regular rhythm at approximately 100 beats/min. The QRS complexes are narrow. There are P waves evident buried within the ST segment (demonstrated by asterisks in the figure); the P waves are inverted in leads II, III, and aVF, suggesting atrial depolarization moving from inferior to superior. The RP interval (the distance from the R wave to the next P wave, demonstrated in the figure) is shorter than the PR interval (the distance from the P wave to the next sequential R wave, demonstrated in the figure), thus we can categorize this as a short RP tachycardia. The differential includes atrial tachycardia with an extremely prolonged PR interval, AV nodal and AV reentrant tachycardias, and accelerated junctional tachycardias. Reentrant tachycardias and atrial tachycardias usually occur at faster rates than seen in this tracing, and an atrial tachycardia with such a prolonged PR interval would be rare. In the setting of the other abnormalities on this tracing described below, the most likely diagnosis is an accelerated junctional rhythm with retrograde atrial activation explaining the P waves.

115-2. What other abnormality is present?

Pathologic Q waves, ST-segment elevation, and T-wave inversion are seen in the inferior leads II, III, and aVF. There is slight ST depression in aVL that is reciprocal to the inferior ischemia. Arrhythmia in the setting of acute myocardial infarction and inotrope use is common. In this case, the arrhythmia resolved with treatment of the ischemia and discontinuation of inotropic support.

ANSWERS (Cont.)

Retrograde P waves are demonstrated with asterisks, and the R-P and P-R intervals are demonstrated.

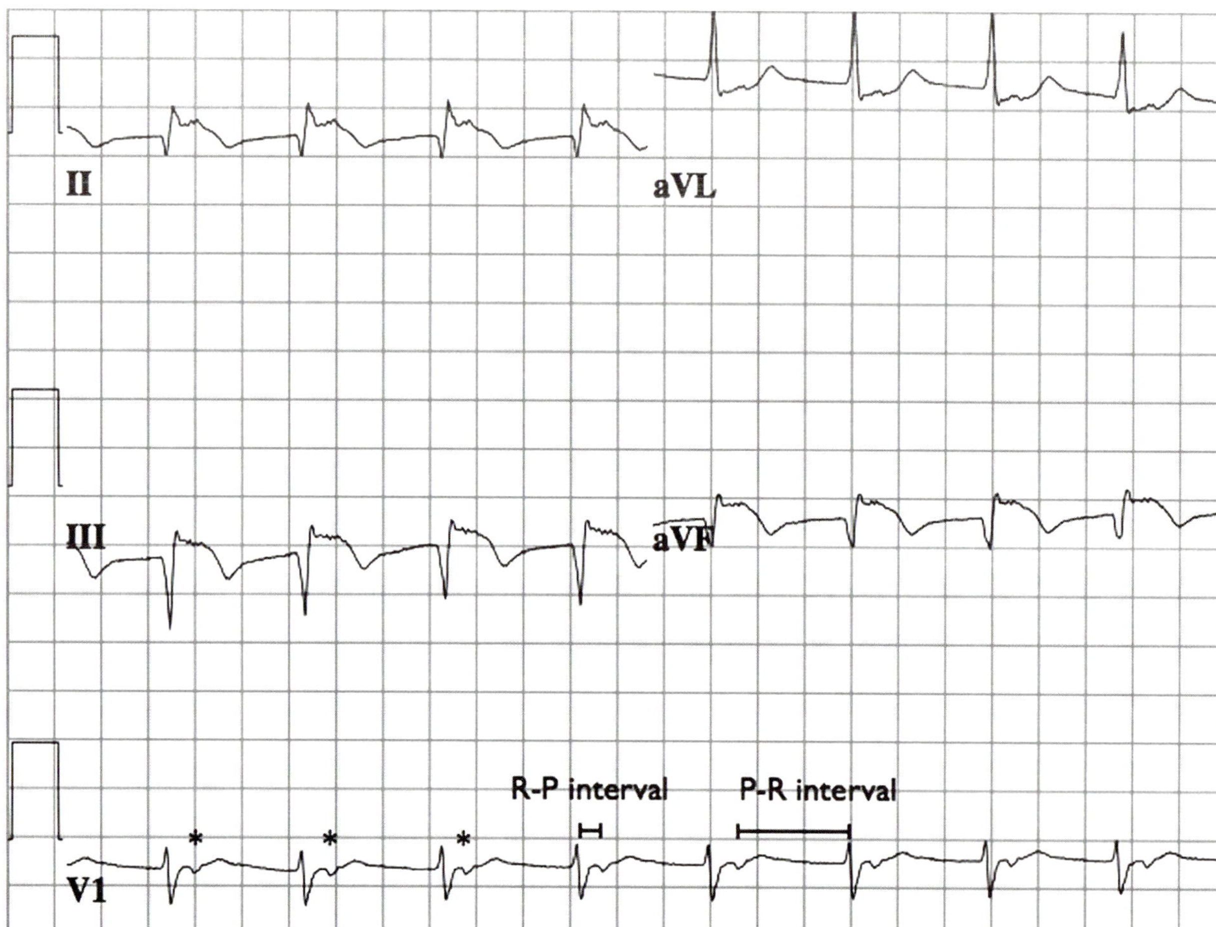

Case #116. The same 78-year-old gentleman, now with this rhythm.

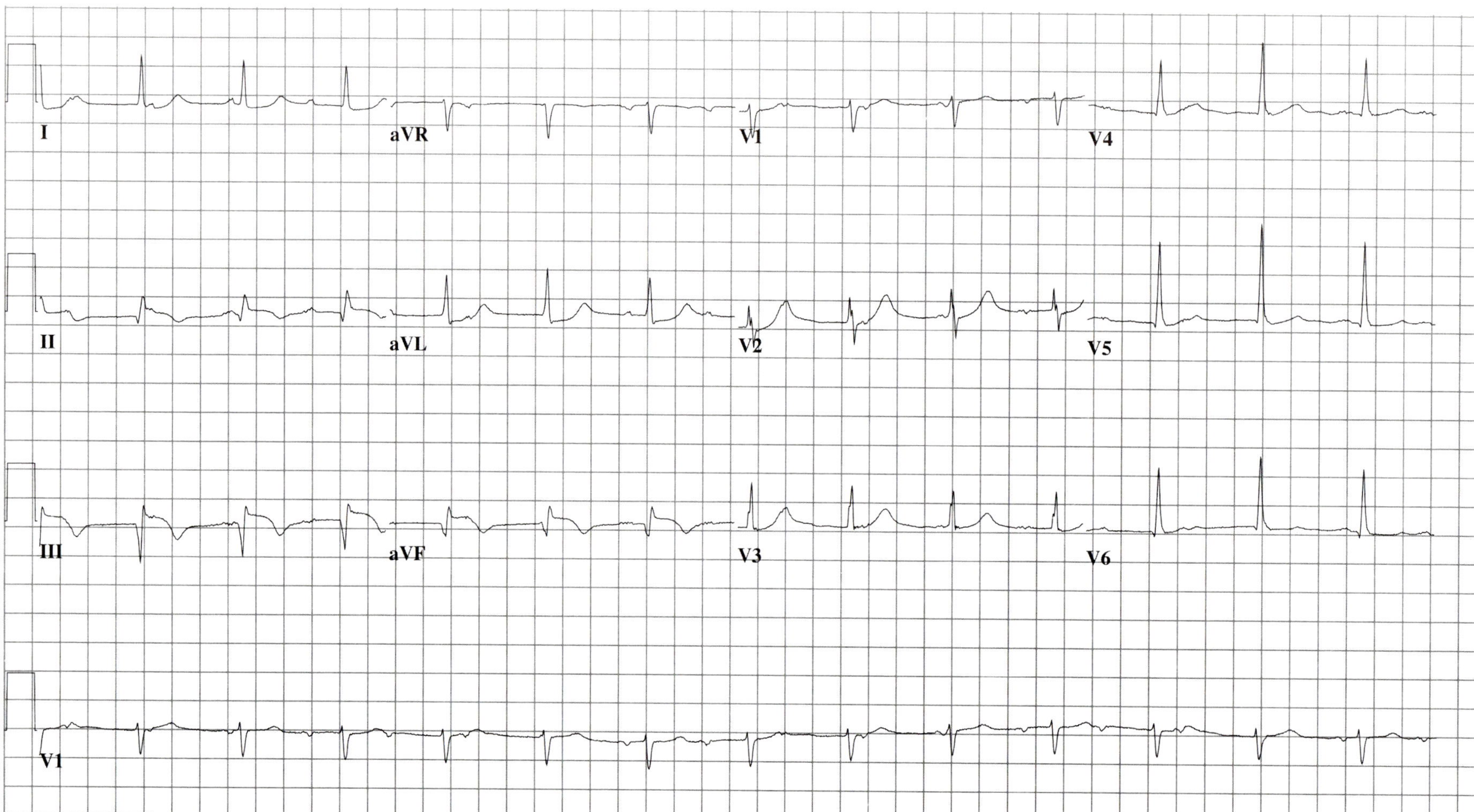

QUESTION

116-1. **What is the rhythm?**

83
P2-4AC
15.0 cm MI 0.9
Gen TIs 1.1
[2d] G78/71 d
FA4/P90
HAR/FS|0
[C] G50/0.80 kHz
FA5/F1/8
TDI
Amplitude (V)
Time (s)
S-T interval
QRS interval
3
2.5

ANSWER

116-1. What is the rhythm?

The patient now is in a narrow complex rhythm slightly slower at approximately 80 beats/min. The R–R interval is regular. Sinus P waves are seen best in lead V1, noted by asterisks in the figure, at a rate of approximately 100 beats/min. There is no clear relationship between the P waves and the QRS complexes. Thus, the diagnosis is complete heart block with an accelerated junctional rhythm (native junctional escape rhythms are usually closer to 40–60 beats/min). The inferior ST elevations persist.

Complete heart block is demonstrated. The P waves are denoted with asterisks. QRS complexes march out at a different rate and rhythm than the P waves.

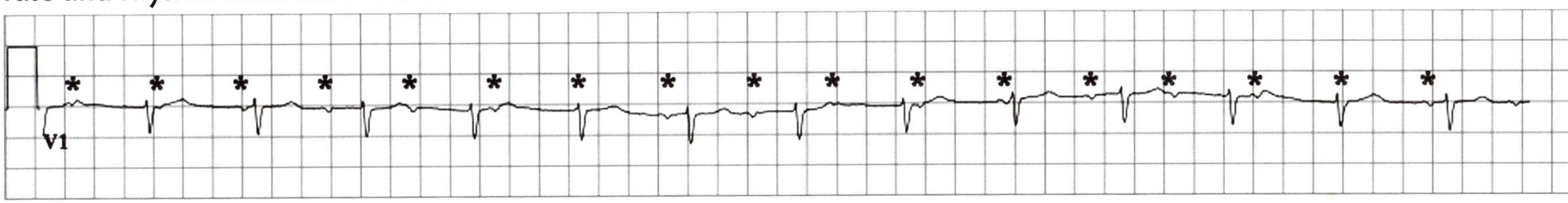

Case #117. A 50-year-old male without cardiac history has an ECG prior to an elective inguinal hernia repair.

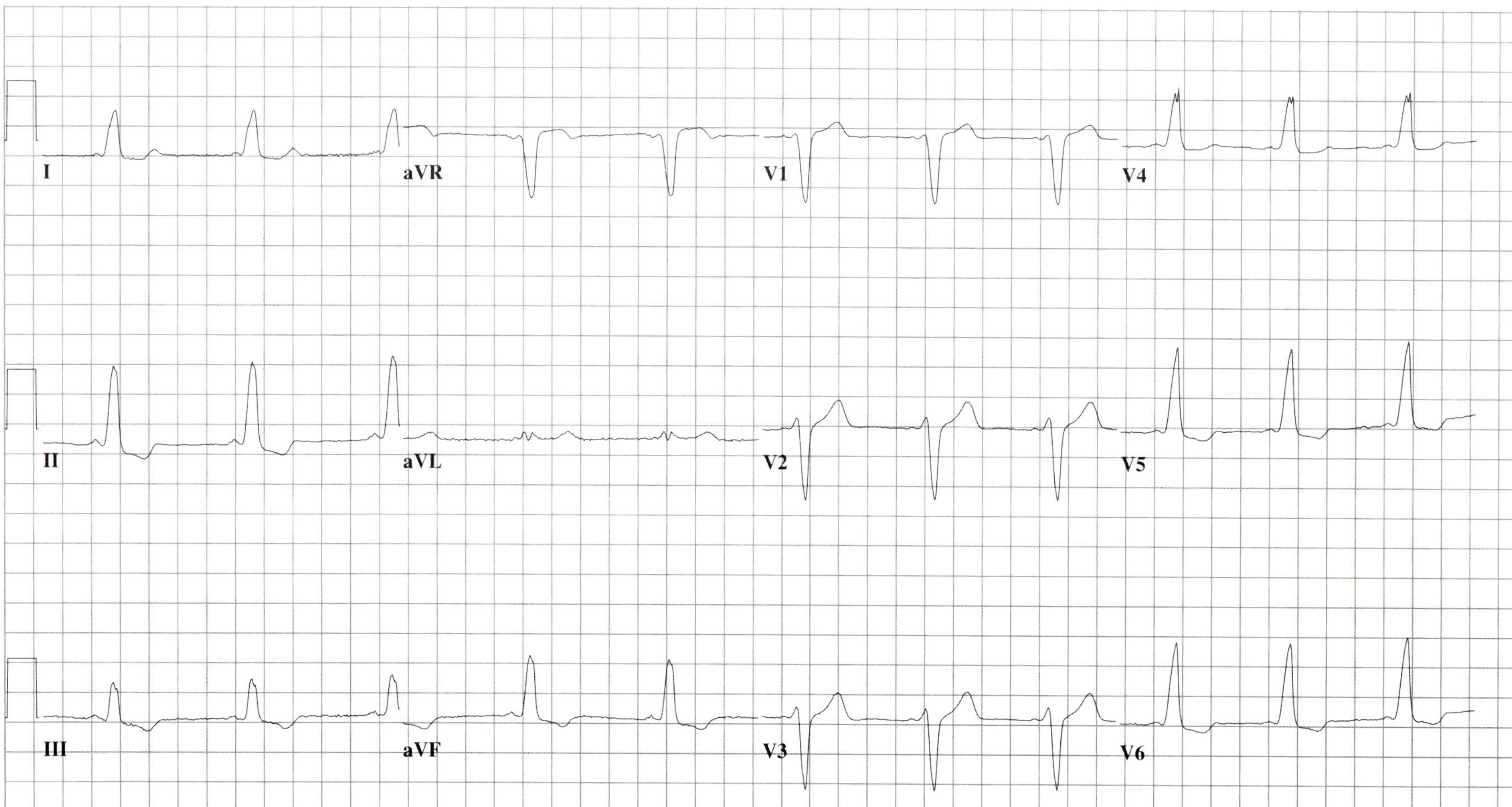

QUESTION

117-1. What abnormalities are present on this ECG? What is the diagnosis?

83
P2-4AC
15.0 cm MI 0.9
Gen TIs 1.1
[2d] G78/71 d
FA4/P90
HAR/FSI0
[C] G50/0.80 kHz
FA5/F1/8
TDI
Amplitude (V)
Time (s)
3
2.5
3.5

ANSWER

117-1. What abnormalities are present on this ECG? What is the diagnosis?

The ventricular rate is 66 beats/min. There is a P wave before every QRS complex and a QRS complex for every P wave. The P waves are upright in leads I, II, aVF, and V6, suggesting sinus origin. However, the PR interval is as short as 100 milliseconds in some leads, and the QRS is quite wide, at over 3.5 small boxes (140 milliseconds). At first glance, there appears to be left bundle branch block with broad QRS, an rS wave in V1 monophasic R wave in leads I and V6. Given the short PR interval, however, closer inspection reveals delta waves in most leads, suggesting that the broad QRS complex is a result of preexcitation and Wolff-Parkinson-White pattern rather than traditional left bundle branch block. The QRS axis is normal, as is the QT interval. There are ST-segment depressions with inverted T waves in the inferior and lateral leads, which are related to the abnormal ventricular depolarization in the setting of Wolff-Parkinson-White.

Presentation:

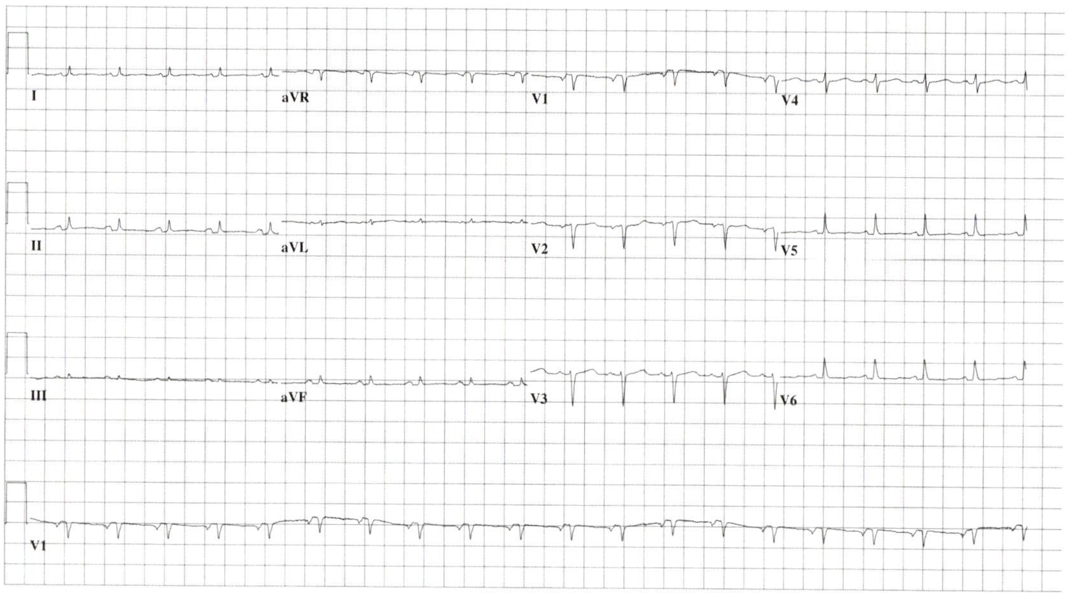

Baseline:

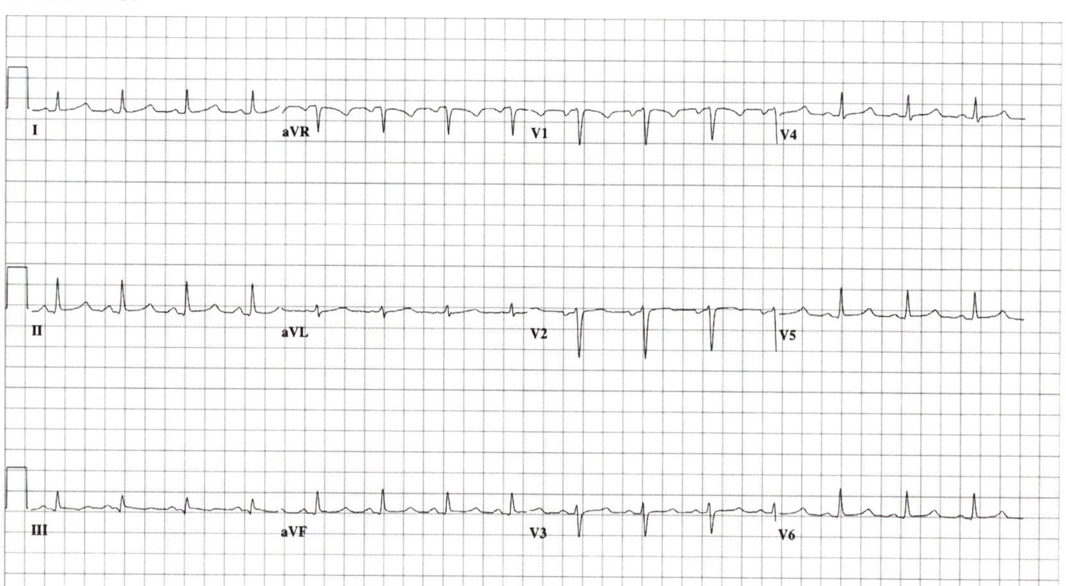

Case #118. **A 76-year-old woman with metastatic breast cancer presents with dyspnea. The presentation and baseline tracings are shown.**

QUESTIONS

118-1. What is the differential diagnosis of dyspnea in a patient with metastatic cancer?

118-2. What abnormalities are present on the ECG?

118-3. What diagnosis is suggested? What bedside maneuver could confirm your suspicion?

83
P2-4AC
15.0 cm MI 0.9
Gen TIs 1.1
[2d] G78/71 d
FA4/P90
HAR/FS10
[C] G50/0.80 kHz
FA5/F1/8
TDI
S-T interval
2.5
3
3.5

ANSWERS

118-1. What is the differential diagnosis of dyspnea in a patient with metastatic cancer?

Dyspnea in a patient with metastatic cancer has a broad differential. "Cancer-related disorders of the nerve and neuromuscular junction can cause dyspnea. There may be dysfunction of the respiratory muscles either due to malignancy itself, paraneoplastic phenomena, or malnutrition". Pleural effusions, tense ascites, and pericardial effusion progressing to tamponade are considerations. Chemotherapeutic medications, particularly anthracyclines and trastuzumab, which are used in breast cancer, can cause cardiomyopathy. Pulmonary embolism, malignant pulmonary parenchymal infiltrates, infections, and anemia are also possible.

118-2. What abnormalities are present on the ECG?

This tracing demonstrates sinus tachycardia at 120 beats/min. The axis is physiologic and intervals are normal. Low voltage is present, defined as total QRS amplitude less than 5 mV in the limb leads and less than 10 mV in the precordial leads. Equally important is the fact that the voltage is strikingly reduced as compared to the baseline tracing. T waves are diffusely flattened, best described as nonspecific T-wave abnormality. There is a hint of PR-segment depression in the limb leads with corresponding PR-segment elevation in lead aVR, which suggests an atrial current of injury.

118-3. What diagnosis is suggested? What bedside maneuver could confirm your suspicion?

Dyspnea on exertion in a patient with metastatic cancer, low ECG voltage, and sinus tachycardia raises concern for pericardial tamponade. Patients with acute onset of pericardial tamponade, as in acute trauma, are generally hypotensive and in shock. In contrast, patients with malignant pericardial tamponade can present more insidiously and subacutely. Over time, the pericardium can stretch to accommodate large volumes of fluid. When a critical limit is reached, intrapericardial pressure becomes greater than intracardiac pressure, limiting diastolic filling and cardiac output. Measuring a pulsus paradoxus at the bedside can provide important diagnostic information while arranging for transthoracic echocardiogram to confirm the diagnosis. The treatment of choice is intravascular volume repletion to maintain preload followed by urgent pericardiocentesis.

Case #119. An 85-year-old woman complains of "skipped beats."

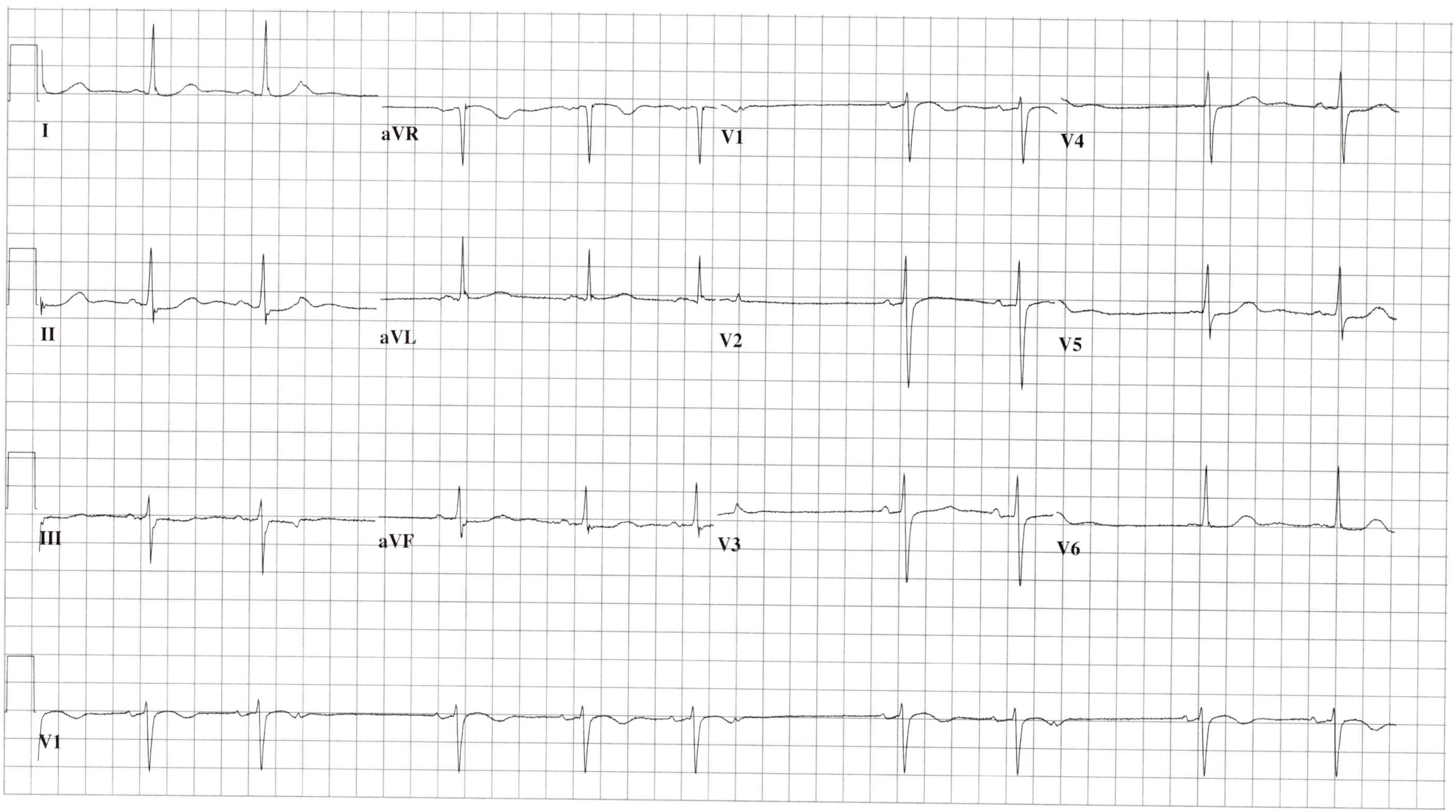

QUESTIONS

119-1. Interpret this ECG.

119-2. Explain the "skipped beats."

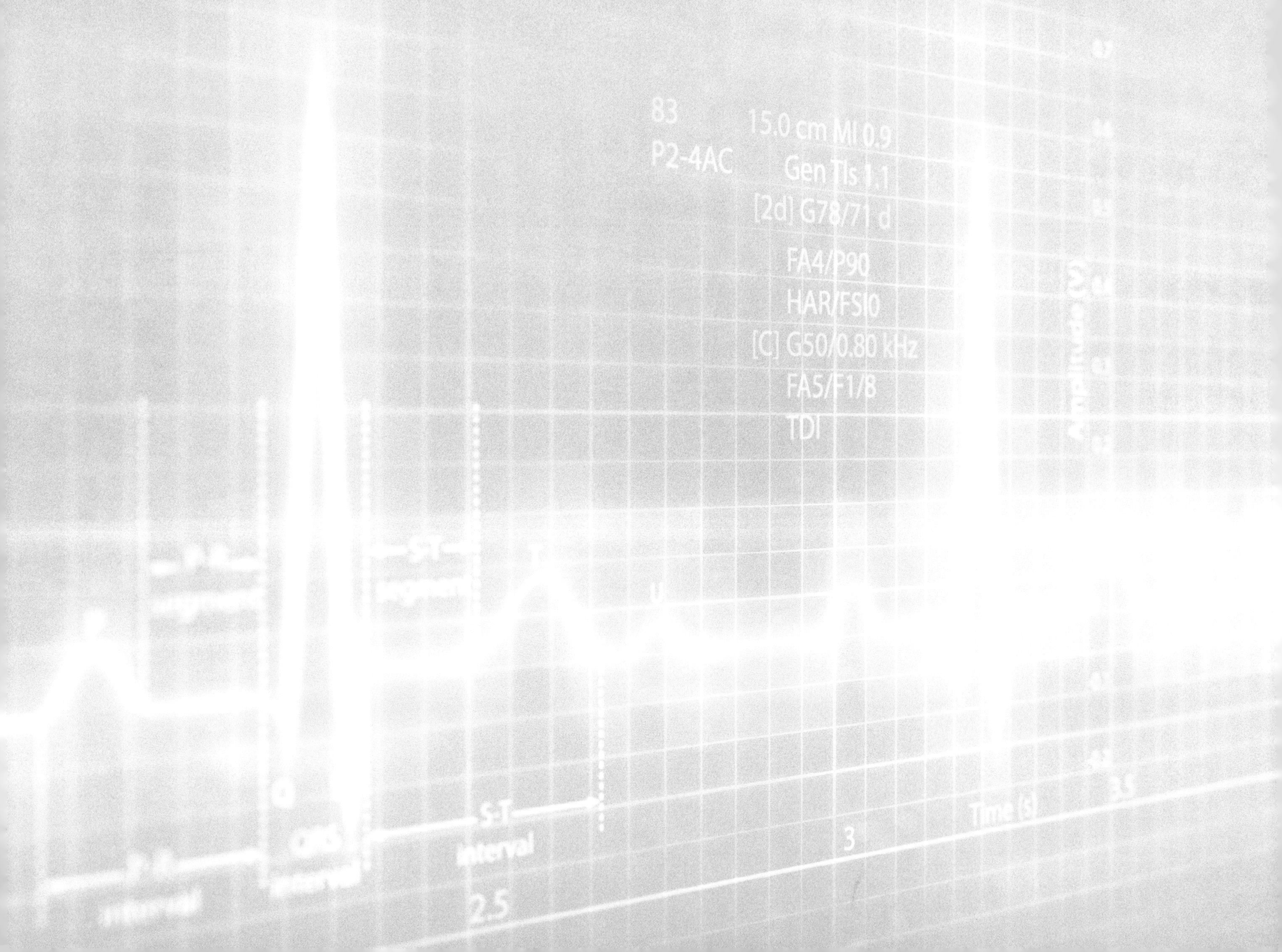
83
P2-4AC
15.0 cm MI 0.9
Gen Tls 1.1
[2d] G78/71 d
FA4/P90
HAR/FSI0
[C] G50/0.80 kHz
FA5/F1/8
TDI
S-T
interval
2.5
3
Time (s)
3.5

ANSWERS

119-1. Interpret this ECG.

There is sinus rhythm with several pauses noted. The axis and intervals are normal and there is no evidence of ischemia or chamber enlargement.

119-2. Explain the "skipped beats."

The differential diagnosis of a pause includes A-V block, sinus arrest, sinus exit block, and a nonconducted premature atrial contraction. Close inspection of the entirety of the pause and the preceding T wave can clarify the diagnosis. In this tracing, the T waves preceding each pause contain a sharp inflection, which represents a nonconducted P wave (figure). The P wave occurs earlier than would be predicted on the basis of the sinus rate; hence, the pauses are due to nonconducted premature atrial beats.

Sinus P waves are marked with asterisks, and nonconducted premature atrial impulses are marked with arrows. Each nonconducted atrial impulse is followed by a compensatory pause.

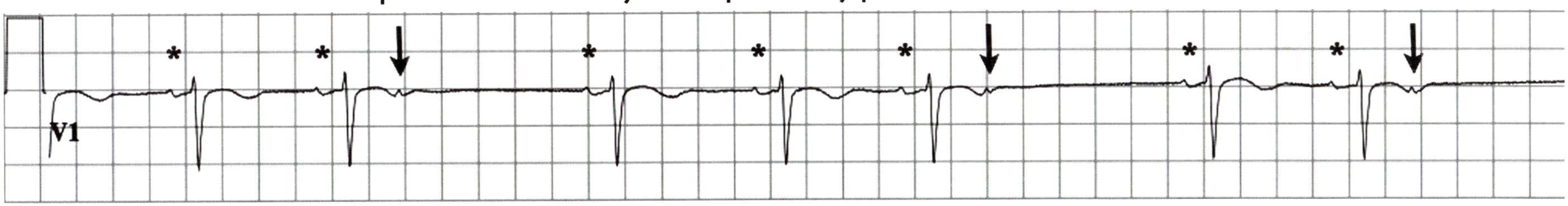

Case #120. A 65-year-old man with history of an anterior MI in the distant past presents with palpitations.

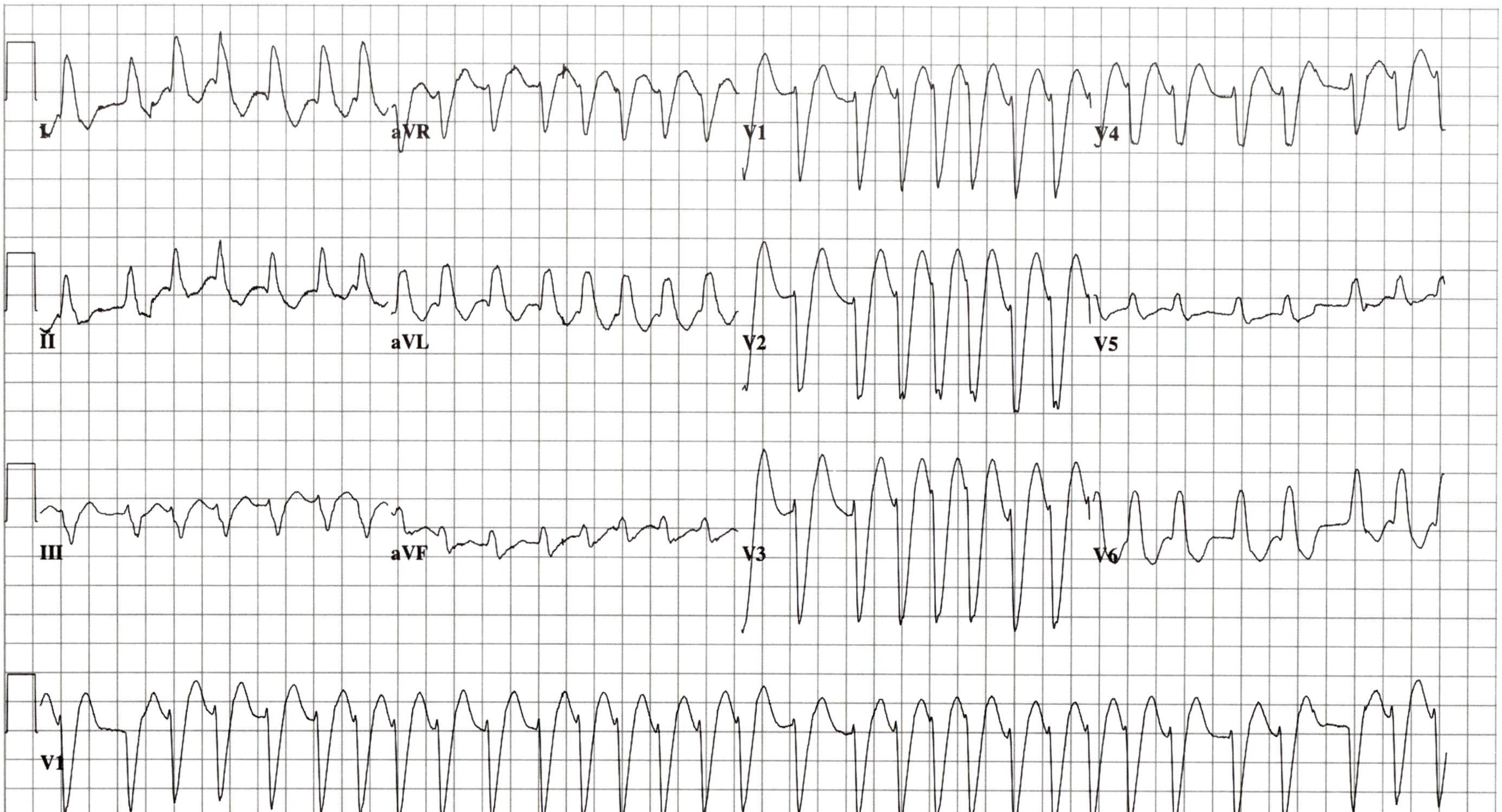

QUESTIONS

120-1. Interpret this tracing.

120-2. Upon presentation, the patient is tachycardic with blood pressure 130/70. How would you proceed?

83
P2-4AC
15.0 cm MI 0.9
Gen TIs 1.1
[2d] G78/71 d
FA4/P90
HAR/FS0
[C] G50/0.80 kHz
FA5/F1/8
TDI
Amplitude (V)
S-T
interval
Time (s)
2.5
3
3.5

ANSWERS

120-1. Interpret this tracing.

This tracing demonstrates an irregularly irregular wide-complex tachycardia with a rate of approximately 186 beats/min. There is no discernible atrial activity. The QRS interval is 140 milliseconds and the morphology is that of a left bundle branch block (LBBB), as evidenced by the small r wave and broad S wave in lead V1 and broad R wave in leads I and V6. It is critical to distinguish a ventricular tachycardia (VT) from a supraventricular tachycardia. VT is rarely so irregular as seen in this case. Given that the morphology of the QRS complex is consistent with that of a typical bundle branch block, the diagnosis is atrial fibrillation with rapid ventricular response and LBBB.

120-2. Upon presentation, the patient is tachycardic with blood pressure 130/70. How would you proceed?

The underlying rhythm is atrial fibrillation. As the patient is hemodynamically stable, the most prudent immediate course of action would be to proceed with pharmacologic rate control. β-Blockers or calcium channel blockers would be reasonable initial options. β-Blockers should be used with caution if severe obstructive lung disease is present, whereas calcium channel blockers should be used with caution if heart failure is present.

Case #121. A 35-year-old woman found down in a snowstorm.

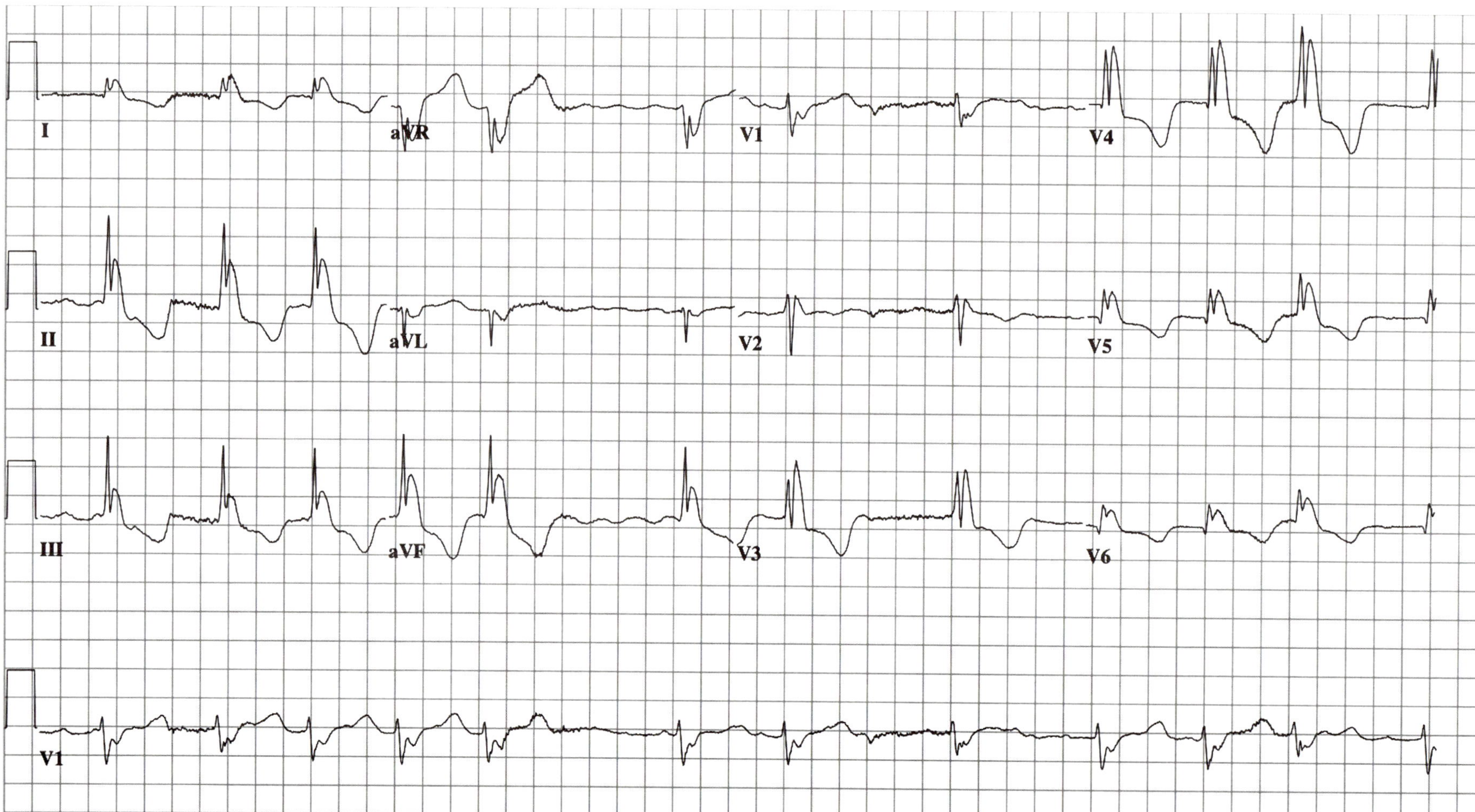

QUESTIONS

121-1. Interpret this tracing.

121-2. What is the differential diagnosis for the observed abnormality?

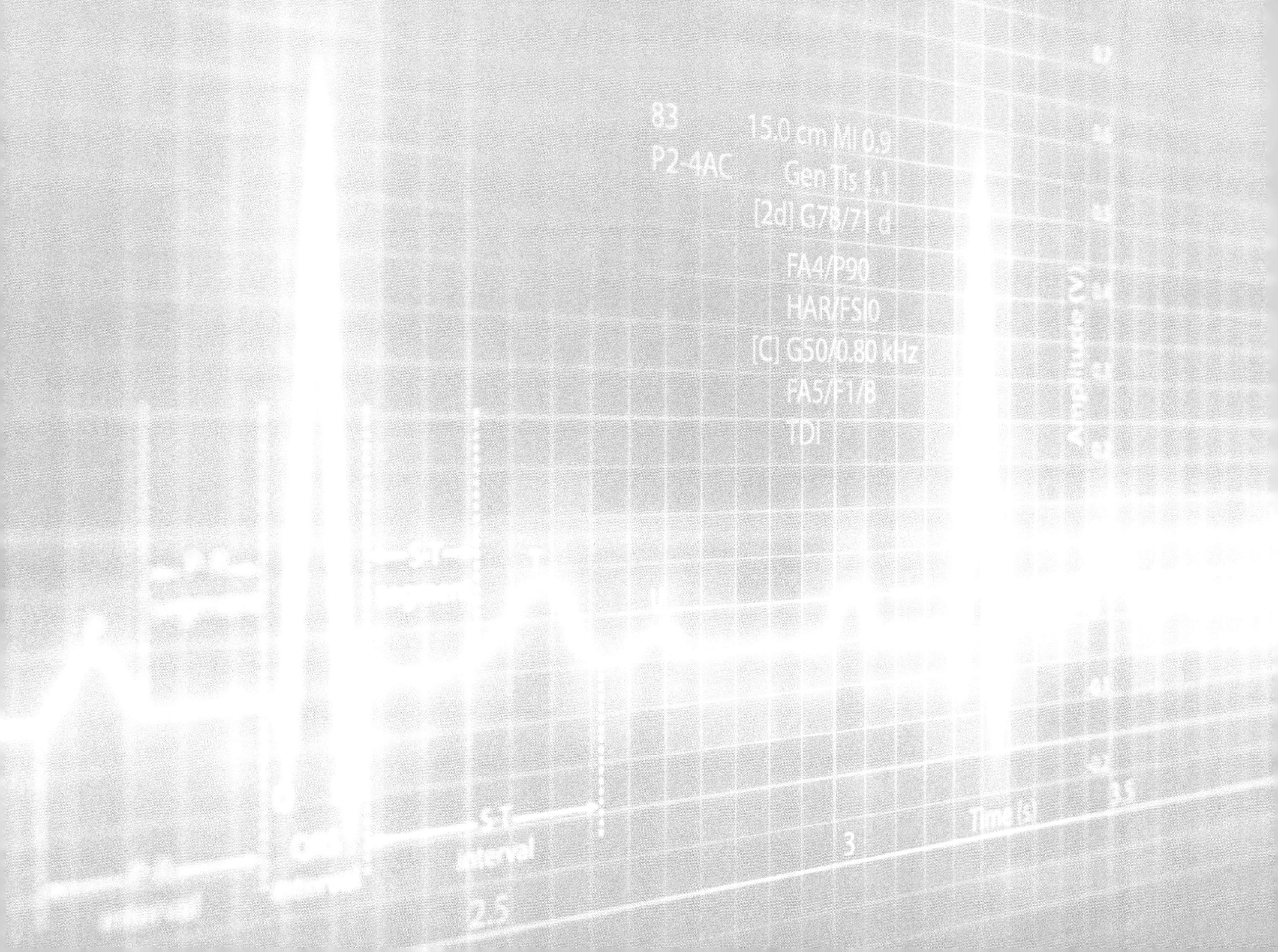
83
P2-4AC
15.0 cm MI 0.9
Gen TIs 1.1
[2d] G78/71 d
FA4/P90
HAR/FSI0
[C] G50/0.80 kHz
FA5/F1/8
TDI
Amplitude (V)
S-T
interval
2.5
3
Time (s)
3.5

ANSWERS

121-1. Interpret this tracing.

This tracing demonstrates an irregularly irregular rhythm at a rate of 72 beats/min. No clear atrial activity is seen, and coarse fibrillatory waves can be visualized best in lead aVF consistent with atrial fibrillation. QRS axis is normal. There are ST-segment depressions and T-wave inversions present in the anterior, lateral, and inferior leads.

The QRS appears widened with a prominent, rounded positive deflection following the QRS at the J point, as shown in the figure. This deflection is consistent with a large Osborn wave, sometimes called a J wave.

ANSWERS (Cont.)

121-2. What is the differential diagnosis for the observed abnormality?

The Osborn wave is classically associated with hypothermia.[1] Other reported associations include central nervous system injury, hypercalcemia, and toxic exposure including cocaine and antipsychotic use.[2]

Rounded elevation at the J point consistent with an Osborn wave.

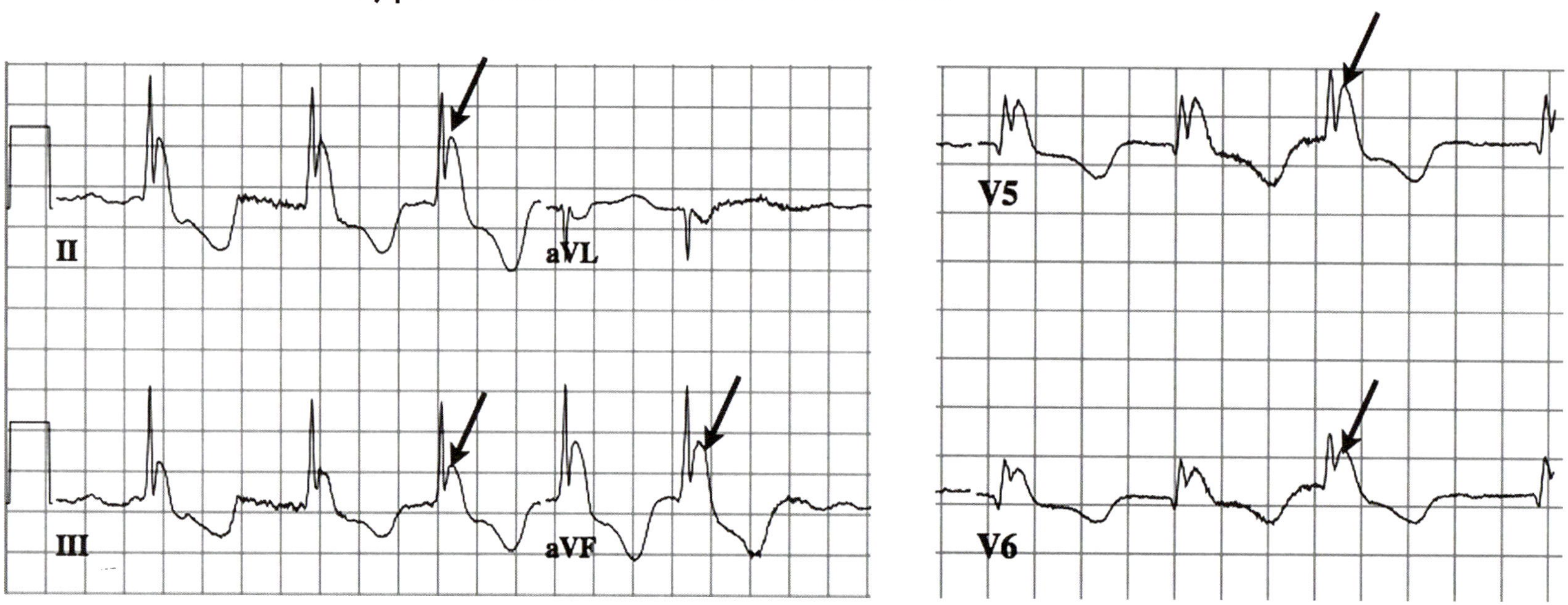

[1]Hurst JW. Naming of the waves in the ECG, with a brief account of their genesis. *Circulation* 1998; 98: 1937-1942.
[2]Dutto L, Allione A, Ricca M, et al. A spiked arrowhead in severe hypothermia: the Osborn wave. *BMJ Case Rep* 2009. Epub 6 Mar 2009.

Case #122. A 79-year-old woman presents with syncope.

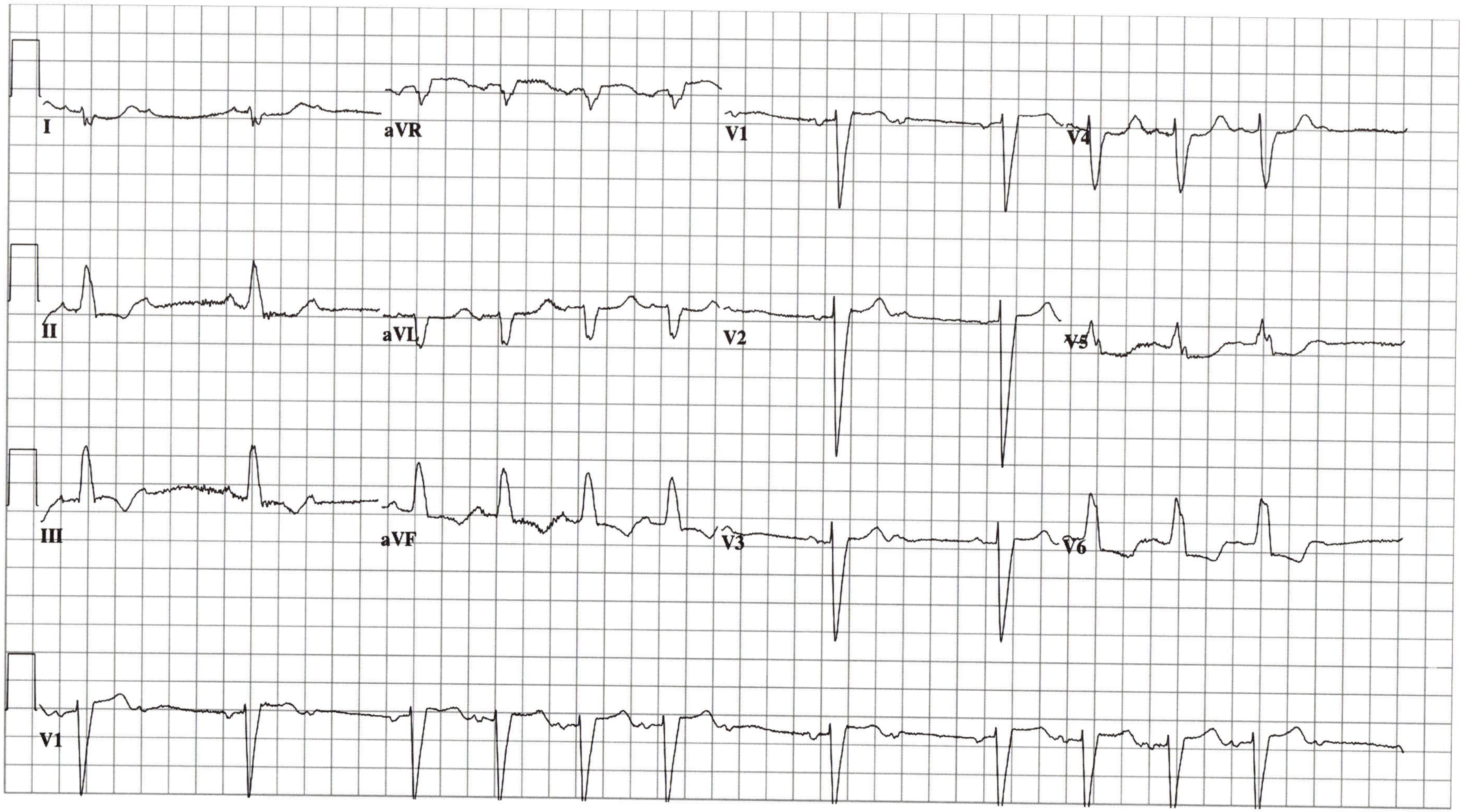

QUESTIONS

122-1. What is the diagnosis?

122-2. What treatment is recommended?

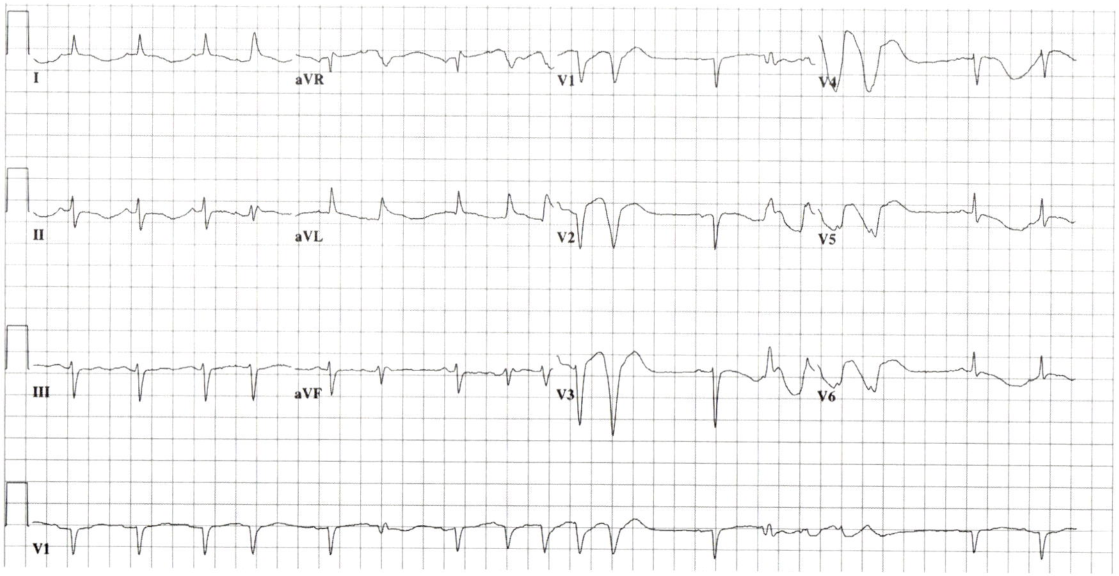

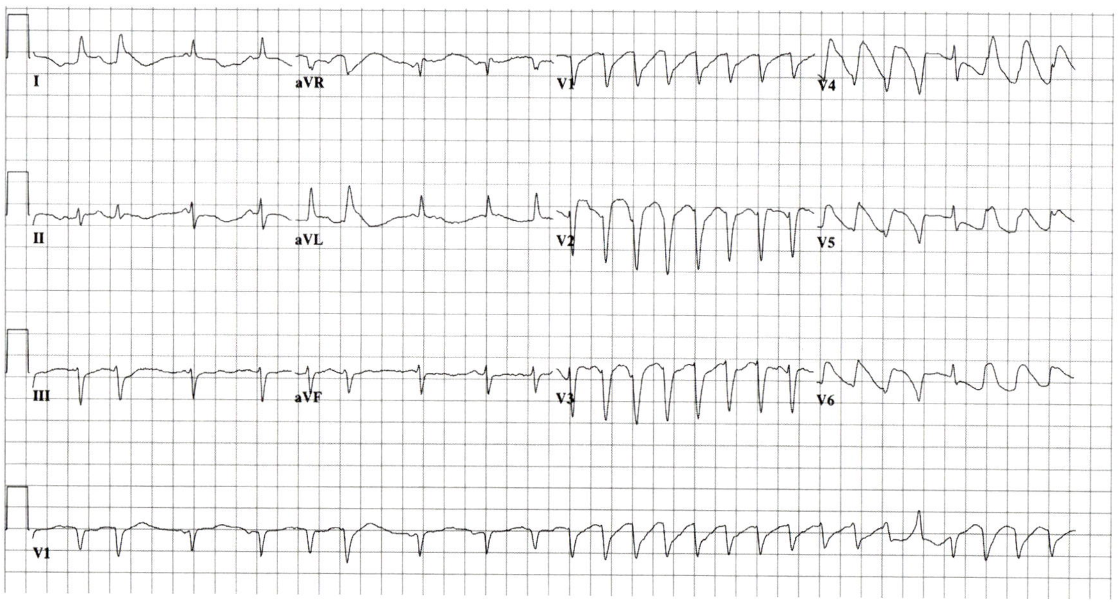

Case #123. **An 82-year-old woman admitted to the intensive care unit with sepsis, yesterday initiated on haloperidol for agitation, now with these tracings.**

QUESTIONS

123-1. Interpret these tracings: what is the rhythm?

123-2. How do you manage this arrhythmia?

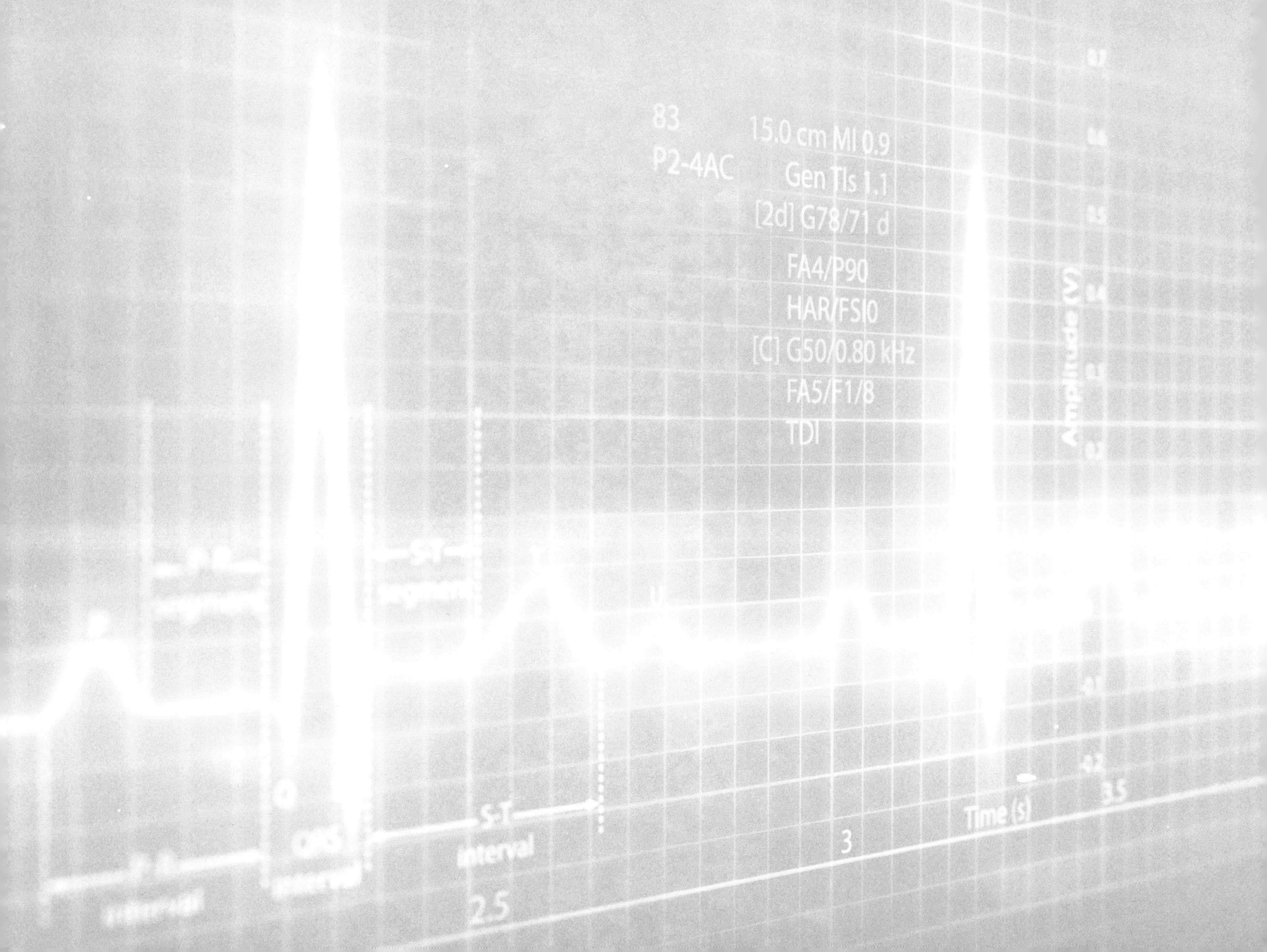
83
P2-4AC
15.0 cm MI 0.9
Gen TIs 1.1
[2d] G78/71 d
FA4/P90
HAR/FSI0
[C] G50/0.80 kHz
FA5/F1/8
TDI
Amplitude (V)
S-T
interval
2.5
3
Time (s)
3.5

ANSWERS

123-1. Interpret these tracings: what is the rhythm?

These tracings are complex and best assessed systematically. First, the rate: the R–R interval is variable throughout the tracings; hence, an assessment of the overall rate is best done by counting the number of QRS complexes in the 10-second rhythm strip and multiplying by 6. For the first tracing, the overall rate by this method is 108 beats/min; for the second tracing, the overall rate is 150 beats/min. There are 2 distinct rhythms: one wide complex and the other narrow complex. The first 3 beats of the first tracing are sinus beats at a rate of approximately 100 beats/min with clear P waves preceding each QRS in lead II. The fourth beat is a premature atrial contraction followed by another sinus beat. Hence, sinus rhythm is present for at least a portion of the tracing. The middle portion of the first tracing reveals short run of a wide complex tachycardia with subtly variable QRS morphology. This is followed by a pause, a sinus beat, another short run of wide complex tachycardia with variable QRS morphology, another pause, and 2 sinus beats. A very prolonged QT interval with deeply inverted T wave is evident, most obvious in leads I, II, and V4.

The second tracing is similar, starting in sinus rhythm with premature atrial and ventricular contractions. The second half of the tracing reveals a long run of wide complex tachycardia with variable QRS morphology and QRS axis—polymorphic ventricular tachycardia. Now, inspecting the sinus rhythm beats again, best seen on the first tracing: the axis is leftward. The QT interval, best visualized in lead II, is prolonged to almost 600 milliseconds. The T waves of the sinus beats are inverted. Note that the QT interval depends on the R–R interval: the QT interval prolongs even further after a pause, seen best examining the second to last QRS complex of the first tracing in leads V4 through V6.

Synthesizing the findings: There are runs of polymorphic ventricular tachycardia with shifting axis seen in the setting of a grossly prolonged QT. These findings suggest a type of polymorphic ventricular tachycardia called torsades de pointes or "twisting of the points." The rhythm is commonly initiated by a premature beat followed by a pause, which causes the QT interval to prolong further as seen here.

123-2. How do you manage this arrhythmia?

Causes of QT-interval prolongation and polymorphic ventricular tachycardia include electrolyte disturbance (hypokalemia, hypocalcemia, and hypomagnesemia), medication effect (antipsychotics, methadone, quinolone, and macrolide antibiotics), and genetic abnormalities. Electrolyte abnormalities should be corrected and offending medications withdrawn immediately. Infusions of magnesium, even in the absence of hypomagesemia, can terminate torsades. Given that the QT interval is longer at slower heart rates (longer R–R intervals), β-agonists or transvenous pacing can be used to avoid bradycardia. If the rhythm is sustained and hemodynamically unstable, ACLS measures should be initiated.

Case #124. A 22-year-old patient with complex cyanotic congenital heart disease seen in follow-up.

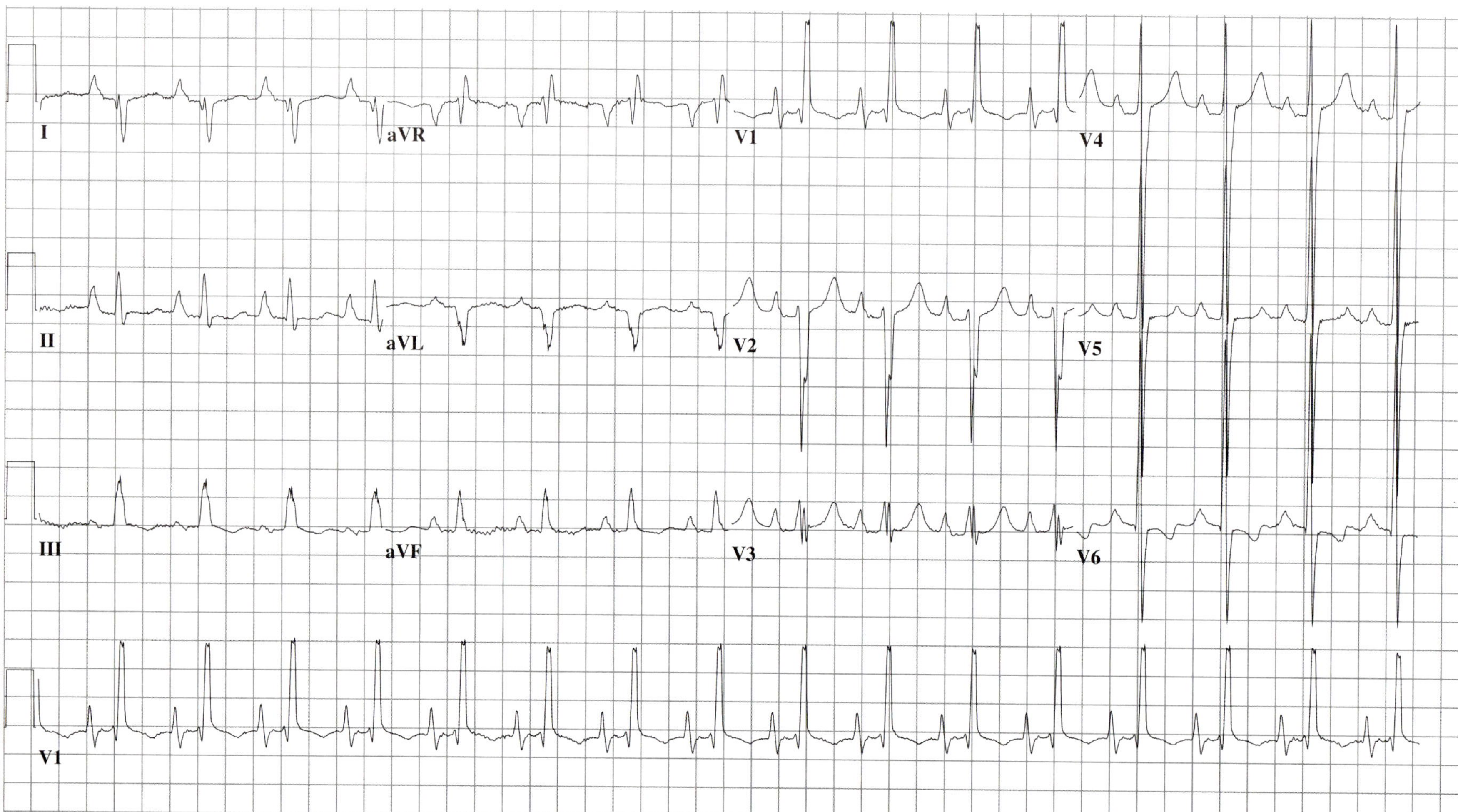

QUESTIONS

124-1. What are the abnormalities on the tracing?

124-2. What are some of the electrocardiographic clues that suggest biventricular hypertrophy?

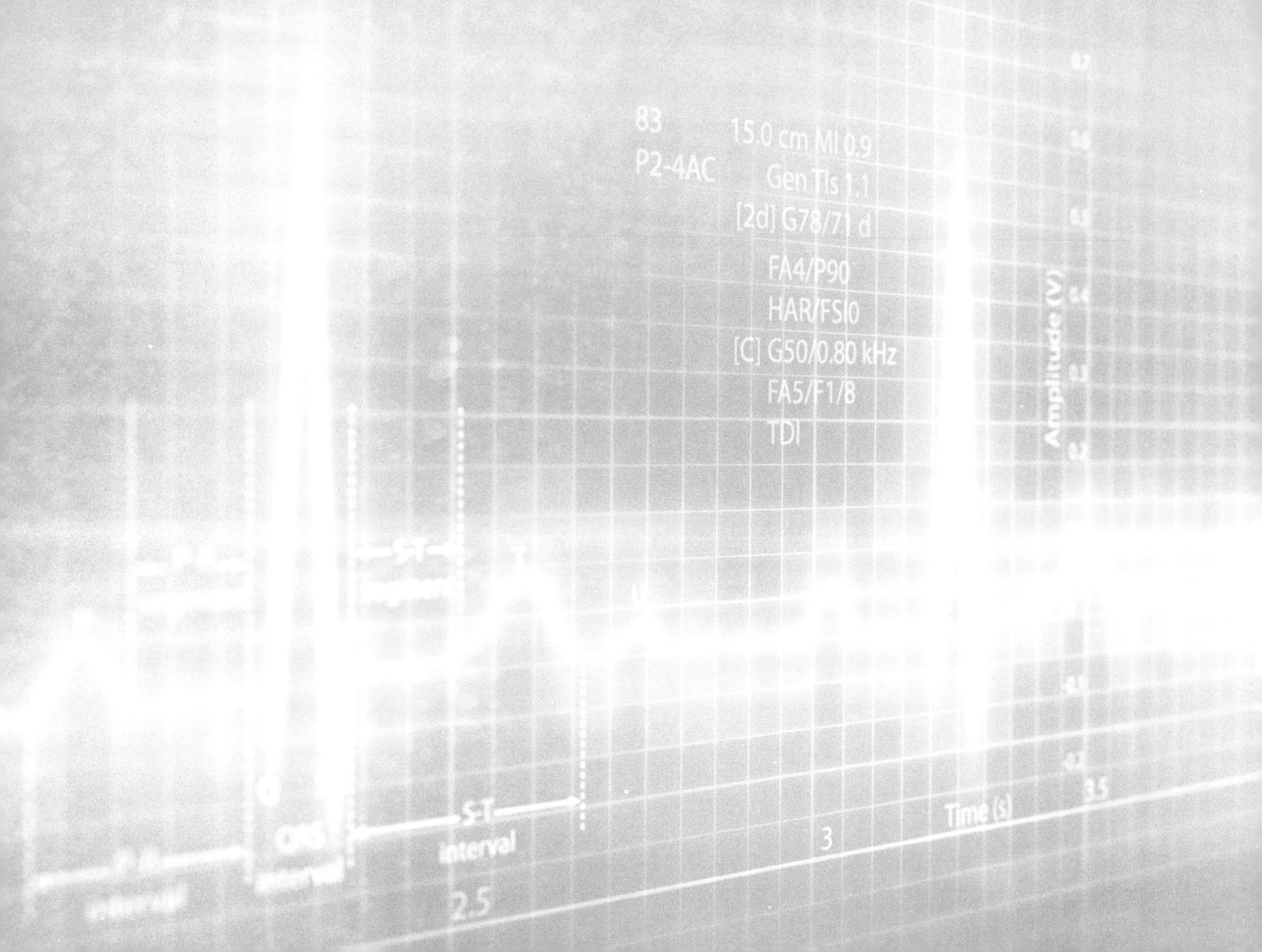
83
P2-4AC
15.0 cm MI 0.9
Gen TIs 1.1
[2d] G78/71 d
FA4/P90
HAR/FSI0
[C] G50/0.80 kHz
FA5/F1/8
TDI
Amplitude (V)
S-T
interval
Time (s)
2.5
3
3.5

ANSWERS

124-1. What are the abnormalities on the tracing?

This tracing demonstrates normal sinus rhythm at approximately 100 beats/min. There is right-axis deviation. The QRS has a right bundle branch block morphology with RSR′ in lead V1. There is evidence of both right and left atrial abnormality, left ventricular hypertrophy (LVH), and right ventricular hypertrophy.

124-2. What are some of the electrocardiographic clues that suggest biventricular hypertrophy?

Biventricular hypertrophy can be suggested by the presence of voltage criteria for LVH in the precordial leads coupled with right-axis deviation or a tall R wave in V1. Right ventricular hypertrophy in combination with left atrial enlargement is also suggestive. This patient had tetralogy of Fallot with pulmonary hypertension and Eisenmenger syndrome. The tetralogy of Fallot consists of a ventricular septal defect, overriding aorta, pulmonary stenosis, and right ventricular hypertrophy.

Case #125. An 18-year-old man with weakness.

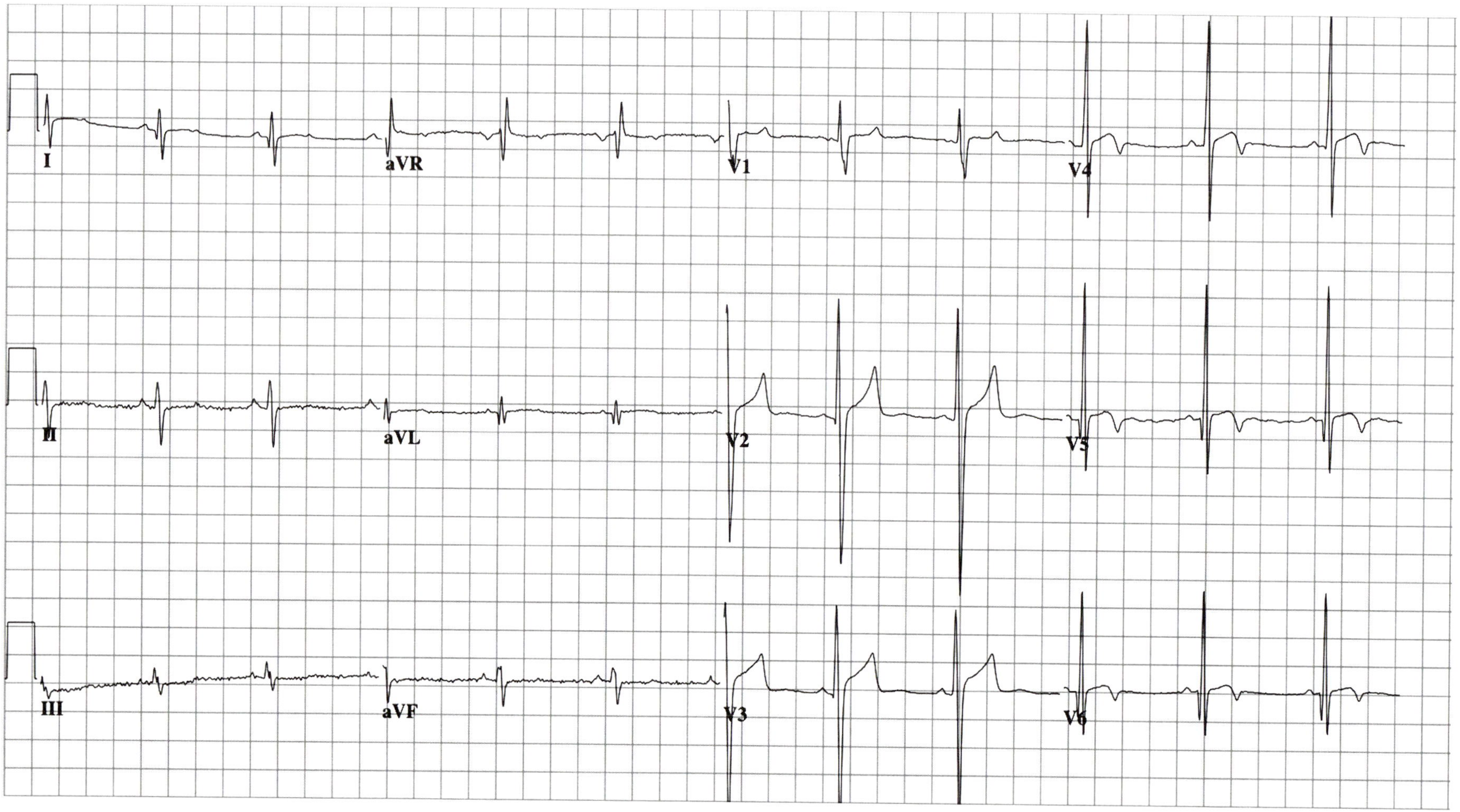

QUESTIONS

125-1. Interpret this ECG.

125-2. What is the differential diagnosis of a tall R wave in V1?

125-3. What systemic disease would cause these ECG findings?

83
P2-4AC
15.0 cm MI 0.9
Gen TIs 1.1
[2d] G78/71 d
FA4/P90
HAR/FSI0
[C] G50/0.80 kHz
FA5/F1/8
TDI
Amplitude (V)
Time (s)
2.5
3
3.5

ANSWERS

125-1. Interpret this ECG.

Sinus rhythm is present at a rate of 70 beats/min. The QRS axis is in the northwest quadrant, approximately −120 degrees. Narrow Q waves are present in leads I, aVL, V5, and V6 with biphasic T waves in V4 through V6. A tall R wave in present in leads V1 and V2.

125-2. What is the differential diagnosis of a tall R wave in V1?

A tall R wave in lead V1 can be secondary to right ventricular hypertrophy, posterior myocardial infarction, or Wolff-Parkinson-White syndrome. A tall R wave in lead V1 is also characteristic of patients with muscular dystrophy and cardiac involvement.

125-3. What systemic disease would cause these ECG findings?

This patient has muscular dystrophy. The muscular dystrophies can involve the myocardium and cardiac conduction system producing fibrosis in a characteristic posterobasal distribution, leading to the observed abnormalities in axis, R-wave progression, and the narrow lateral Q waves. An echocardiogram would be useful to screen for systolic dysfunction and guide appropriate therapies for heart failure.

Case #126. A 78-year-old gentleman with a history of coronary artery disease presents with 30 seconds of left-hand weakness consistent with transient ischemic attack.

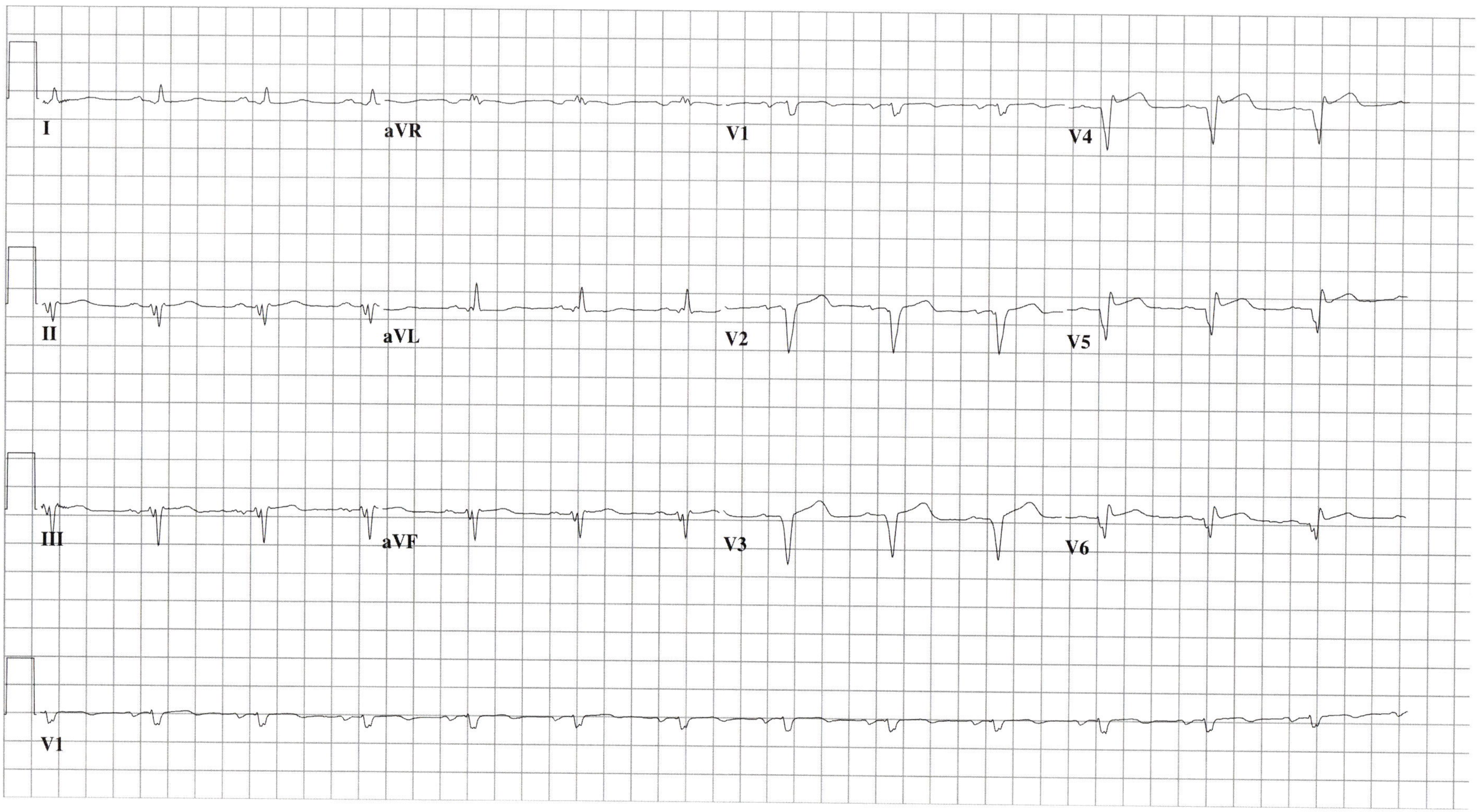

QUESTIONS

126-1. Interpret this ECG.

126-2. What is the differential diagnosis for the ECG abnormalities? Are there clues as to the possible reason for the patient's transient ischemic attack?

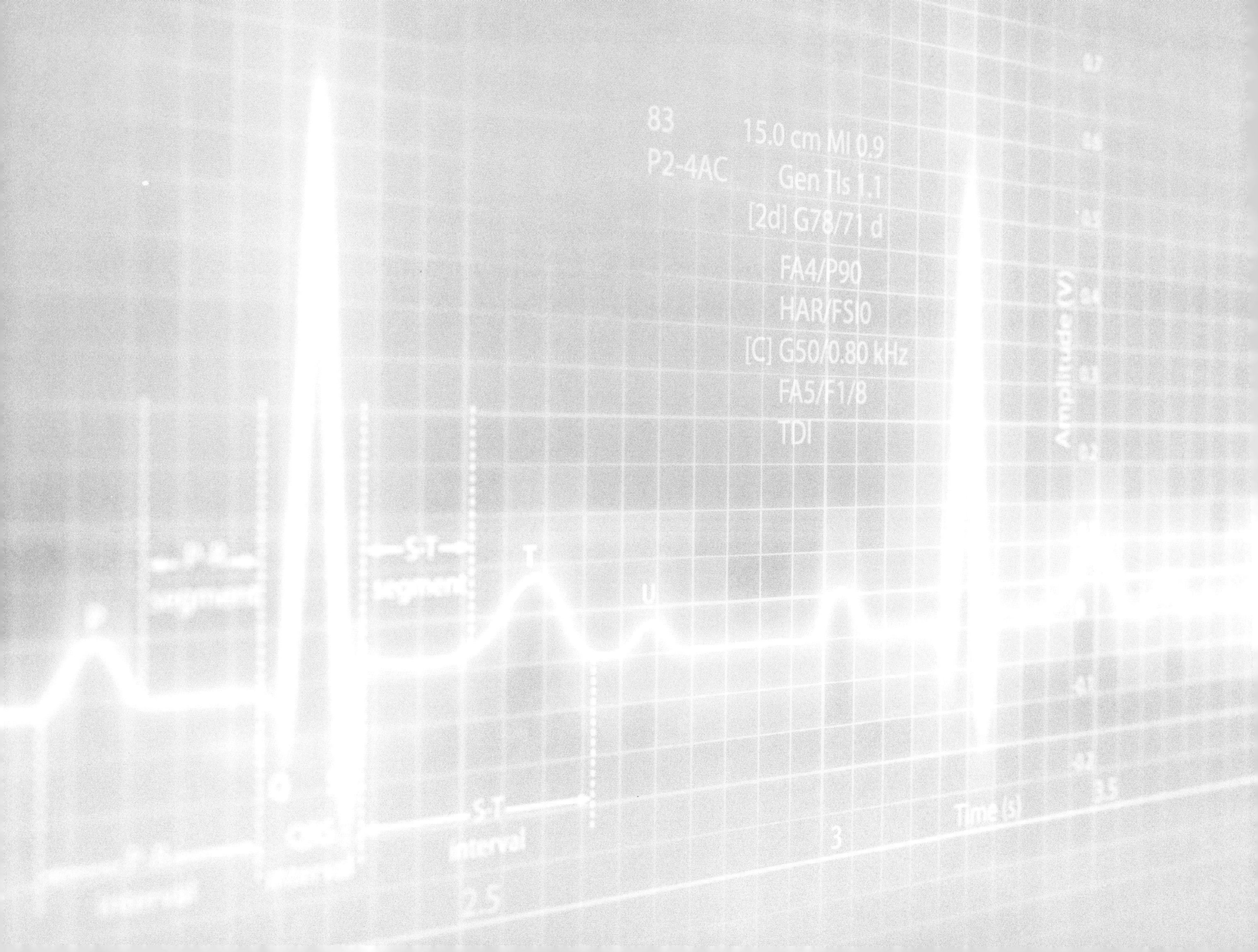
83
P2-4AC
15.0 cm MI 0.9
Gen TIs 1.1
[2d] G78/71 d
FA4/P90
HAR/FS|0
[C] G50/0.80 kHz
FA5/F1/8
TDI
Amplitude (V)
S-T segment
T
U
S-T interval
Time (s)
3
3.5
2.5

ANSWERS

126-1. Interpret this ECG.

Sinus rhythm is present at a rate of approximately 80 beats/min. The QRS is positive in lead I and negative in leads aVF and II consistent with leftward axis. The PR interval is at the upper limit of normal at 200 milliseconds. The QRS complex is widened to 120 milliseconds; however, the morphology of the QRS is not consistent with either right or left bundle branch block. Hence, a nonspecific interventricular conduction delay is diagnosed. There are broad, pathologic Q waves present in the anterior leads V2, V3, V4, V5, and V6. In leads V4, V5, and V6, there is 2 mm of ST-segment elevation with upright T waves.

126-2. What is the differential diagnosis for the ECG abnormalities? Are there clues as to the possible reason for the patient's transient ischemic attack?

Differential diagnosis of ST-segment elevation on the ECG includes ischemia and many other causes including repolarization abnormalities, pericarditis, electrolyte abnormalities, and left ventricular aneurysm.[1] In this case, the constellation of a history of coronary disease but absence of an ischemic syndrome, Q waves on the ECG with ST elevation, and upright T waves is consistent with left ventricular aneurysm, which was confirmed on echocardiogram. Left ventricular aneurysms can induce stasis of blood and thrombus formation, which cause TIA or ischemic stroke if embolization occurs.

[1]Wang K, Asinger RW, Marriott HJL. ST-segment elevation in conditions other than acute myocardial infarction. *New Engl J Med* 2003; 349: 2128-2135.

Case #127. A 55-year-old man undergoing therapeutic hypothermia after cardiac arrest.

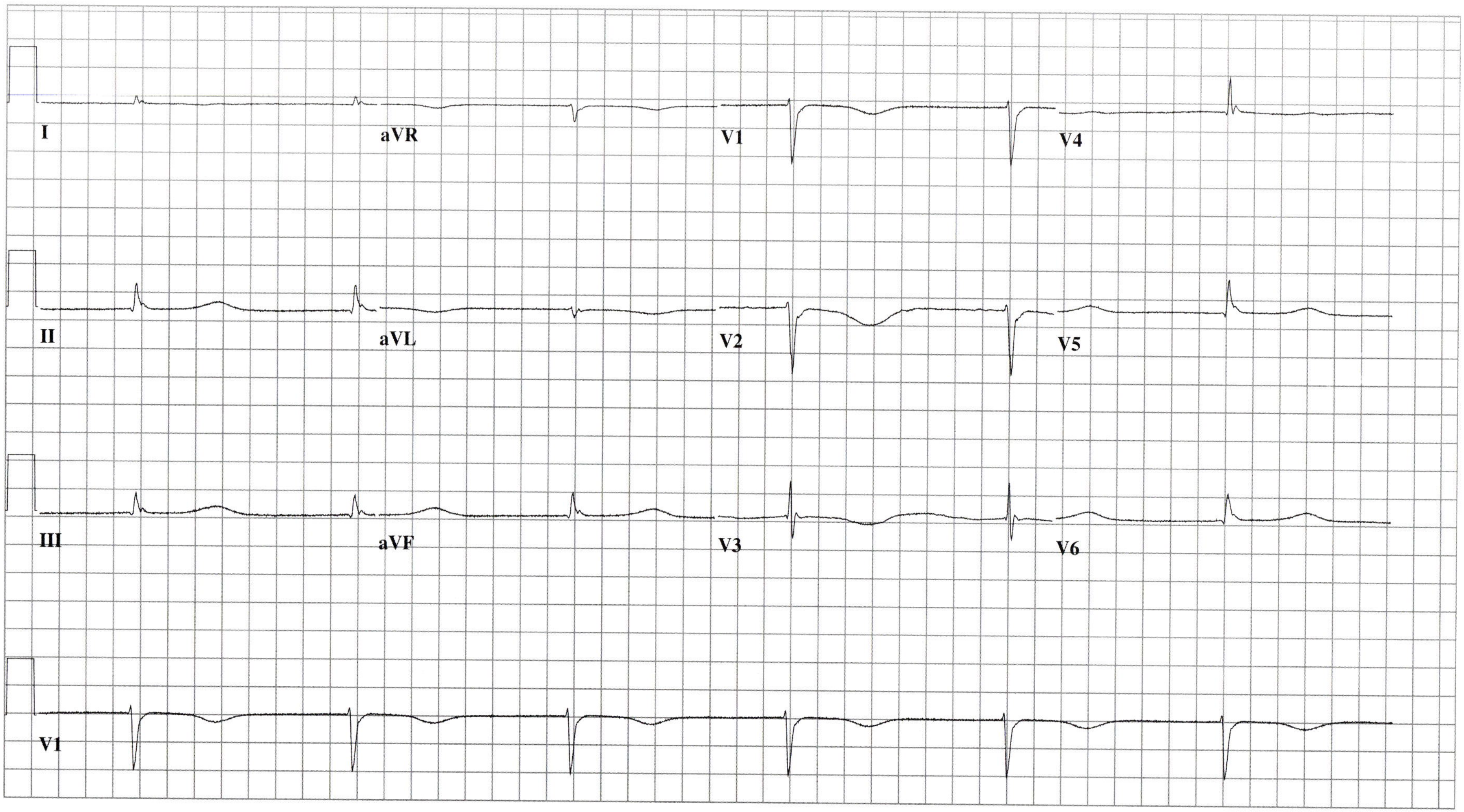

QUESTIONS

127-1. Interpret this ECG. What is the rhythm?

127-2. How many abnormalities can you identify on this ECG?

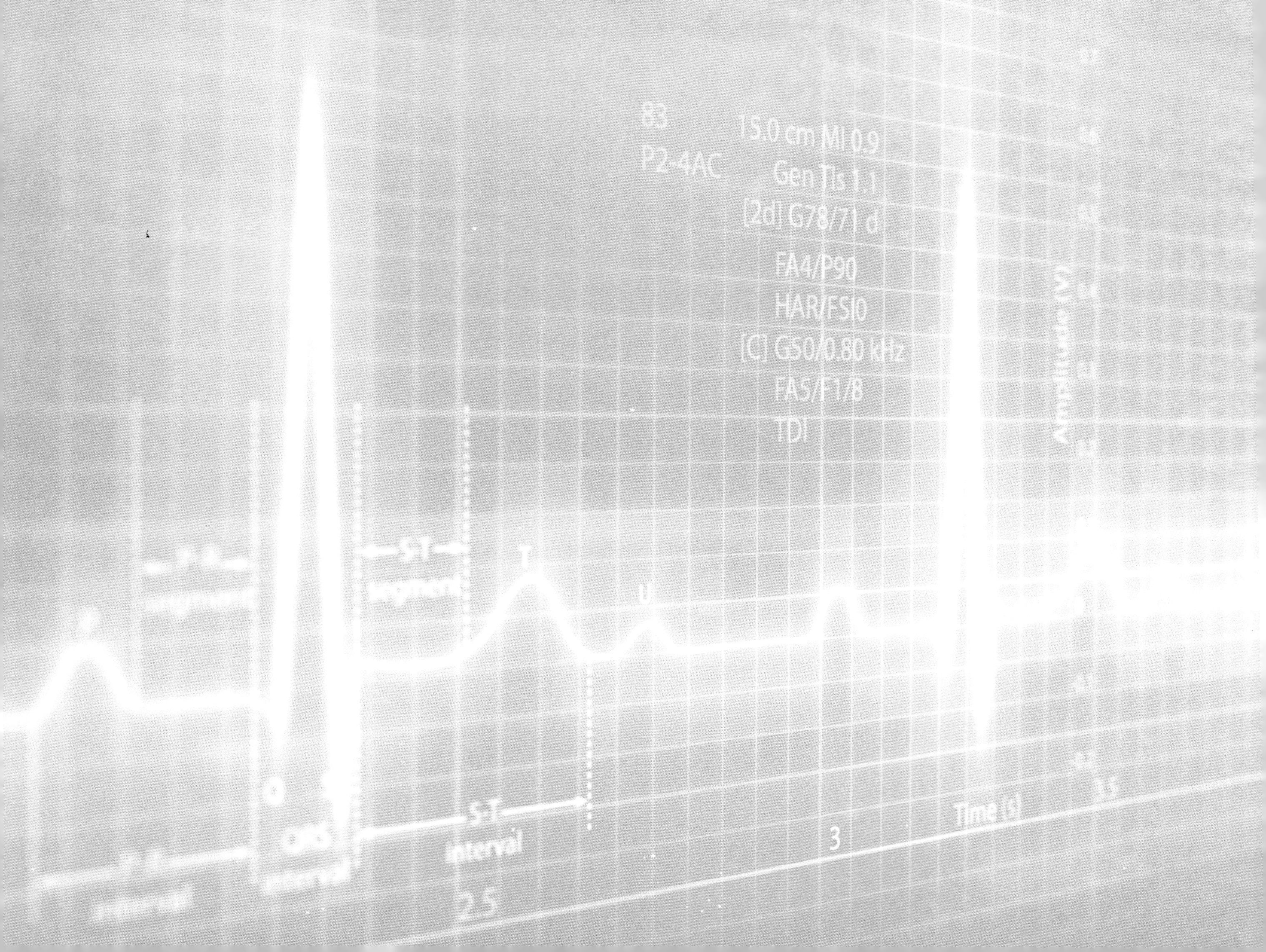
83
P2-4AC
15.0 cm MI 0.9
Gen Tls 1.1
[2d] G78/71 d
FA4/P90
HAR/FSI0
[C] G50/0.80 kHz
FA5/F1/8
TDI
Amplitude (V)
S-T
segment
T
U
S-T
interval
QRS
interval
3
3.5
2.5
Time (s)

ANSWERS

127-1. Interpret this ECG. What is the rhythm?

The ECG demonstrates a regular narrow complex bradycardia at 36 beats/min. There is no atrial activity. The differential diagnosis for this rhythm is sinus arrest (complete cessation of sinus node activity) with a bradycardic junctional escape mechanism or underlying fine atrial fibrillation with complete heart block and a junctional escape mechanism. Sinus arrest is favored in this case, as the baseline between QRS complexes is completely isoelectric with no evidence of fibrillatory waves. The QRS axis is normal. The voltage is low in the limb leads (less than 5 mV in all limb leads), but the precordial leads do not meet criteria for low voltage (less than 10 mV in all precordial leads). The QT interval is strikingly prolonged to approximately 800 milliseconds (uncorrected for rate). There are T-wave inversions in leads V1 through V3.

127-2. How many abnormalities can you identify on this ECG?

Sinus arrest, junctional bradycardia, prolonged QT interval, inverted T waves, and low limb-lead voltage are 5 easy-to-spot abnormalities. There is a sixth subtle abnormality—in the figure, close inspection of the terminal portion of the QRS complex reveals a small positive, rounded deflection called an Osborn wave. The Osborn wave is often seen in hypothermic states.[1]

[1]Hurst JW. Naming of the waves in the ECG, with a brief account of their genesis. *Circulation* 1998; 98: 1937-1942.

ANSWERS (Cont.)

Subtle Osborn waves are visualized as positive deflections after the QRS complex. Osborn waves can be seen in states of hypothermia.

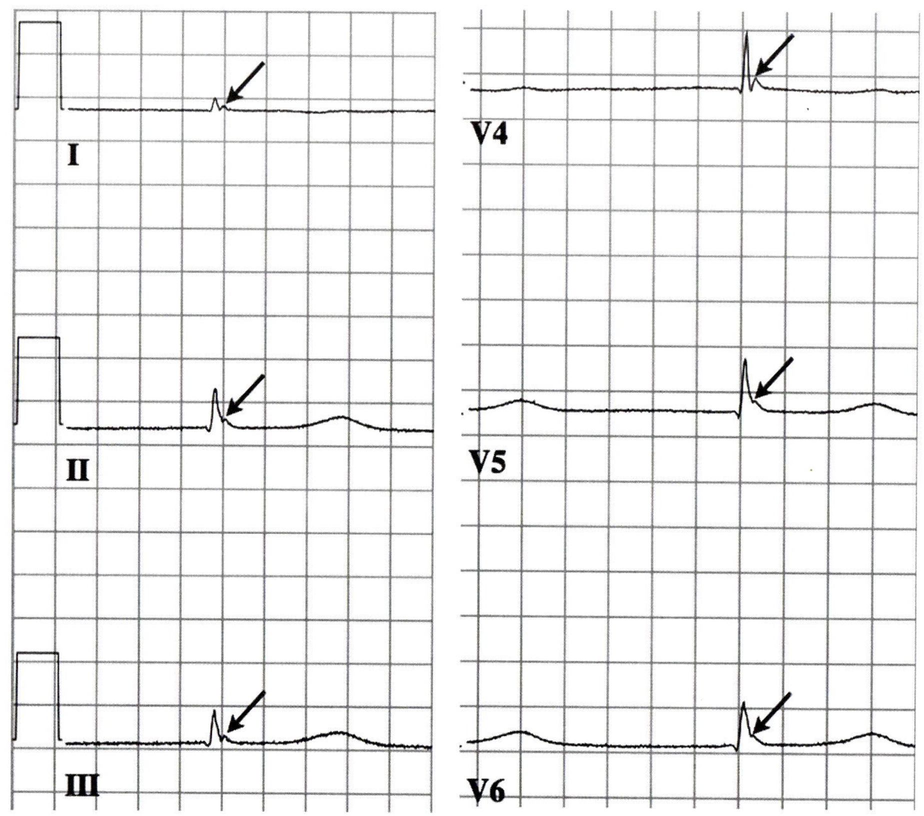

Case #128. A 67-year-old woman presents with palpitations.

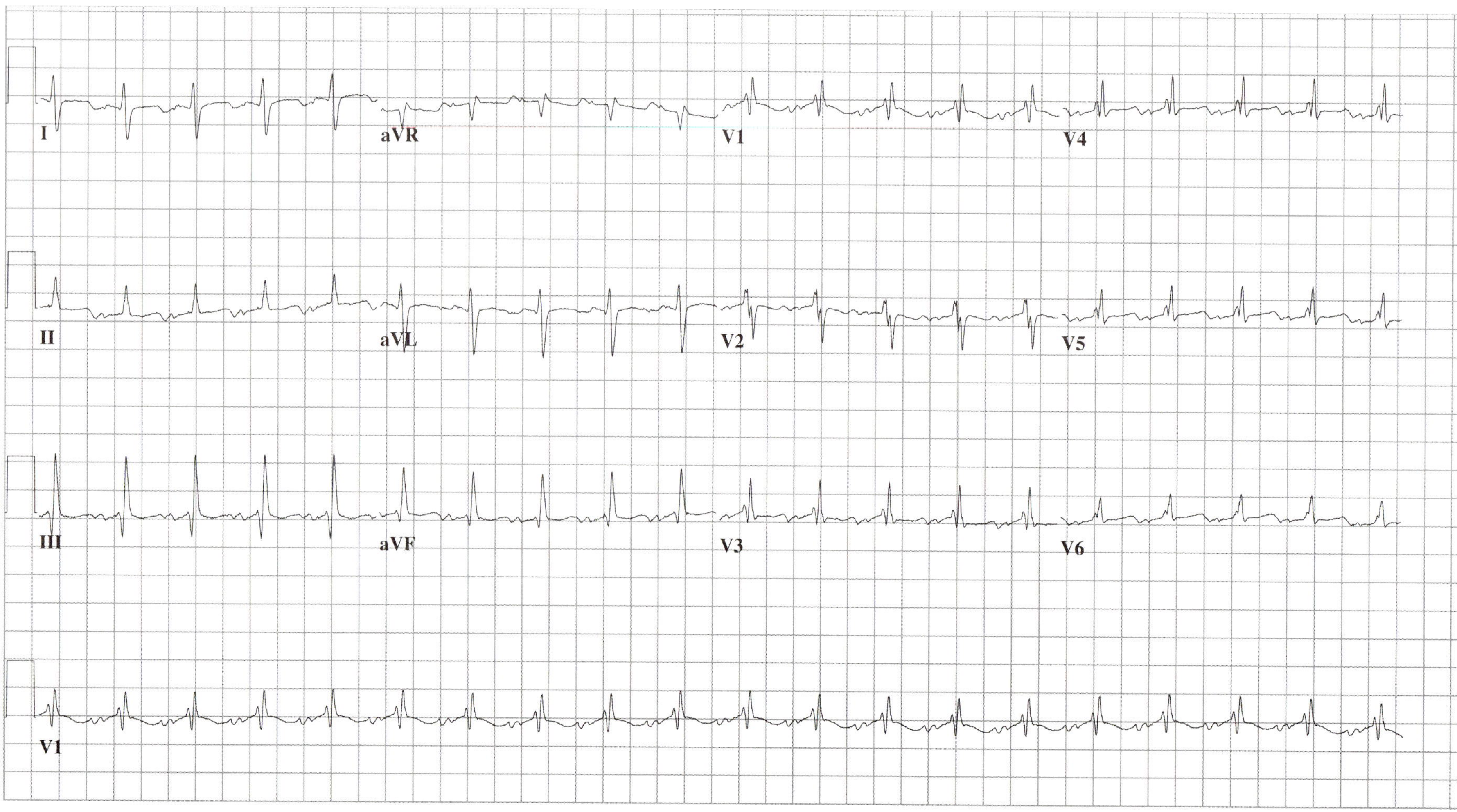

QUESTION

128-1. Interpret this ECG.

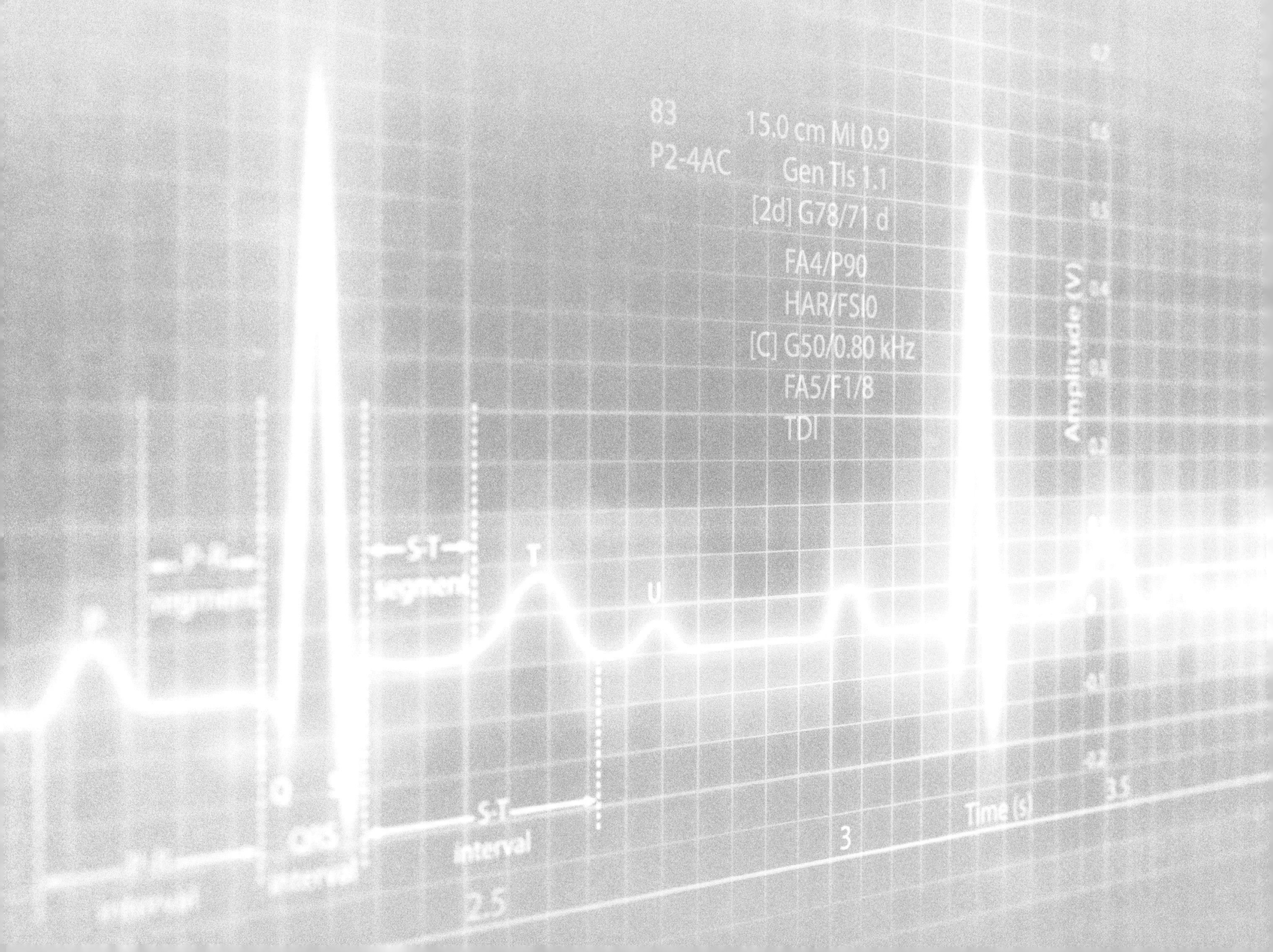
83
15.0 cm MI 0.9
P2-4AC
Gen Tls 1.1
[2d] G78/71 d
FA4/P90
HAR/FSI0
[C] G50/0.80 kHz
FA5/F1/8
TDI
Amplitude (V)
S-T
segment
T
U
S-T
interval
QRS
interval
Time (s)
2.5
3
3.5

ANSWER

128-1. Interpret this ECG.

This tracing reveals a regular tachycardia at a rate of 120 beats/min. Axis is rightward. P waves precede each QRS complex with a prolonged PR interval over 200 milliseconds. The P waves have an abnormal morphology—triphasic in lead V1, predominantly negative in lead I, and triphasic in the inferior leads including lead II. In contrast, recall that normal sinus P waves are upright in leads II, III, and aVF and biphasic in lead V1. The figure demonstrates P waves in this tracing contrasted with normal sinus P waves. This rhythm thus represents an ectopic atrial tachycardia. Other findings include an incomplete right bundle branch block, with an RSR′ morphology in lead V1 but total QRS duration less than 120 milliseconds. There are diffuse ST-segment abnormalities that are nonspecific.

This patient's P waves compared to normal sinus P waves.

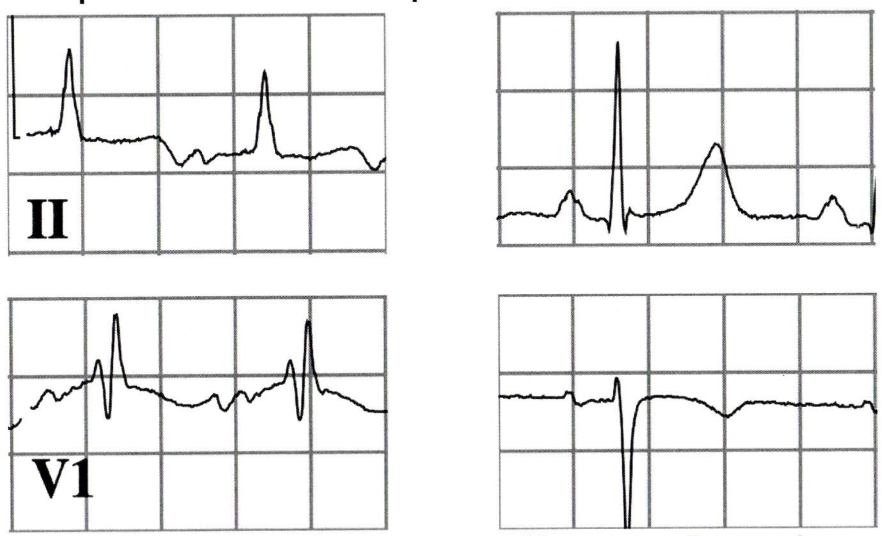

This patient's P waves are triphasic in leads II and V1

Normal sinus P waves that are positive in lead II and biphasic in lead V1

Case #129. A 22-year-old asymptomatic woman with a family history of sudden unexplained death.

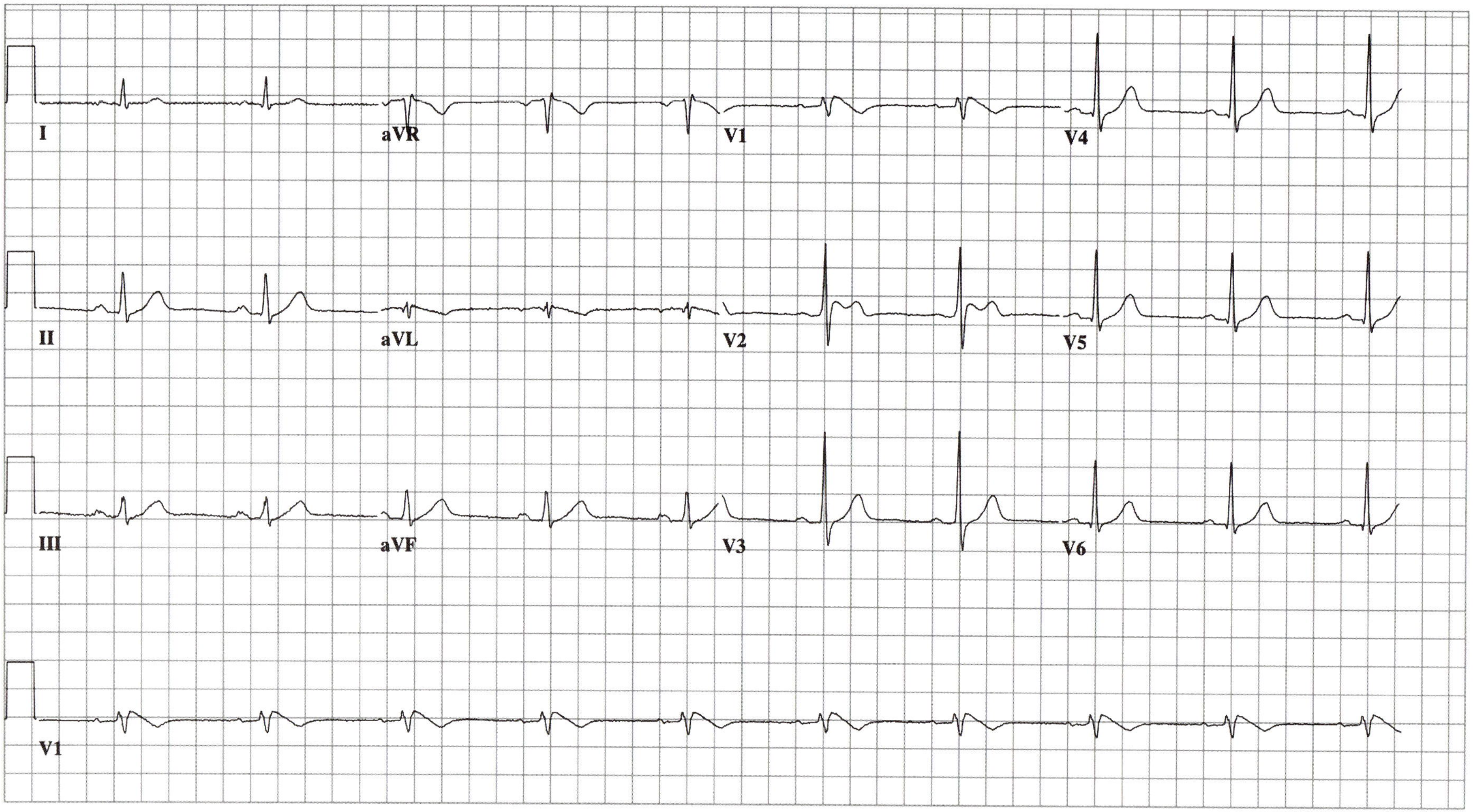

QUESTIONS

129-1. Interpret this ECG.

129-2. What is the diagnosis?

83
P2-4AC
15.0 cm MI 0.9
Gen TIs 1.1
[2d] G78/71 d
FA4/P90
HAR/FSI0
[C] G50/0.80 kHz
FA5/F1/8
TDI
S-T
interval
QRS
interval
2.5
3
3.5
Time (s)
Amplitude (V)

ANSWERS

129-1. Interpret this ECG.

This tracing reveals sinus rhythm at 60 beats/min. The intervals and axis are normal, and there is no evidence of chamber enlargement. Close inspection of V1 reveals 2 mm of downsloping, coved ST-segment elevation leading into an inverted T wave; in V2, there is ST-segment elevation with a biphasic or "saddleback" pattern to the ST segment.

129-2. What is the diagnosis?

This ECG is consistent with Brugada type II pattern. Criteria include the "saddleback"-type ST segment and ST elevation in the precordial leads. This ECG pattern can be considered suggestive of Brugada syndrome, in contrast to the type I pattern, which is considered diagnostic given a suggestive clinical circumstance. The appropriate evaluation of an asymptomatic patient with a Brugada type II ECG is controversial.

Case #130. A 38-year-old gentleman presents with progressive dyspnea on exertion for the past 6 months.

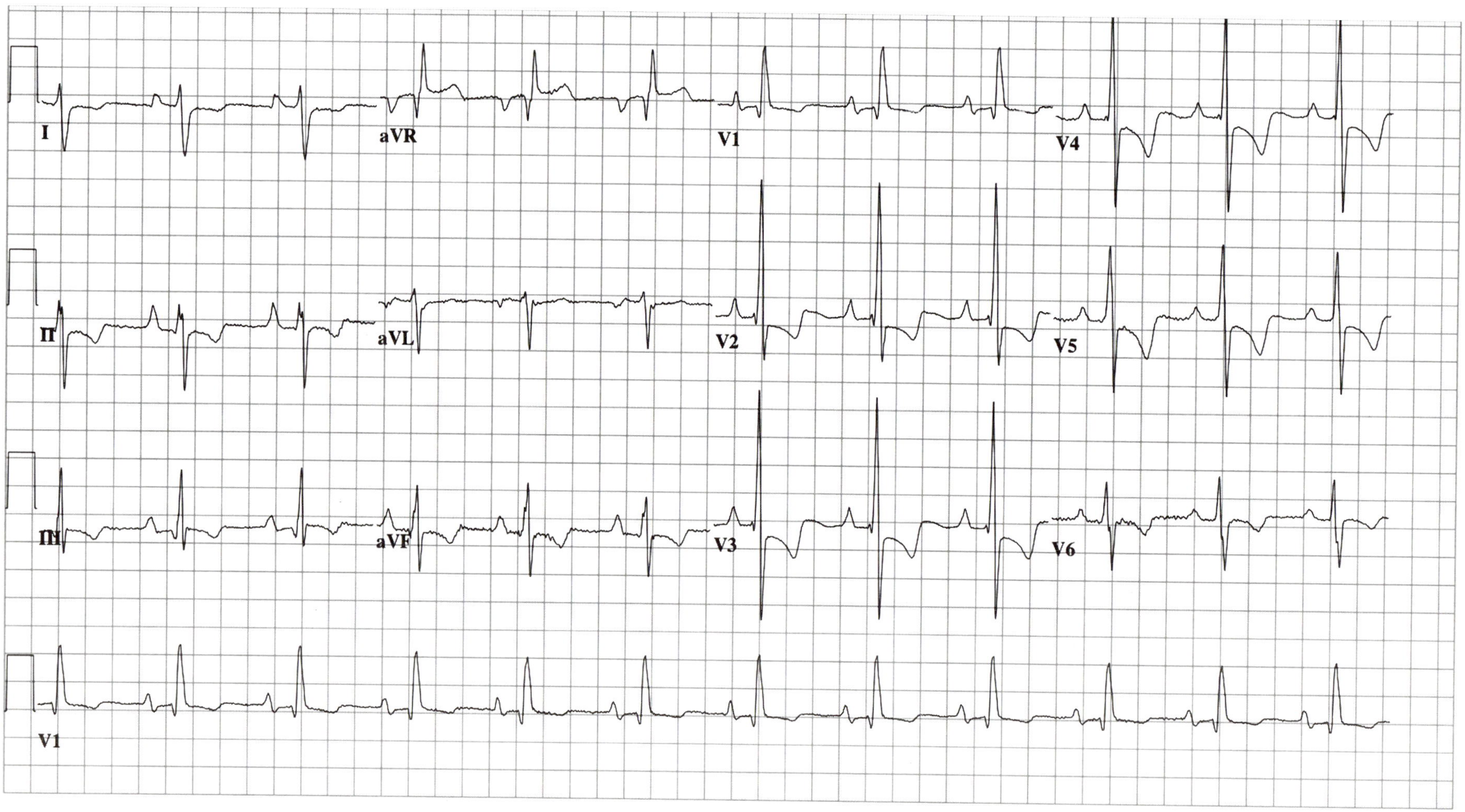

QUESTIONS

130-1. What abnormalities are present?

130-2. What are some of the physical exam findings that may be present in this patient?

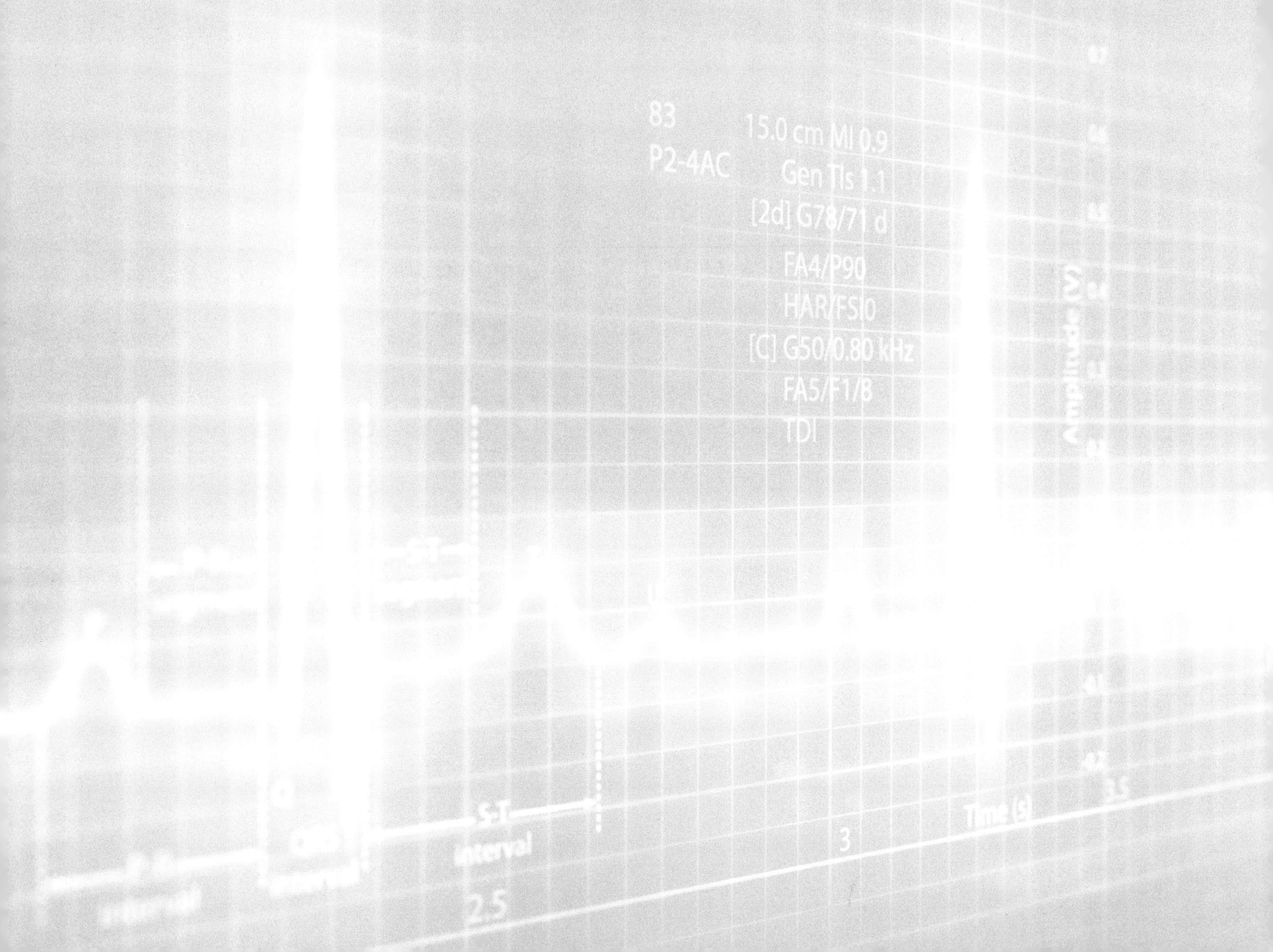
83
P2-4AC
15.0 cm MI 0.9
Gen Tls 1.1
[2d] G78/71 d
FA4/P90
HAR/FSI0
[C] G50/0.80 kHz
FA5/F1/8
TDI
Amplitude (V)
S-T
interval
Time (s)
2.5
3
3.5

ANSWERS

130-1. What abnormalities are present?

This tracing demonstrates normal sinus rhythm at a rate of 70 beats/min. There is right-axis deviation. There is evidence of right atrial abnormality based on P-wave amplitude greater than 2.5 mV in lead II and P-wave amplitude in lead V1 greater than 1.5 mV. There is also evidence of right ventricular hypertrophy. Finally, there are T-wave inversions and ST-segment depressions most notable in the anterior leads, consistent with right ventricular strain.

130-2. What are some of the physical exam findings that may be present in this patient?

This patient's ECG demonstrates multiple abnormalities of the right heart. Pulmonary hypertension was confirmed with echocardiogram and right heart catheterization. The classic physical exam findings in patients with pulmonary hypertension include increased loudness of the pulmonic component of the second heart sound, pulmonary valve regurgitation, and a right-sided third heart sound if RV failure is present. Significant tricuspid regurgitation is often present, manifesting as a holosystolic murmur at the left lower sternal border with prominent V waves in the jugular venous pulse.

Case #131. A 66-year-old woman presents with syncope and has a procedure performed.

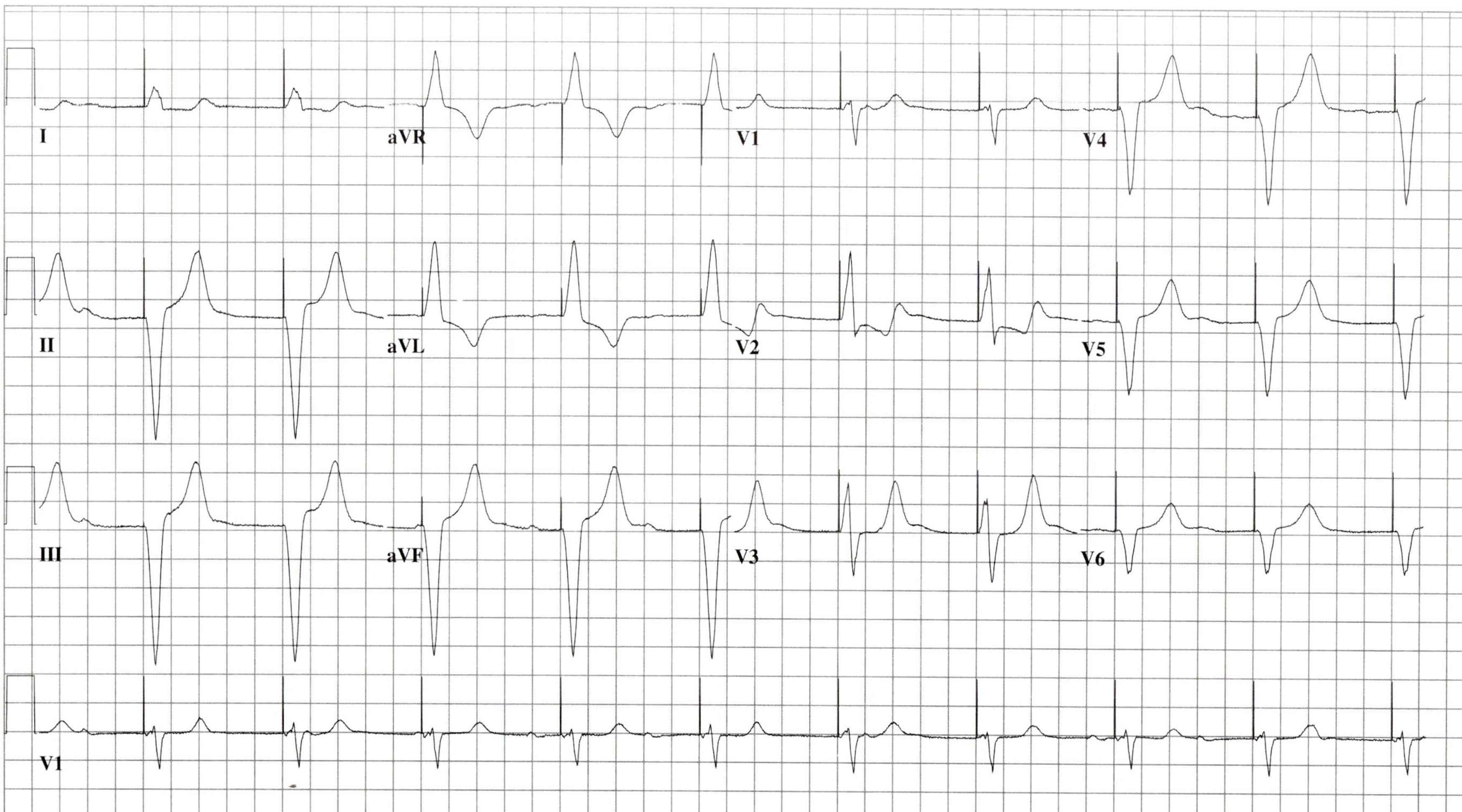

QUESTION

131-1. Interpret this ECG. What is the rhythm? What procedure was performed?

83
15.0 cm MI 0.9
P2-4AC
Gen TIs 1.1
[2d] G78/71 d
FA4/P90
HAR/FSI0
[C] G50/0.80 kHz
FA5/F1/B
TDI
Amplitude (V)
S-T
interval
QRS
interval
P-R
interval
2.5
3
3.5
Time (s)

ANSWER

131-1. Interpret this ECG. What is the rhythm? What procedure was performed?

The ventricular rate is 60 beats/min. QRS complexes are wide and each QRS is preceded by a pacemaker impulse consistent with ventricular pacing. Close inspection of the rhythm strip reveals P waves marching through the QRS complexes without any A-V synchrony. This is consistent with complete heart block and placement of a single pacemaker lead in the ventricle providing ventricular pacing. If there were an atrial pacemaker lead present, the ventricular lead could be programmed to track the atrial impulses restoring A-V synchrony. The figure illustrates the P waves "marching through" the ventricular paced impulses.

P waves, marked with asterisks, are dissociated from the QRS complexes: Complete heart block with a single-lead ventricular pacemaker is present.

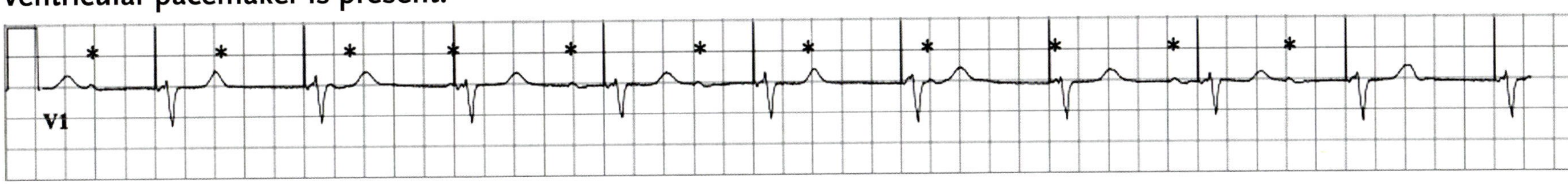

Case #132. A 77-year-old patient with known rheumatic mitral stenosis, maintained on digoxin, presents with palpitations.

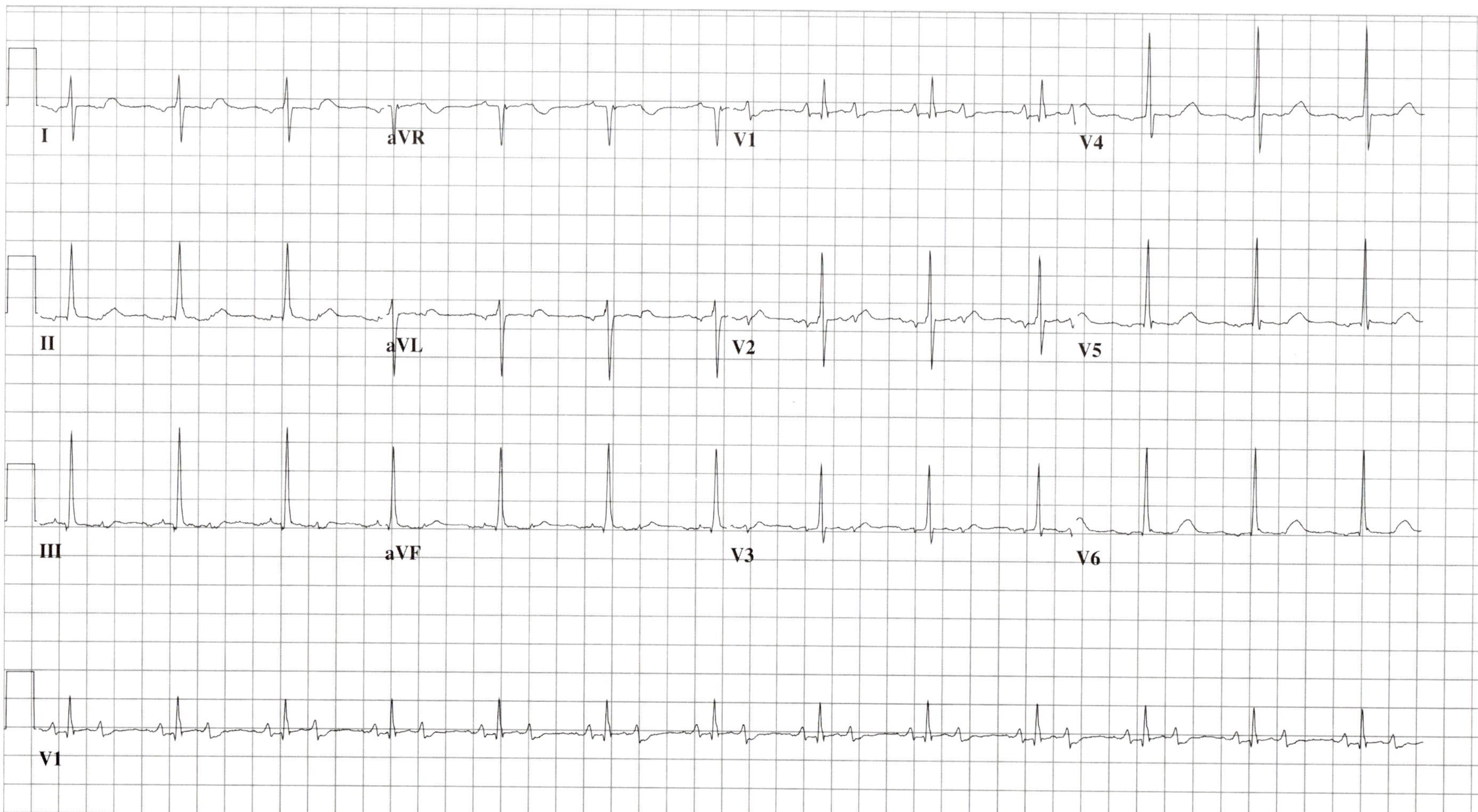

QUESTIONS

132-1. Interpret this tracing.

132-2. What are the common rhythms seen in digoxin toxicity?

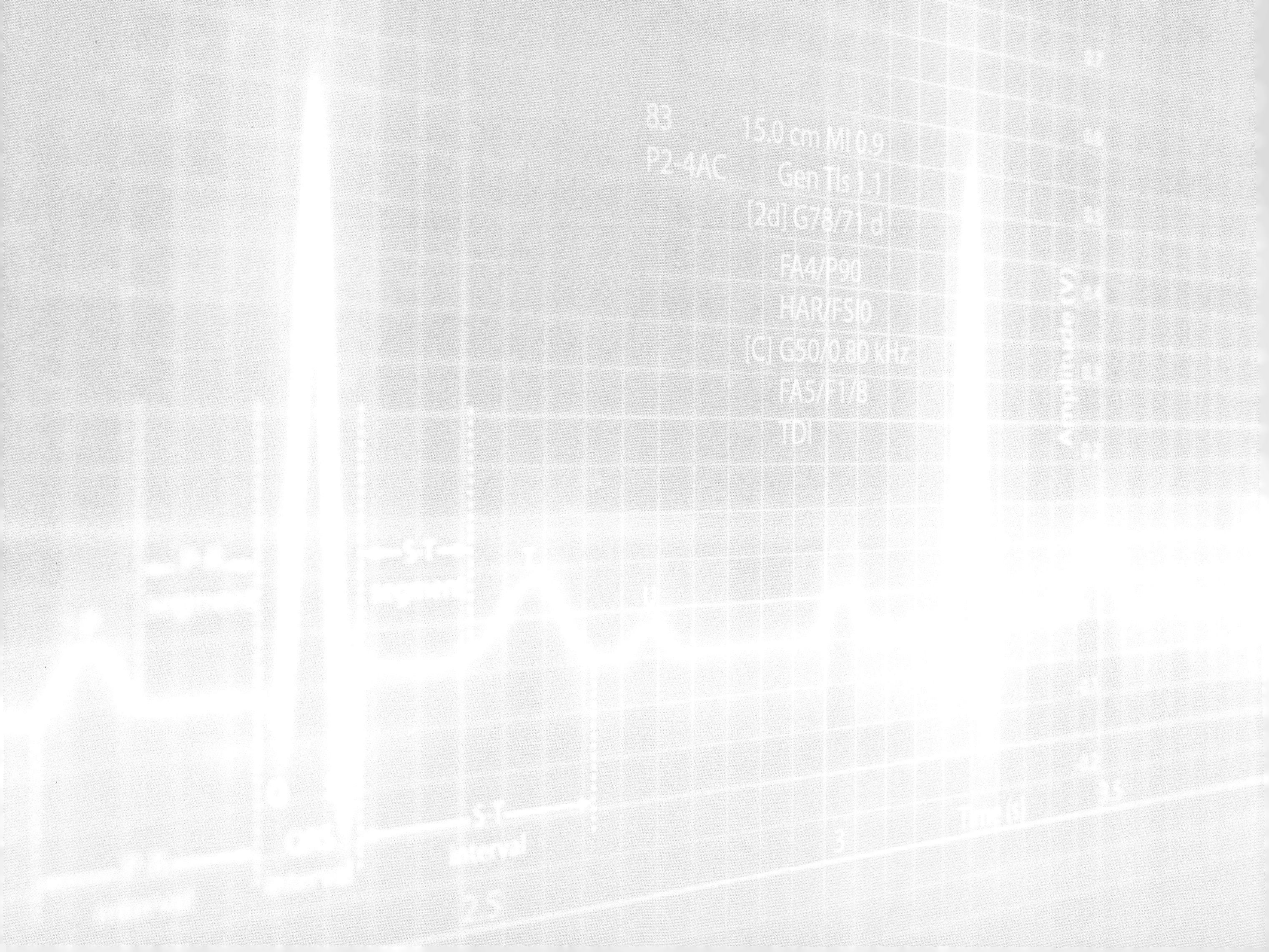
83
P2-4AC
15.0 cm MI 0.9
Gen TIs 1.1
[2d] G78/71 d
FA4/P90
HAR/FSI0
[C] G50/0.80 kHz
FA5/F1/8
TDI
S-T
interval
2.5
3

ANSWERS

132-1. Interpret this tracing.

This is a complex ECG with multiple abnormalities. The ventricular rate is approximately 75 beats/min. There are 2 P waves for each QRS complex, consistent with 2-to-1 AV block. The P waves have an abnormal morphology, negative polarity in leads II and I, consistent with a nonsinus origin. The atrial rate is approximately 150 beats/min. The rhythm is thus ectopic atrial tachycardia with 2-to-1 AV block. The axis is rightward with a tall R wave in V1 consistent with right ventricular hypertrophy from the patient's known mitral stenosis. Subtle downsloping ST-segment depression is seen throughout consistent with digoxin effect.

132-2. What are the common rhythms seen in digoxin toxicity?

One must distinguish between digoxin effect and digoxin toxicity. Digoxin effect manifests as downsloping ST-segment depression with a "scooped" configuration. This is not pathologic, but rather an expected finding when digoxin is used. Digoxin toxicity, in contrast, can cause both increased cardiac automaticity and AV block. Atrial tachycardia with block is one of several rhythms classically observed in the setting of digoxin toxicity. Other classic rhythms include bidirectional ventricular tachycardia (ventricular tachycardia with alternating QRS axis), and atrial fibrillation with complete heart block and an accelerated junctional escape, which results in "regularization" of atrial fibrillation.

Case #133. A 62-year-old man presents with cardiac arrest. Tracings pre and post defibrillation are shown.

Pre-defibrillation:

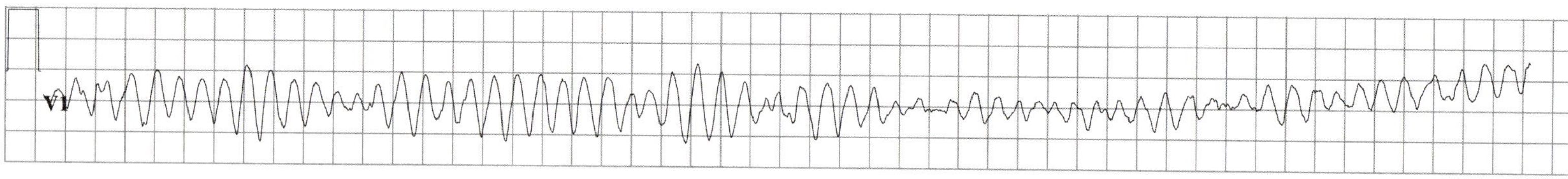

Post-defibrillation:

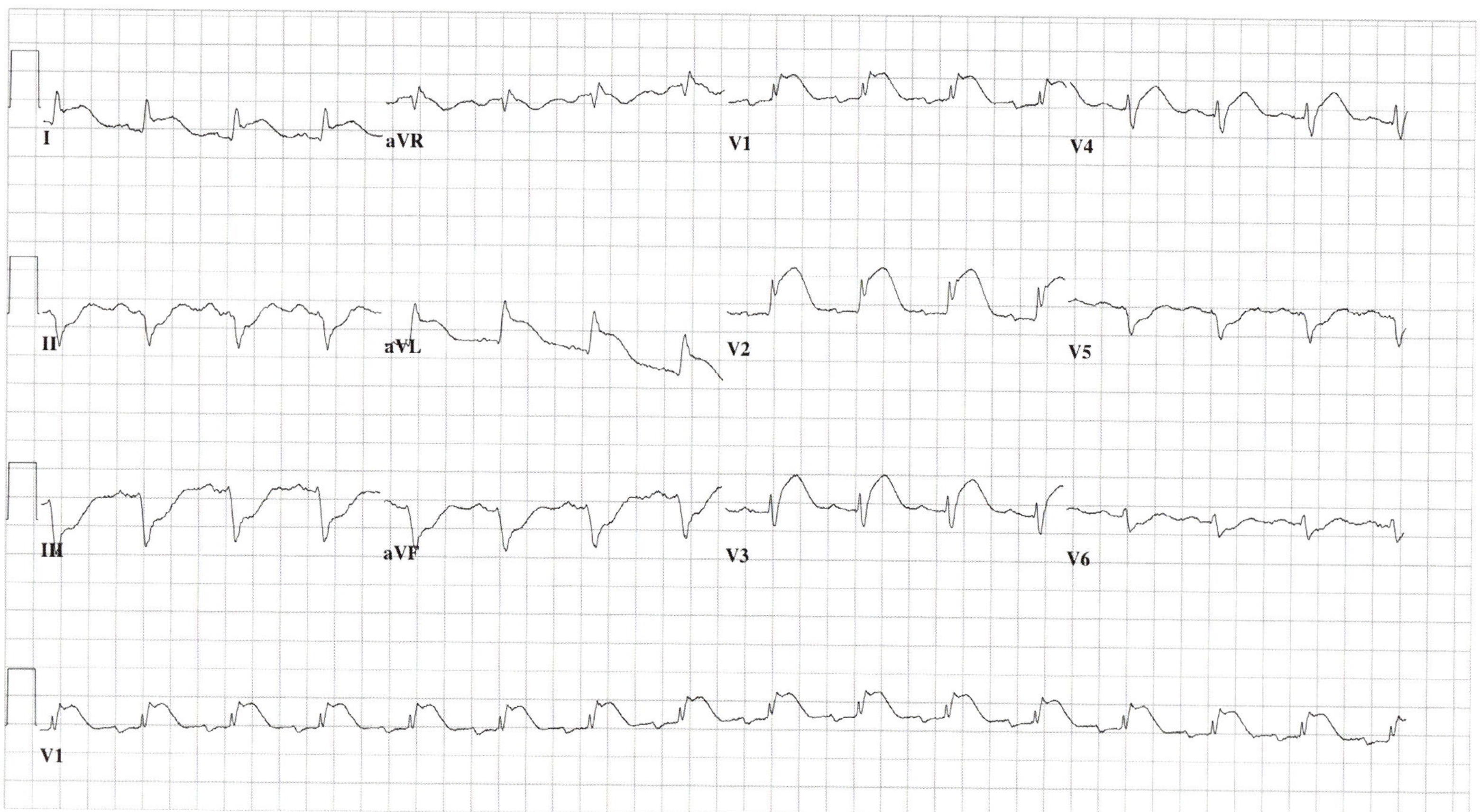

QUESTIONS

133-1. What does the pre-defibrillation ECG strip demonstrate?

133-2. What are the findings of the post-defibrillation ECG?

83
P2-4AC
15.0 cm MI 0.9
Gen TIs 1.1
[2d] G78/71 d
FA4/P90
HAR/FSI0
[C] G50/0.80 kHz
FA5/F1/B
TDI
Amplitude (V)
3
2.5

ANSWERS

133-1. What does the pre-defibrillation ECG strip demonstrate?

The first portion of the strip demonstrates a very fast polymorphic VT, which then degenerates into a chaotic, rapid rhythm with no discernible, regular electrical activity. The rate is unphysiologic at greater than 300 beats/min. This is an example of ventricular fibrillation.

133-2. What are the findings of the post-defibrillation ECG?

Post defibrillation, there is sinus rhythm with first-degree AV block. The axis is leftward. There is an RSR′ wave in lead V1 consistent with incomplete right bundle branch block. There are ST-segment elevations in leads I, aVL, and V1 through V4 with reciprocal depressions in the inferior leads. Thus, the diagnosis is proximal occlusion of the left anterior descending coronary artery leading to ventricular fibrillation. After defibrillation, this patient underwent successful primary PCI of the occluded LAD.

Case #134. A 66-year-old man presents with syncope and a fall.

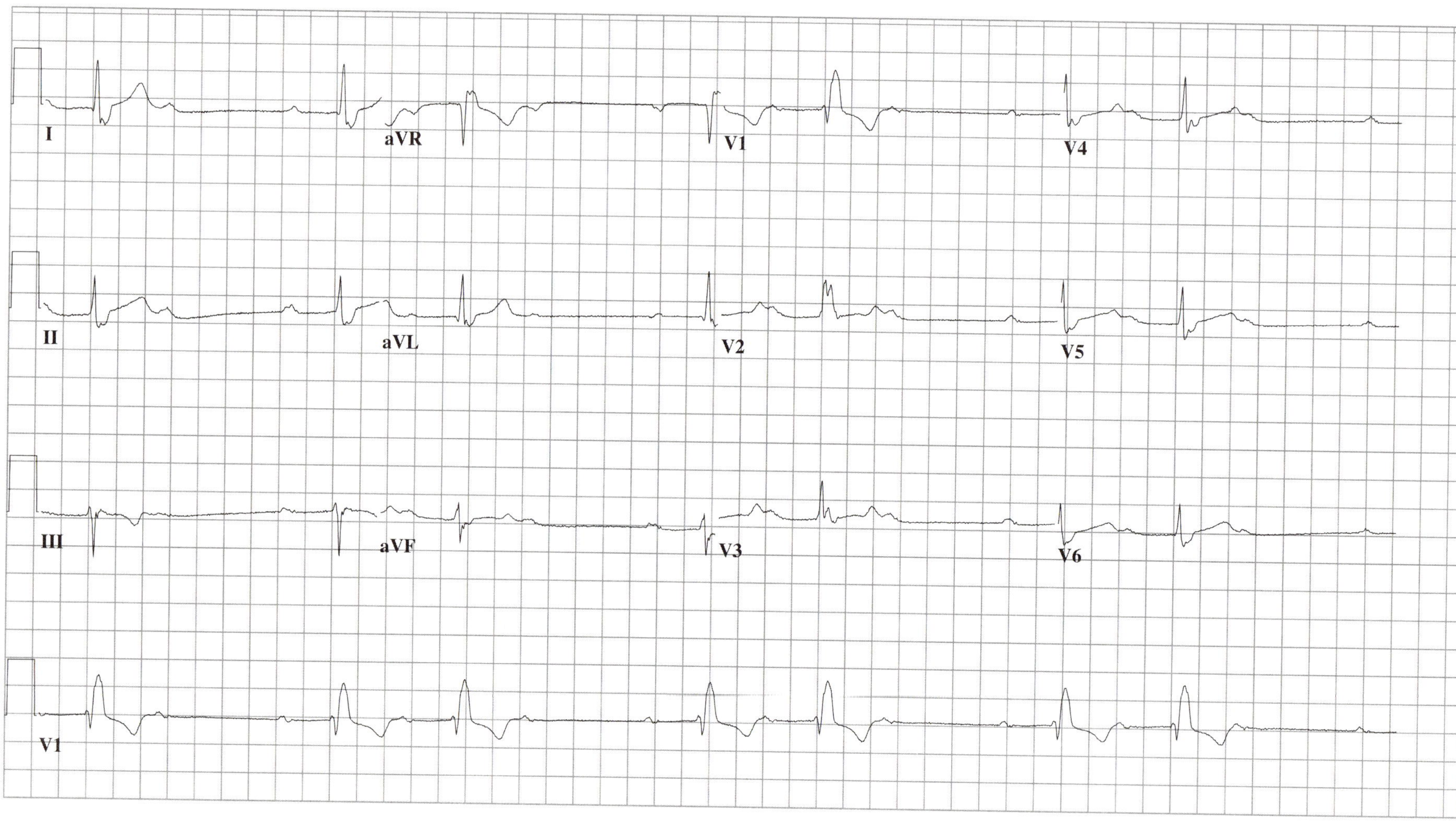

QUESTIONS

134-1. Interpret this ECG. What abnormalities are present?

134-2. Where in the cardiac conduction system is the block most likely to be located?

83
P2-4AC
15.0 cm MI 0.9
Gen TIs 1.1
[2d] G78/71 d
FA4/P90
HAR/FSI0
[C] G50/0.80 kHz
FA5/F1/8
TDI
2.5
3
3.5

ANSWERS

134-1. Interpret this ECG. What abnormalities are present?

This tracing reveals a regularly irregular wide complex rhythm at a rate of 45 beats/min. Every QRS complex is preceded by a P wave, but not every P wave is followed by a QRS complex, suggesting that some form of AV block is present. The PR interval before the second QRS complex in the rhythm strip is prolonged at 390 milliseconds. The subsequent PR interval is the same. Next, a nonconducted P wave follows. The pattern of 2 conducted P waves with the same PR interval followed by a nonconducted P wave then repeats. This pattern of blocked P waves without progressive PR-interval prolongation is consistent with Mobitz type II second-degree AV block. The frontal plane axis of the QRS complex is normal at approximately 0 degree (the QRS complex is isoelectric in lead aVF). The QRS duration is prolonged at 150 milliseconds with a right bundle branch block morphology. Differentiation between Mobitz type I and Mobitz type II second-degree AV block can be challenging—one helpful strategy is to compare the PR interval of the QRS complex directly after a nonconducted P wave with the PR interval of the QRS complex immediately preceding the nonconducted P wave. If the PR interval of the QRS complex preceding the nonconducted P wave is longer than the PR interval of the QRS complex directly following the nonconducted P wave, Mobitz I is present. If the PR intervals are the same, Mobitz II is present.[1]

134-2. Where in the cardiac conduction system is the block most likely to be located?

When Mobitz type II AV block is present, the anatomic location of the diseased conduction system is below the AV node, deep in the His–Purkinje system. Infra-Hisian disease is further suggested by the presence of right bundle branch block. In contrast, when Mobitz type I (Wenckebach) is present, the block could be either at the level of the AV node or deeper in the His–Purkinje system. Mobitz I with a narrow QRS in a young patient without comorbid heart disease is likely to represent AV nodal block. In contrast, Mobitz I with a wide QRS in an older patient with heart disease may represent either disease at the level of the AV node or infra-Hisian disease.[1]

[1]Barold SS, Hayes DL. Second-degree atrioventricular block: a reappraisal. *Mayo Clin Proc* 2001; 76: 44-57.

Baseline tracing:

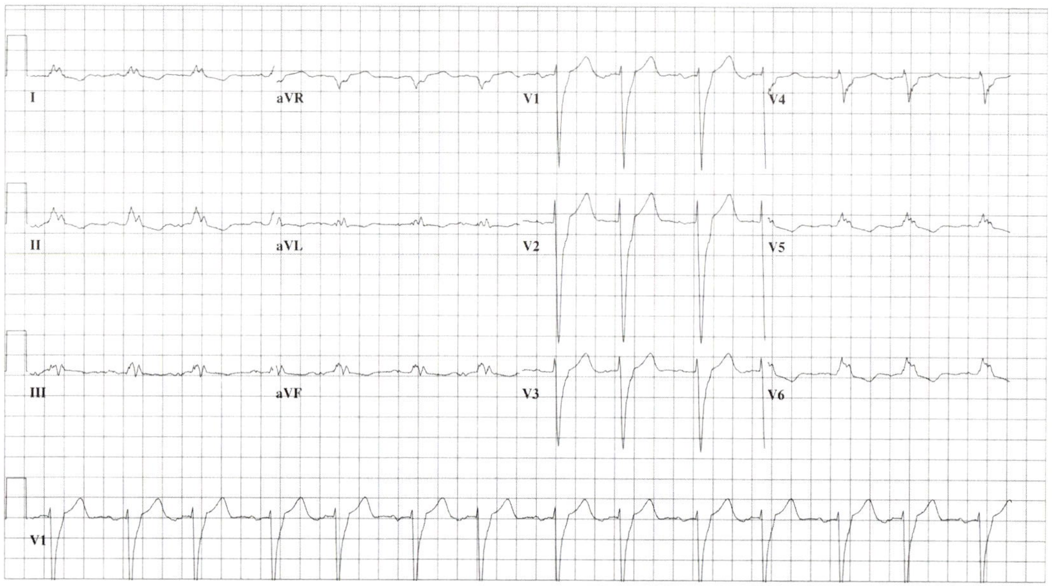

Tracing postprocedure:

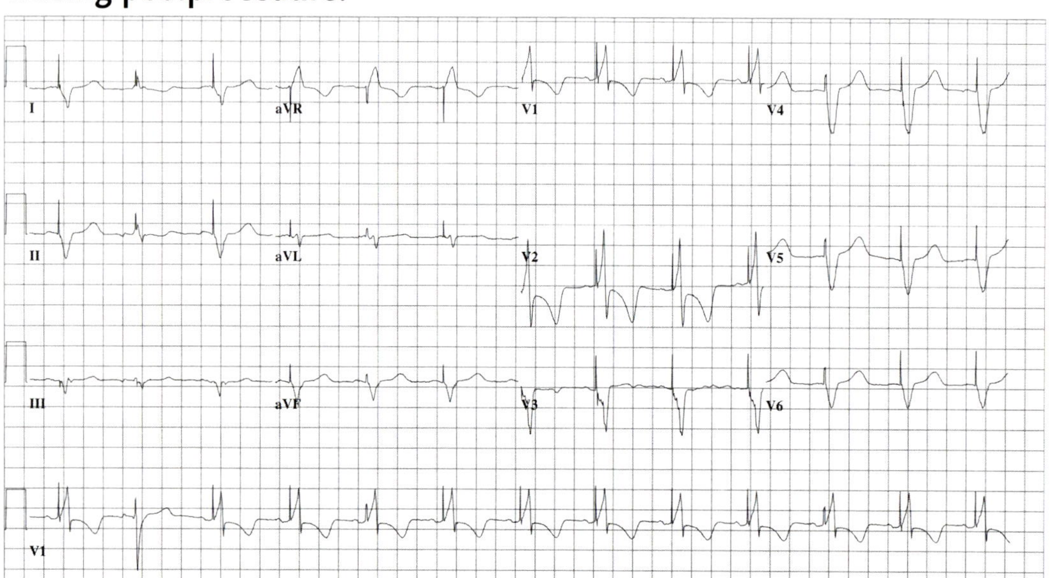

Case #135. A 73-year-old man underwent a cardiac procedure.

QUESTIONS

135-1. What abnormalities are present on the baseline tracing?

135-2. Interpret the postprocedure tracing: What type of pacemaker was placed?

135-3. What clinical information can you surmise about the patient?

83
P2-4AC
15.0 cm MI 0.9
Gen TIs 1.1
[2d] G78/71 d
FA4/P90
HAR/FS10
[C] G50/0.80 kHz
FA5/F1/8
TDI
Amplitude (V)
P-R
S-T
QRS interval
S-T interval
P-R interval
2.5
3
3.5
Time (s)

ANSWERS

135-1. What abnormalities are present on the baseline tracing?

This tracing reveals sinus rhythm with very subtle irregularity of the R–R intervals. Closely examining P-wave morphology in lead II and the lead V1 rhythm strip, this irregularity is due to premature atrial beats in a pattern of atrial bigeminy. The QRS axis is normal. There is left atrial abnormality diagnosed in the sinus beats with a broad, slurred P wave broader than 120 milliseconds visible in lead II. The QRS duration is prolonged to greater than 120 milliseconds and has a left bundle branch block morphology (with an rS wave in lead V1, and a broad, notched R wave in leads I and V6). The ST segments are displaced and T waves are inverted opposite the major deflection of the QRS. These repolarization abnormalities are secondary to the left bundle branch block and are not due to ischemia.

135-2. Interpret the postprocedure tracing: What type of pacemaker was placed?

The rate is slightly faster than 75 beats/min. The rhythm is sinus with ventricular pacing present. The ventricular pacemaker is tracking the intrinsic atrial rhythm with a constant PR interval of approximately 150 milliseconds. The QRS axis is extreme rightward, with a negative QRS in I and a negative QRS in aVF. The QRS complex is positive in V1, hence has "right bundle branch morphology." The second beat of the rhythm strip is a fusion beat, or a combination of native conduction and a simultaneous paced beat.

This pattern of paced beats with rightward axis and right bundle branch block morphology is not consistent with a normal right ventricular apical; in that case, the QRS polarity should be positive in lead I because depolarization moves from right to left. When right ventricular pacing is present, the QRS has a downward polarity in lead V1, because the right ventricle is anterior to the left ventricle. In this tracing, the QRS morphology has a different pattern, suggesting that depolarization is moving from left to right and posterior to anterior. This QRS vector is consistent with biventricular pacing, also called cardiac resynchronization therapy. When a biventricular pacemaker is placed, a ventricular lead is secured in the right ventricle and a second ventricular lead is placed in the coronary sinus to provide synchronous pacing of the left ventricular myocardium. The coronary sinus is a posterolateral structure, although there is significant individual variability. When simultaneously pacing via both these leads, the left ventricular mass generates more voltage than the right ventricular mass and hence the QRS vector on the 12-lead ECG is consistent with the majority of depolarization moving from posterior to anterior and from left to right.

135-3. What clinical information can you surmise about the patient?

The theory of biventricular pacing is predicated on the idea of restoring synchronous ventricular contraction. In patients with left bundle branch block, the left ventricular free wall contracts later than the septum. In patients with comorbid systolic dysfunction and heart failure, this ventricular dyssynchrony and inefficiency can contribute significantly to impaired cardiac output. Therefore, patients with a wide QRS complex and left bundle branch block, low ejection fraction, and a history of heart failure symptom despite maximal medical therapy should be considered for implantation of a biventricular pacemaker.

Case #136. A 76-year-old patient with chronic kidney disease presents with cardiac arrest.

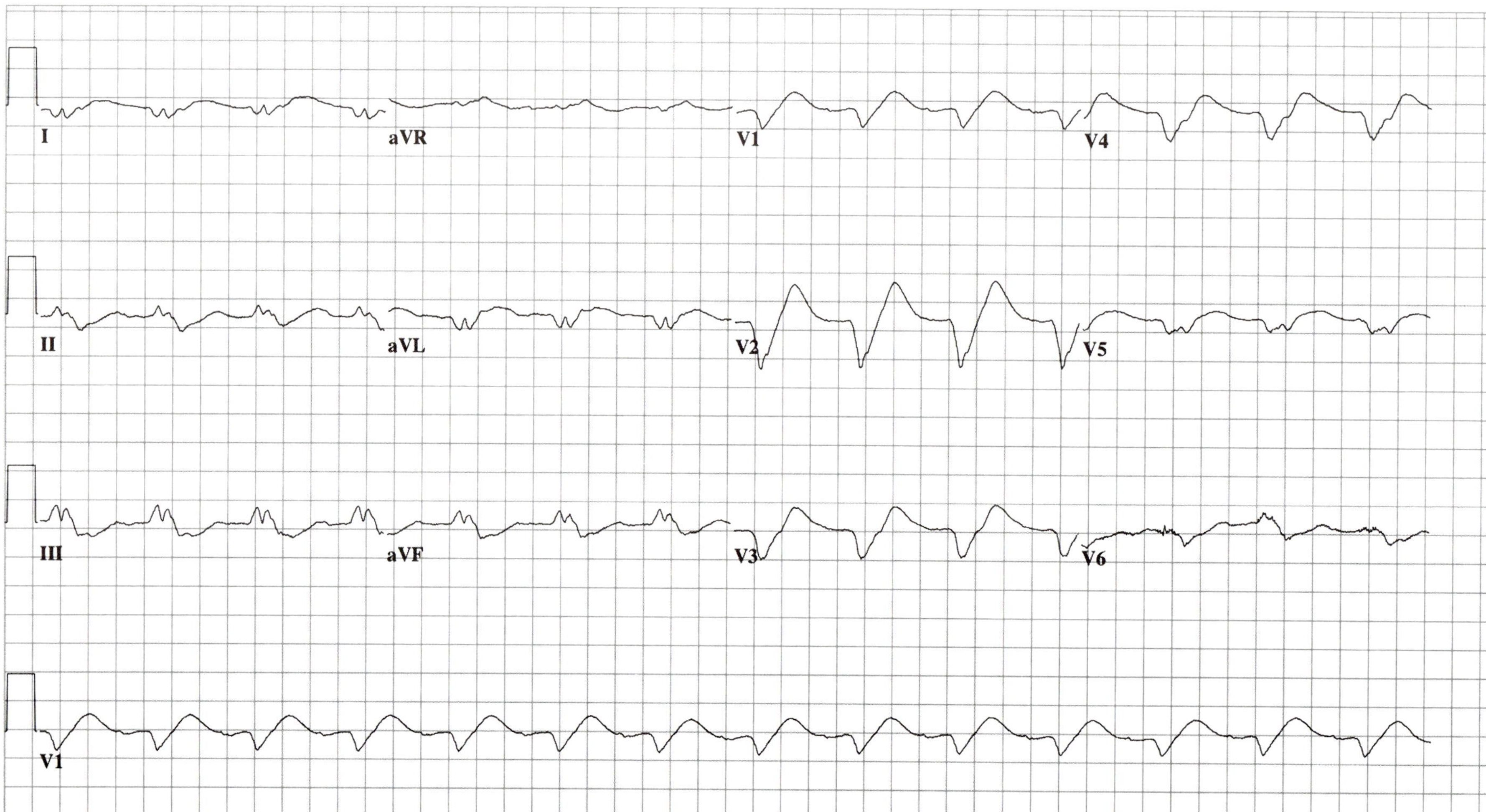

QUESTIONS

136-1. What are the salient findings on this ECG?

136-2. What would you do next?

83
P2-4AC
15.0 cm MI 0.9
Gen TIs 1.1
[2d] G78/71 d
FA4/P90
HAR/FSlo
[C] G50/0.80 kHz
FA5/F1/B
TDI
Amplitude (V)

ANSWERS

136-1. What are the salient findings on this ECG?

The ventricular rate is approximately 75 beats/min. Small P waves of low amplitude are barely visible prior to each QRS complex in lead V1. First-degree AV block is present. The QRS complex is extremely wide and bizarre with a nonspecific intraventricular conduction delay. T waves are pointed and peaked. Wide, bizarre QRS complexes with pointed T waves suggest hyperkalemia as the cause of cardiac arrest.

136-2. What would you do next?

Empiric treatment for hyperkalemia would be indicated prior to any lab checks. Intravenous calcium should be given to stabilize the cardiac membrane. Rapid narrowing of the QRS complex can be seen after administration of IV calcium. Other treatments to decrease serum potassium include administration of insulin (with dextrose), bicarbonate, and β-agonists to shift potassium intracellularly and sodium polystyrene or urgent hemodialysis to remove potassium from the body.

Case #137. A 42-year-old gentleman with poorly controlled diabetes presents with stuttering chest pain for up to 15 minutes at a time over 24 hours. He is pain-free at the time of this ECG.

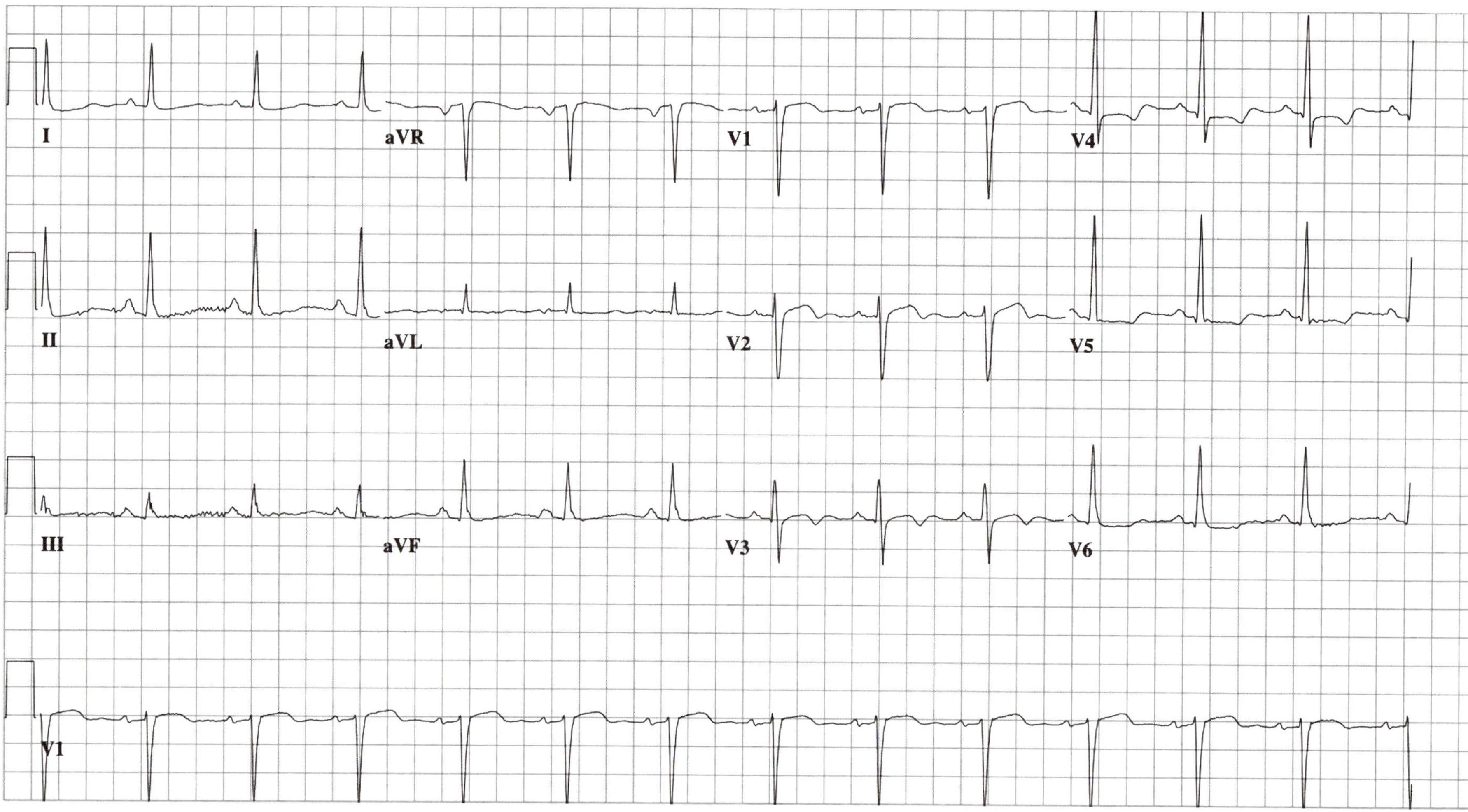

QUESTIONS

137-1. What abnormalities does this ECG demonstrate?

137-2. What is the clinical diagnosis?

83
P2-4AC
15.0 cm MI 0.9
Gen TIs 1.1
[2d] G78/71 d
FA4/P90
HAR/FS10
[C] G50/0.80 kHz
FA5/F1/8
TDI

ANSWERS

137-1. What abnormalities does this ECG demonstrate?

There is sinus rhythm at 75 beats/min. Axis and intervals are normal. There is T-wave flattening in the inferior leads II, III, and aVF and the high-lateral leads I and aVL. In the anterior precordial leads V3 through V6, there are symmetric T-wave inversions and ST-segment depression most notable in lead V4.

137-2. What is the clinical diagnosis?

This patient with risk factors for coronary artery disease presents with chest pain and ECG findings consistent with ischemia. This syndrome could be classified as unstable angina if biomarkers of myocardial necrosis are normal or as non-ST-segment elevation myocardial infarction (NSTEMI) if biomarkers of myocardial necrosis are present. The fact that there are no regional ST-segment elevations on the ECG suggests that the acute coronary syndrome is due to nonocclusive coronary plaque rather than thrombus and plaque leading to a completely occluded coronary artery.

Six hours later, the same patient has acute onset of similar chest pain and this ECG:

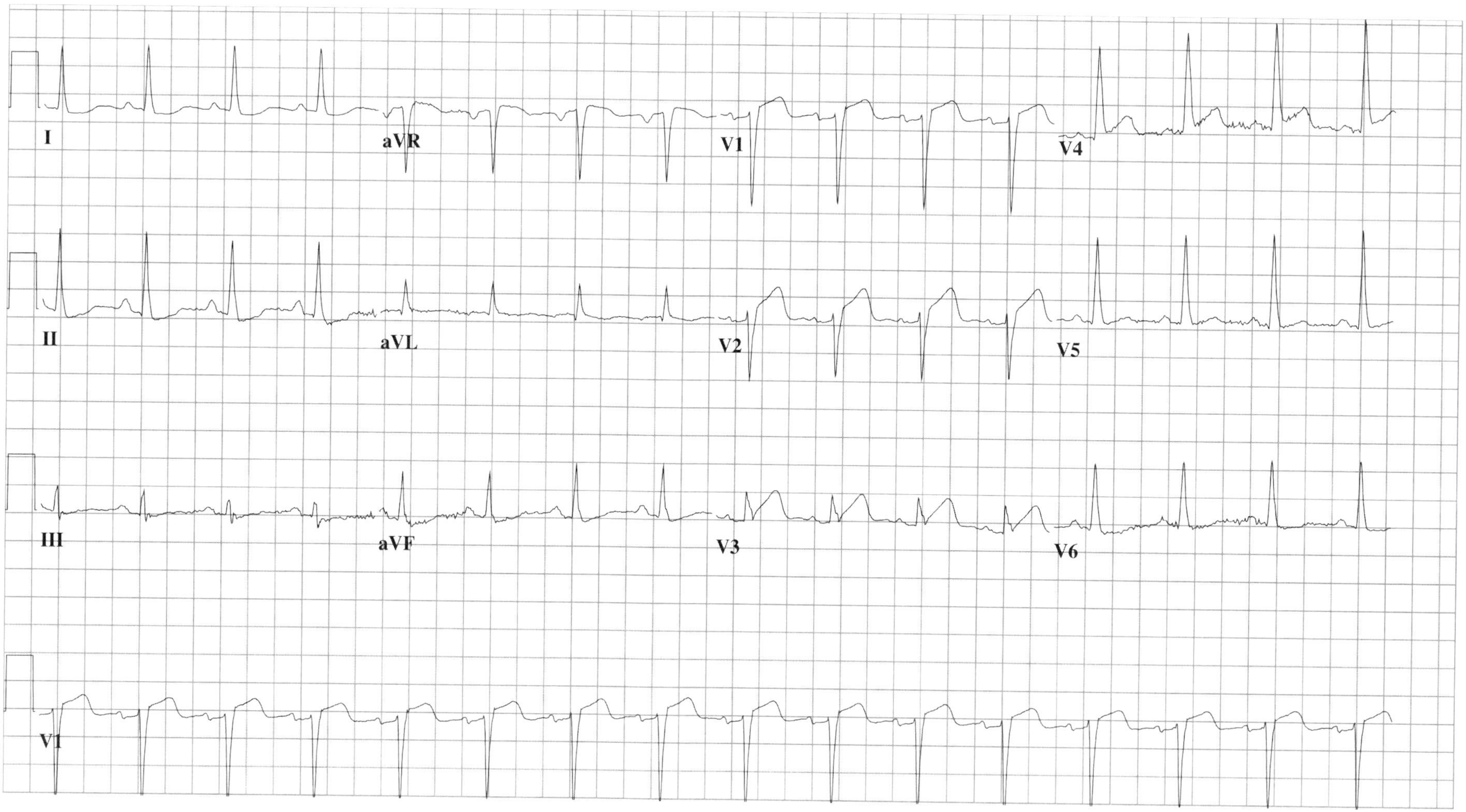

QUESTIONS

137-3. What is the diagnosis?

137-4. Predict what the angiogram will show.

83
P2-4AC
15.0 cm MI 0.9
Gen TIs 1.1
[2d] G78/71 d
FA4/P90
HAR/FSI0
[C] G50/0.80 kHz
FA5/F1/8
TDI
Amplitude (V)
Time (s)
QRS
interval
S-T
interval
2.5
3
3.5

ANSWERS

137-3. What is the diagnosis?

There is sinus rhythm but slightly faster, almost 100 beats/min. Axis and intervals remain normal. Although in the first tracing there were T-wave inversions and ST-segment depressions anteriorly, now the T waves are upright with a broad base. In lead V3 particularly, the T wave is hyperacute, almost taller than the R wave. In leads V3 and V4, there is 1 mm of ST-segment elevation. The transition from inverted T waves to upright T waves is called "pseudonormalization" and occurs when a nonocclusive coronary plaque becomes occlusive in the setting of an acute coronary syndrome. In the figure, the anterior leads of the 2 tracings are shown side by side to illustrate the differences.

The ST and T waves from the 2 tracings are demonstrated side by side. Note the hyperacute, "pseudonormal" T waves and ST-segment elevation in the second tracing compared to the first.

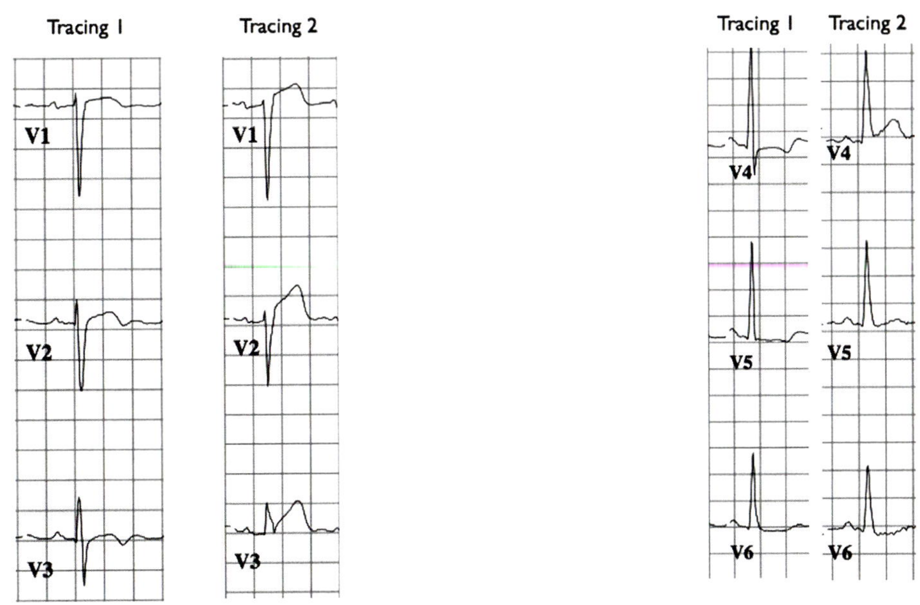

137-4. Predict what the angiogram will show.

The second tracing reveals upright hyperacute T waves with ST-segment elevation in the anterior leads. Also of note are the subtle ST-segment depressions in leads II, III, and aVF, which are consistent with reciprocal change. These changes suggest an occlusive plaque in the left anterior descending artery, which was confirmed and successfully treated at angiography.

Case #138. A 32-year-old male presents with syncope.

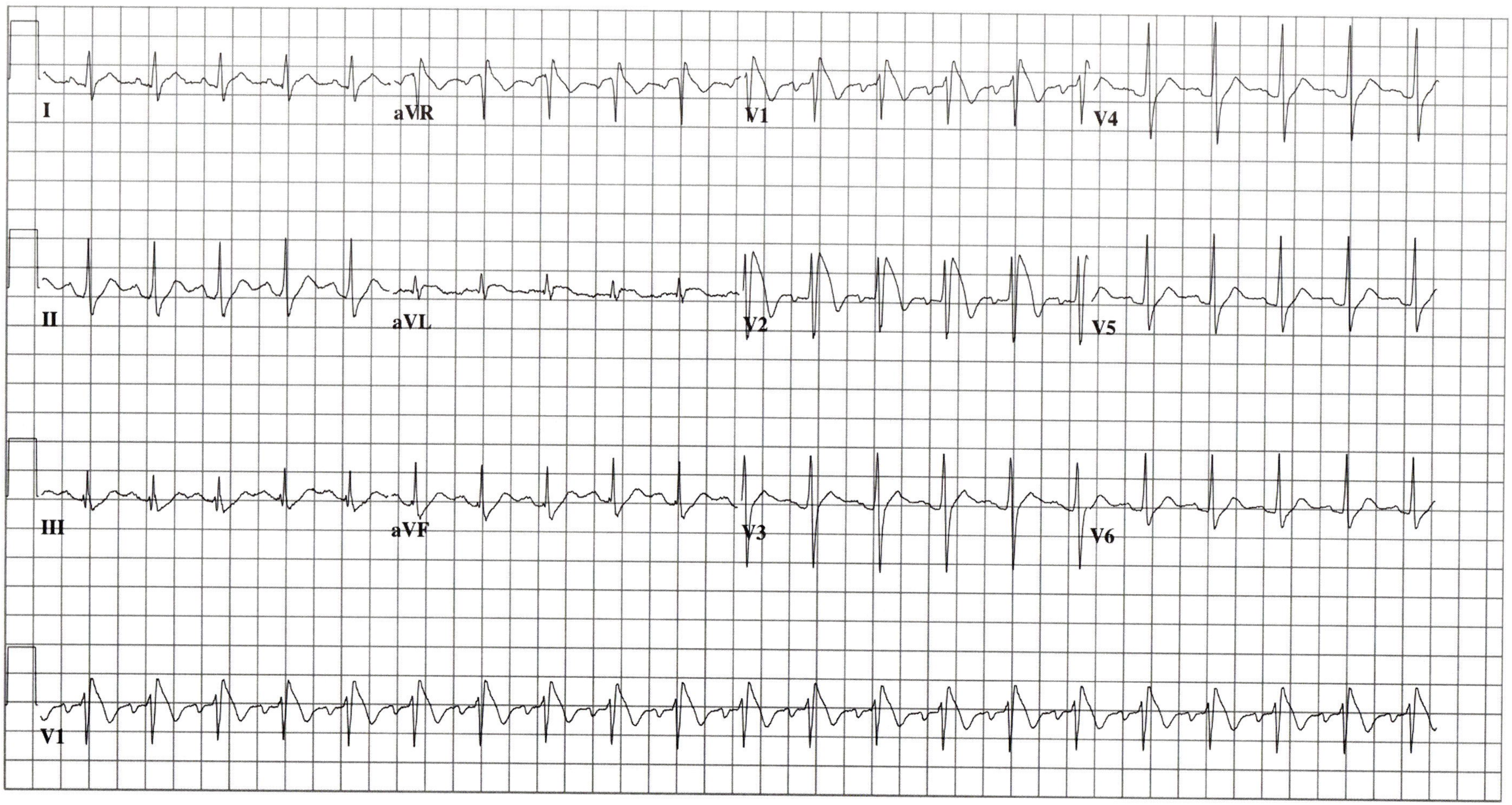

QUESTIONS

138-1. Interpret this ECG. What is the most likely diagnosis?

138-2. What would you do next?

83
P2-4AC
15.0 cm MI 0.9
Gen TIs 1.1
[2d] G78/71 d
FA4/P90
HAR/FSI0
[C] G50/0.80 kHz
FA5/F1/8
TDI
Amplitude (V)
S-T
interval
2.5
3
Time (s)
3.5

ANSWERS

138-1. Interpret this ECG. What is the most likely diagnosis?

There is sinus tachycardia at 120 beats/min. The axis is normal. There is an incomplete right bundle branch block. In leads V1 and V2, there is striking ST-segment elevation with a particular morphology: the ST segments are elevated, downsloping, concave, and coved downward and lead directly into an inverted T wave. This is a typical appearance of the ECG associated with the Brugada syndrome, a syndrome of ventricular tachycardia associated with this ECG morphology. The Brugada syndrome is an inherited syndrome of dysfunction of cardiac sodium channels and consists of this ECG coupled with sudden cardiac death or ventricular tachycardia, syndrome, and a family history.

138-2. What would you do next?

The history of syncope and a Brugada-pattern ECG merits further investigation. Referral to an electrophysiologist and implantation of an implantable cardioverter-defibrillator would be warranted.

Case #139. An 85-year-old male post-op from coronary artery bypass grafting maintained on dobutamine. His ECG is below.

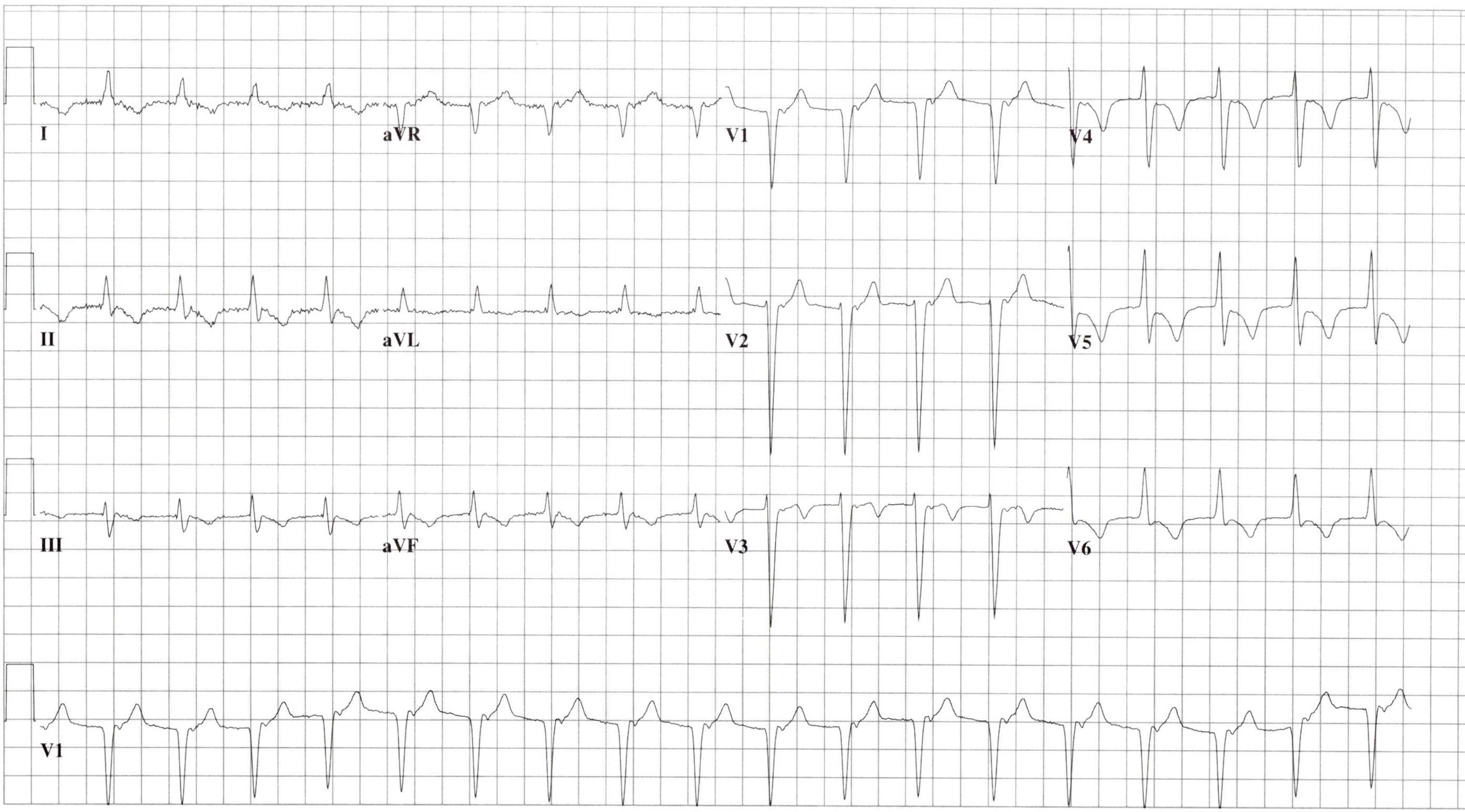

QUESTION

139-1. What abnormalities are present on this ECG?

83
P2-4AC
15.0 cm MI 0.9
Gen TIs 1.1
[2d] G78/71 d
FA4/P90
HAR/FS|0
[C] G50/0.80 kHz
FA5/F1/8
TDI
Amplitude (V)
Time (s)
2.5
3
3.5

ANSWER

139-1. What abnormalities are present on this ECG?

The ventricular rate is approximately 110 beats/min and regular. The QRS duration is approximately 100 milliseconds. The QRS axis is normal. Immediately following each QRS complex, there is a small negative deflection buried in the upstroke of the T wave best seen in lead V1, as shown in the figure. This represents retrograde atrial activation, or a "retrograde P wave," suggesting that activation of the atria occurs after activation of the ventricles. Therefore, the rhythm represents a "short RP tachycardia." The differential diagnosis includes typical AV nodal and AV reentrant tachycardias, atrial tachycardia with an associated first-degree AV block, and junctional tachycardia. AVNRT and AVRT are usually faster than the rate observed here. In this clinical setting of a patient post cardiac surgery maintained on chronotropic and inotropic agents, this tracing represents a junctional tachycardia. In this case, the AV node demonstrates increased automaticity and subsumes the pacemaker function of the sinus node. This rhythm is observed after cardiac surgery, in states of digoxin toxicity, in patients maintained on inotropic and chronotropic medications such as dobutamine, and in patients with congenital heart disease. The remainder of the tracing reveals T-wave inversions in the limb leads and anterior and lateral precordial leads with ST-segment depressions most prominent in the anterior V4 through V6, which suggest myocardial ischemia. Finally, there is fine baseline artifact in the limb leads.

Retrograde atrial activation is seen in lead V1.

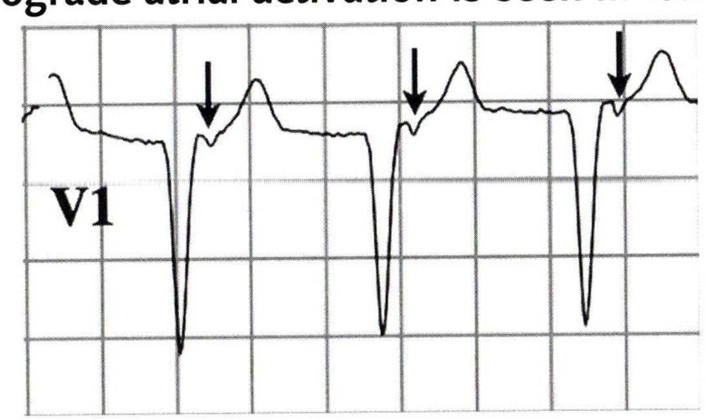

Case #140. A 59-year-old male with hypertension presents to the emergency department with 2 episodes of syncope.

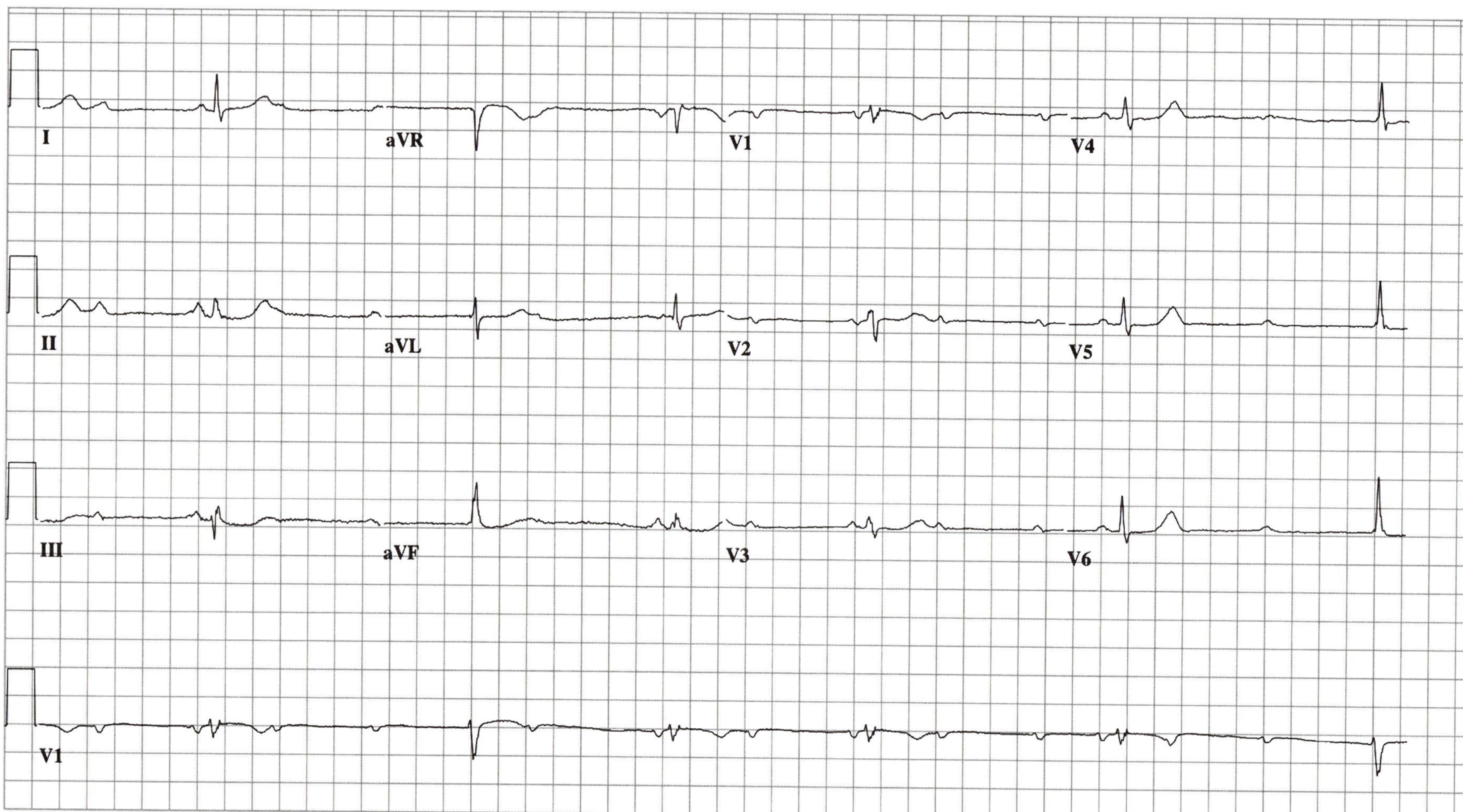

QUESTIONS

140-1. Interpret this ECG. What rhythm is present?

140-2. What treatment is indicated?

83
P2-4AC
15.0 cm MI 0.9
Gen Tls 1.1
[2d] G78/71 d
FA4/P90
HAR/FSI0
[C] G50/0.80 kHz
FA5/F1/B
TDI
interval
2.5
3

ANSWERS

140-1. Interpret this ECG. What rhythm is present?

This ECG shows an irregular bradycardia with a ventricular rate of 36 beats/min. Assess the V1 rhythm strip, as shown in the figure, to determine the rhythm: Starting at the left of the tracing, there is a P wave (marked by an asterisk) that is not conducted, followed by a P wave that is conducted with a PR interval of just over 120 milliseconds (the QRS complex that results from this conducted P wave is marked with an arrow). The QRS complex associated with this P wave is narrow, with a duration of 90 to 100 milliseconds. After this first QRS complex, we see 2 nonconducted P waves, a narrow QRS complex with a different morphology (marked with a circle), another nonconducted P wave, and then a P wave that is again conducted with PR interval of approximately 120 milliseconds. Because there are more P waves than QRS complexes, AV block is present. There is no progressive lengthening of the PR interval as seen with Mobitz type I, and there are periods where multiple sequential P waves do not conduct. Given this intermittent AV conduction and multiple consecutive nonconducted P waves, this rhythm is best termed high-grade AV block. The second and sixth QRS complexes (marked in the figure with circles) are junctional escape beats that occur after a long pause. The QRS complexes have normal axes and normal QT and QRS intervals. The QRS has an RSR′ morphology in lead V1.

140-2. What treatment is indicated?

This patient has high-grade A-V block and syncope. Placement of a permanent pacemaker is indicated.

Asterisks identify P waves. Pointed arrows denote QRS complexes with A-V conduction. The circles denote junctional escape beats.

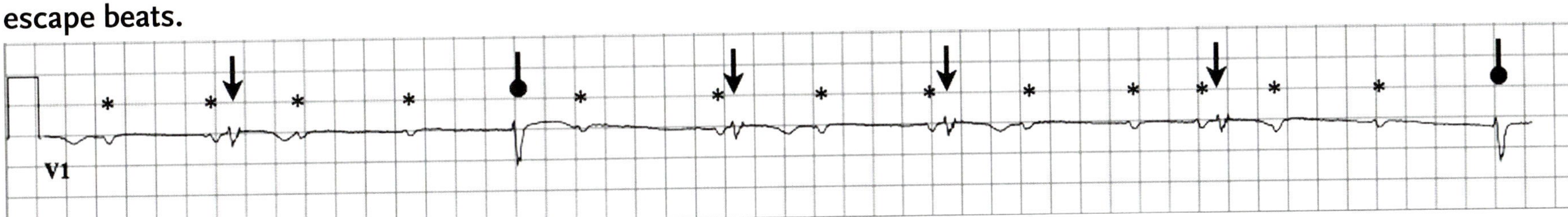

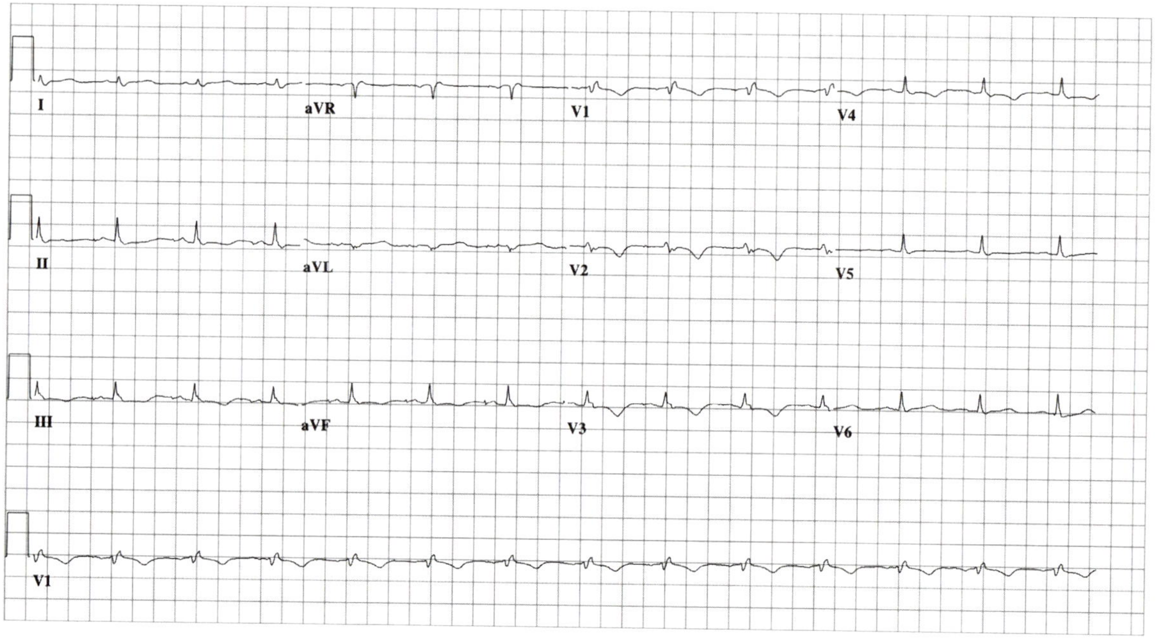

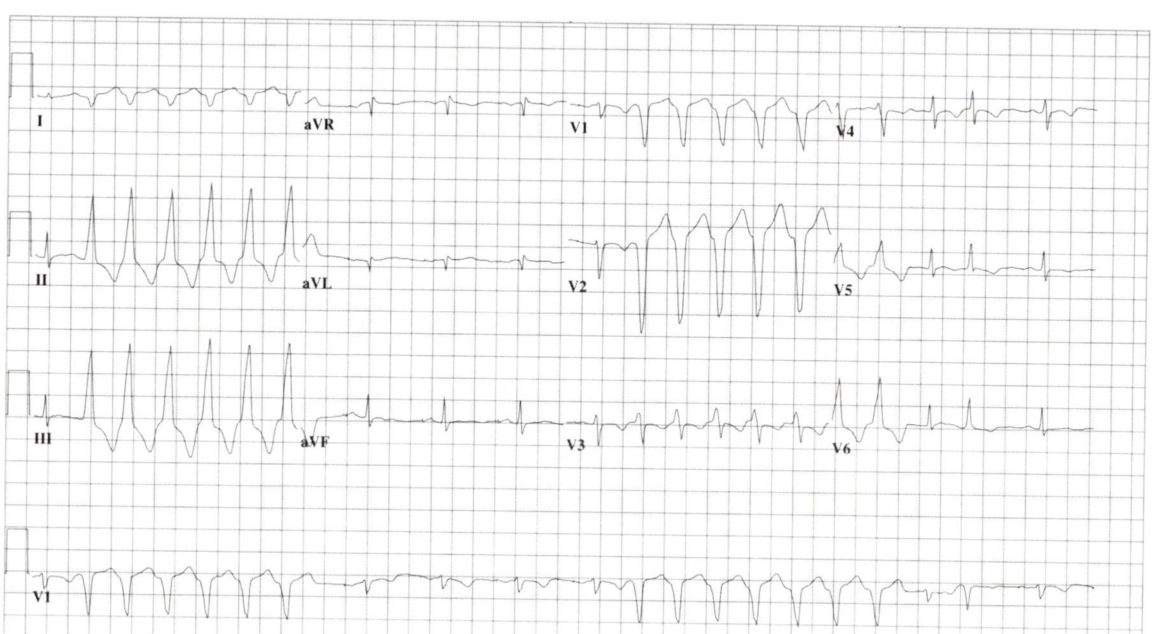

Case #141. A 23-year-old with a history of syncope. Two tracings are shown.

QUESTIONS

141-1. What are the notable findings?

141-2. What is the most likely diagnosis?

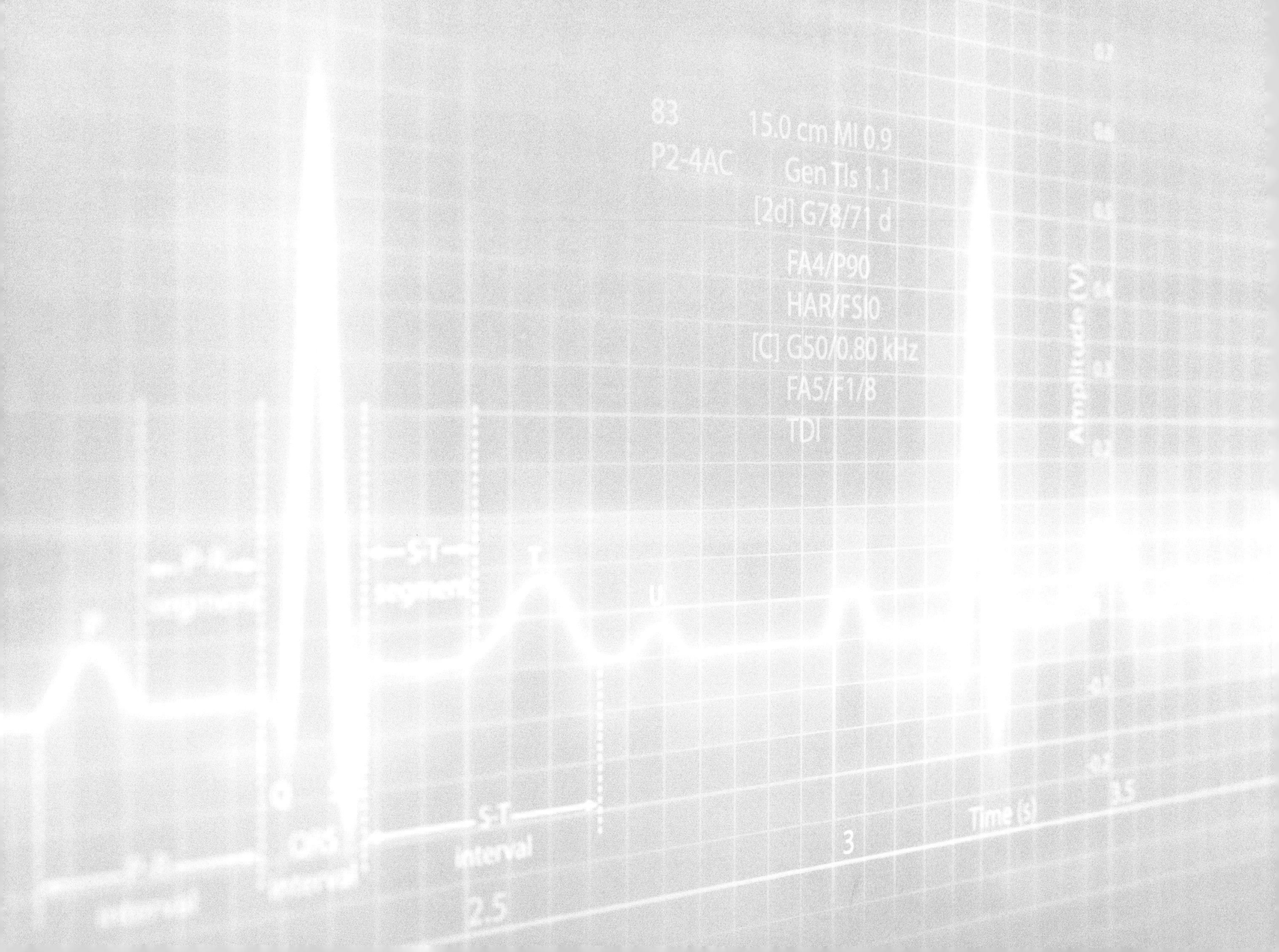
83
P2-4AC
15.0 cm MI 0.9
Gen TIs 1.1
[2d] G78/71 d
FA4/P90
HAR/FS10
[C] G50/0.80 kHz
FA5/F1/8
TDI
Amplitude (V)
S-T
segment
T
U
S-T
interval
QRS
interval
2.5
3
Time (s)
3.5

ANSWERS

141-1. What are the notable findings?

The first tracing reveals atrial pacing (pacer spikes are very subtle but can be visualized just prior to the P wave in leads II, III, and aVF). Axis is normal. There is low voltage present with incomplete right bundle branch block. There are diffusely flat T waves with inversions present inferiorly and in leads V1 through V3. The second tracing reveals runs of nonsustained monomorphic wide complex tachycardia interspersed with the native beats most consistent with ventricular tachycardia.

141-2. What is the most likely diagnosis?

This is a young person with syncope due to ventricular tachycardia. The baseline ECG is abnormal with low voltage, incomplete right bundle branch block, and T-wave inversions. These findings are consistent with a diagnosis of arrhythmogenic right ventricular cardiomyopathy (ARVC), a genetic condition whereupon the ventricular myocardium is replaced by fibro-fatty tissue leading to malignant arrhythmias. It is a rare disease but responsible for a significant number of sudden cardiac deaths in young athletes. Additional ECG features may include a "notch" inscribed within the ST segment, sometimes visualized in the precordial leads, called an epsilon wave. An example of an epsilon wave is shown in Figure 1. If suspected, the diagnosis of ARVC can be further investigated with detailed family screening, echocardiography, cardiac MRI, and signal averaged ECG.[1]

Epsilon waves are noted after depolarizations within the ST segment.

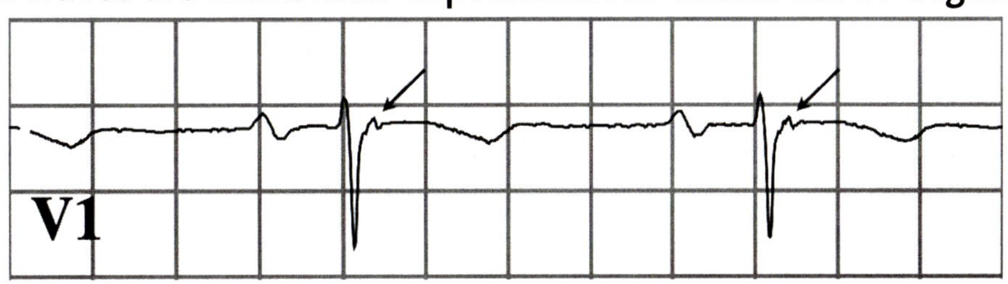

[1]Marcus F, McKenna W, Sherril D, et al. Diagnosis of arrhythmogenic right ventricular cardiomyopathy/dysplasia: proposed modification of the task force criteria. *Circulation* 2010; 12: 1533-1541.

Case #142. A 76-year-old woman presenting with vomiting and upper epigastric "pressure" coupled with "heart fluttering."

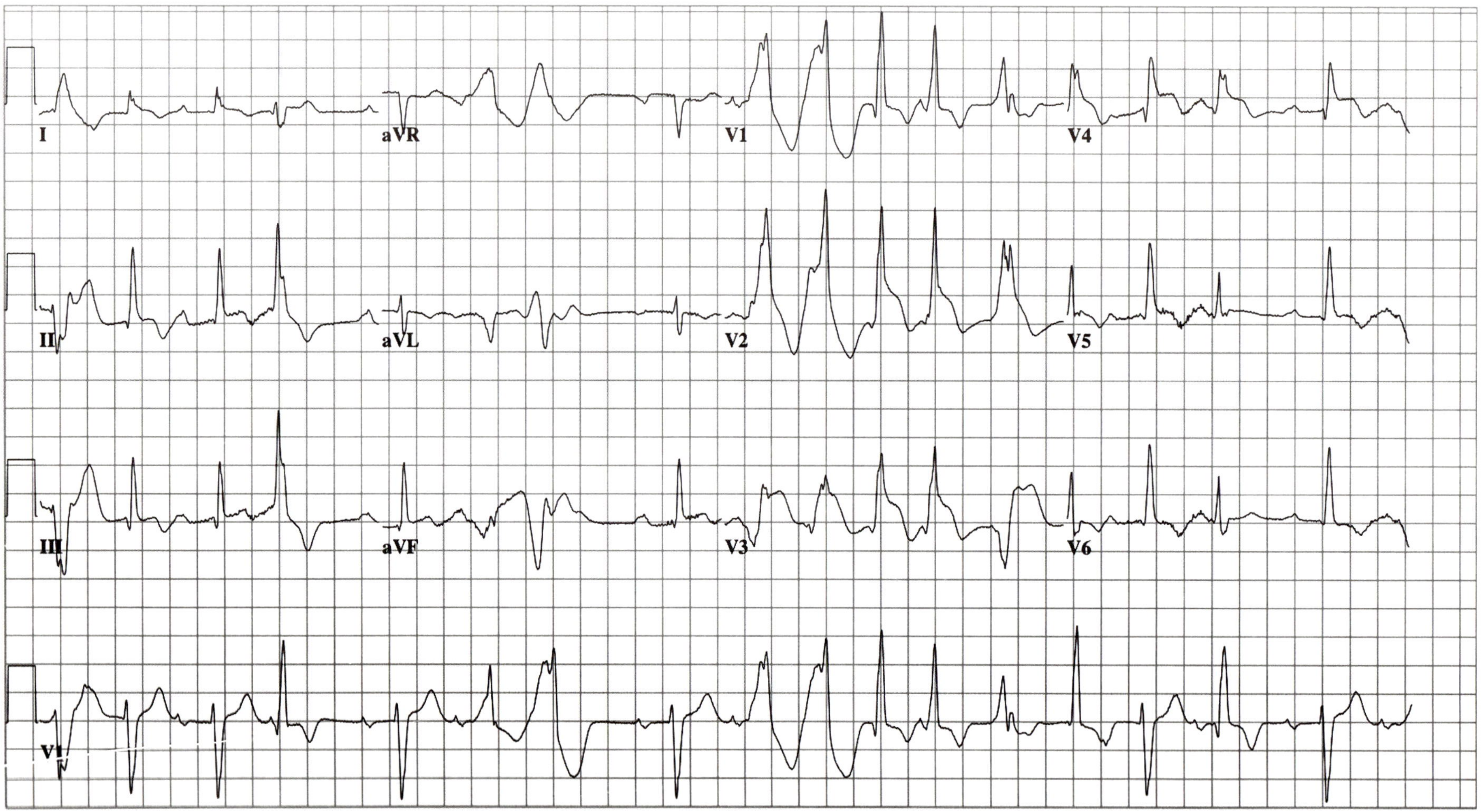

QUESTION

142-1. Interpret this ECG.

83
15.0 cm MI 0.9
P2-4AC
Gen TIs 1.1
[2d] G78/71 d
FA4/P90
HAR/FSI0
[C] G50/0.80 kHz
FA5/F1/8
TDI
Time (s)
3
2.5
3.5

ANSWER

142-1. Interpret this ECG.

This is a complex tracing. The overall rate is approximately 100 beats/min. To assess the rhythm, examine the rhythm strip and find the P waves, which are shown using asterisks in the figure. The second, third, fifth, eighth, and seventeenth QRS complexes, shown using arrows in the figure, have similar morphology and are preceded by sinus P waves with the same PR interval. These are the sinus beats conducted with a first-degree AV block. Interspersed are several junctional and ventricular ectopic beats and, in the middle of the tracing, a 5-beat salvo of polymorphic ventricular tachycardia. Polymorphic ventricular tachycardia is associated with ischemia; the inspection of the sinus beats for ischemic changes reveals 1 mm of ST-segment elevation in leads I and II, III and aVF as well as 3 mm of ST-segment elevation with a small Q wave in the anterior precordial leads. The overall impression is antero-infero-lateral ST-segment elevation myocardial infarction leading to polymorphic VT. Urgent reperfusion therapy is indicated.

P waves are seen marked with asterisks marching through the rhythm strip. Arrows denote beats that are conducted from atria to ventricle. Polymorphic VT is seen between conducted sinus beats with A-V dissociation.

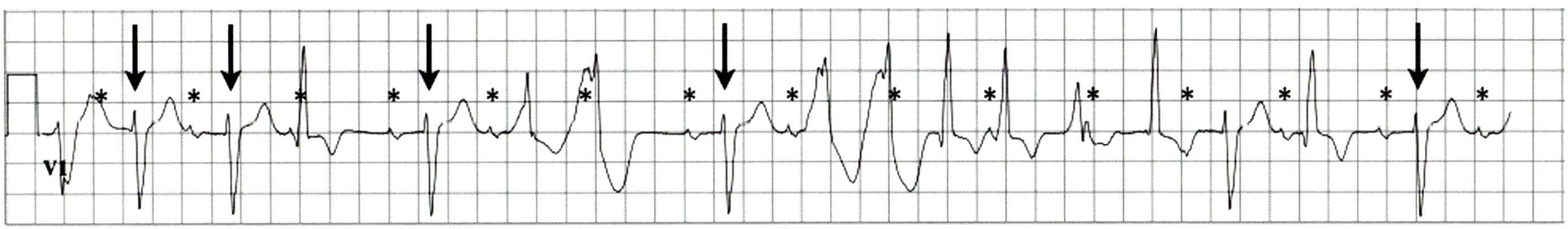

Case #143. An 89-year-old woman with intermittent palpitations and dizziness.

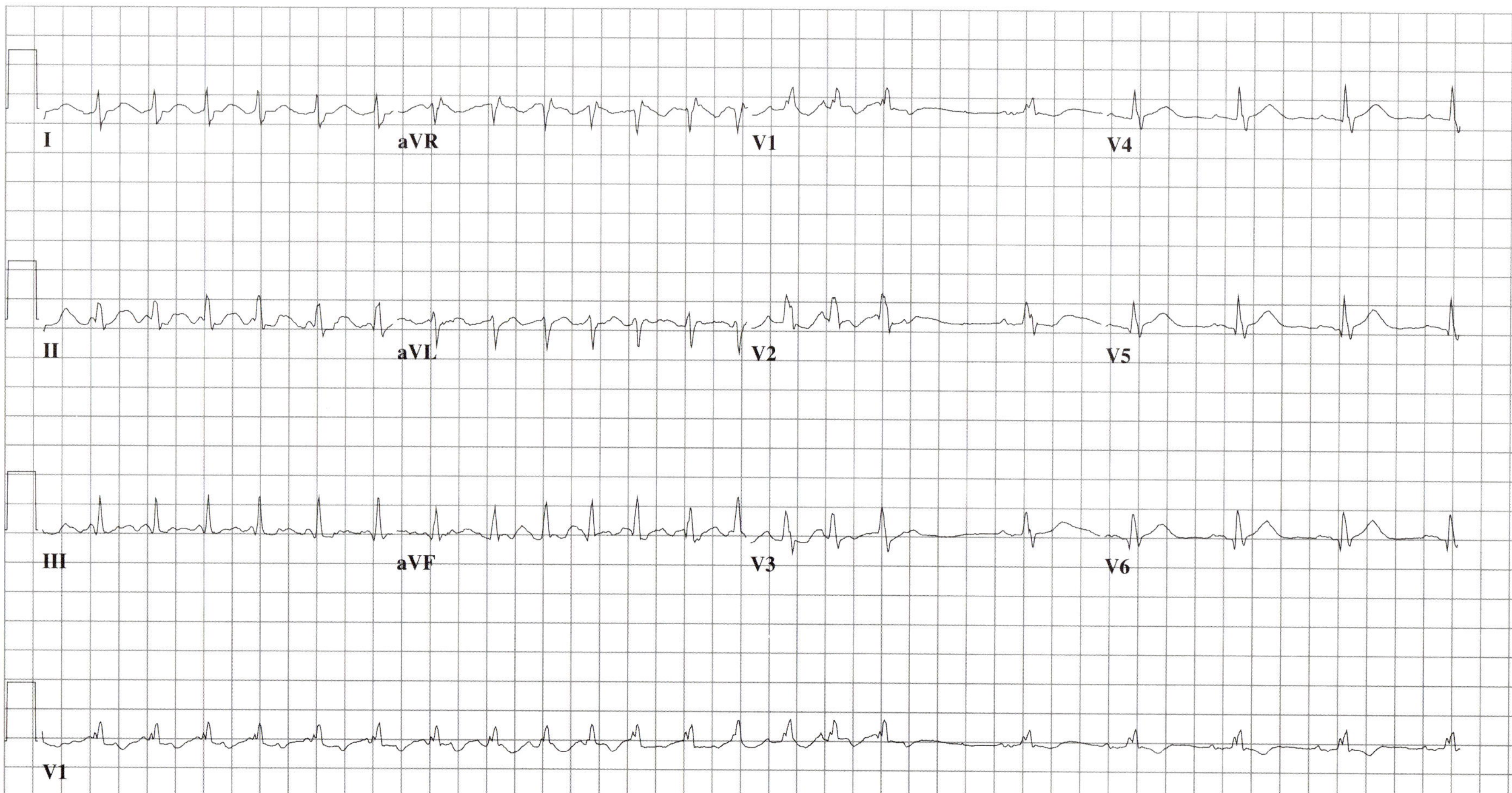

QUESTION

143-1. Interpret this ECG: what rhythm abnormalities are present?

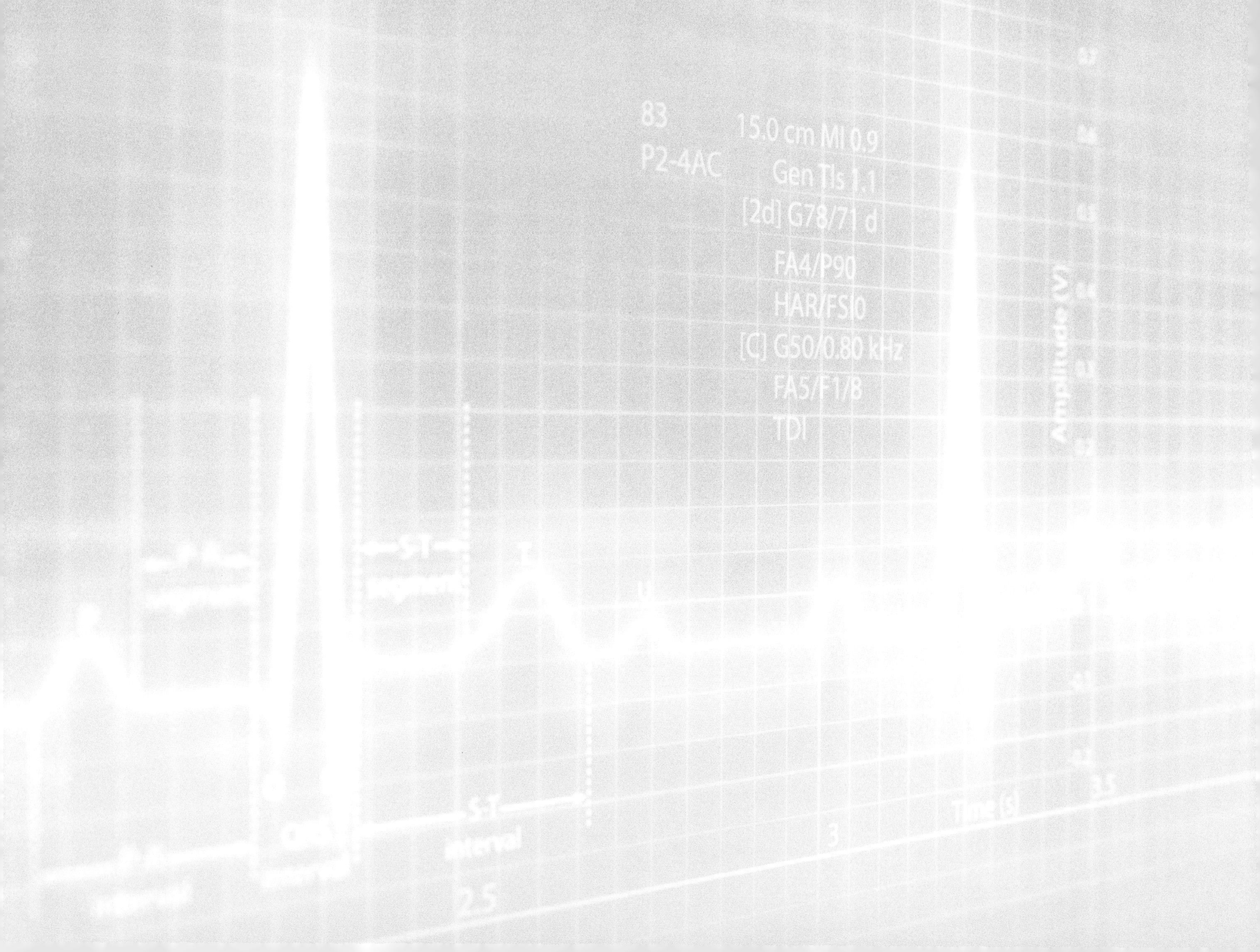
83
P2-4AC
15.0 cm MI 0.9
Gen TIs 1.1
[2d] G78/71 d
FA4/P90
HAR/FS|0
[C] G50/0.80 kHz
FA5/F1/8
TDI
Amplitude (V)
S-T
interval
2.5
3
3.5
Time (s)

ANSWER

143-1. Interpret this ECG: what rhythm abnormalities are present?

There are 2 distinct rhythms seen on this ECG. The first portion of the tracing reveals an irregularly irregular tachycardia with a very fast rate. Next, there is a pause followed by 5 beats of sinus rhythm, which conclude the rhythm strip. The QRS voltage is low with an RSR′ morphology in leads V1 and V2 consistent with an incomplete right bundle branch block because the QRS width is narrow. This ECG is diagnostic of paroxysmal atrial fibrillation as a cause of the patient's intermittent symptoms.

Case #144. A 49-year-old woman presents with cardiac arrest. On examination, warm, dry, flushed skin, and dilated pupils are noted.

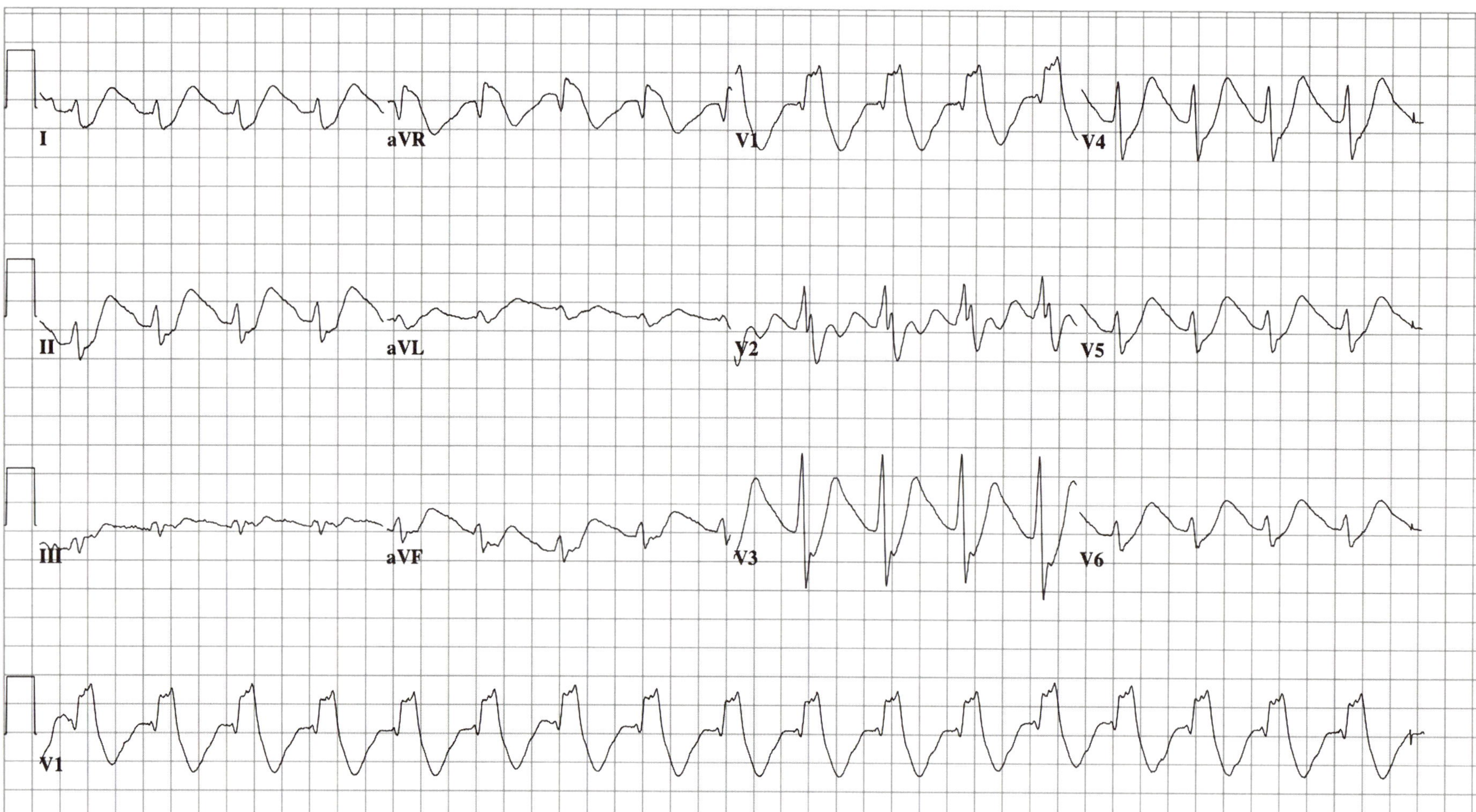

QUESTIONS

144-1. Interpret this ECG.

144-2. What is the differential diagnosis of these abnormalities?

83
P2-4AC
15.0 cm MI 0.9
Gen TIs 1.1
[2d] G78/71 d
FA4/P90
HAR/FS0
[C] G50/0.80 kHz
FA5/F1/8
TDI
3
2.5

ANSWERS

144-1. Interpret this ECG.

The rate is 100 beats/min. The rhythm is indeterminate, with no clear P waves seen. The QRS complex is extremely wide and bizarre appearing with a right bundle branch block pattern. The axis is extreme rightward. The QT interval is extremely prolonged.

144-2. What is the differential diagnosis of these abnormalities?

The differential diagnosis of a wide, bizarre QRS complex with prolonged QT and extreme rightward axis should include a ventricular rhythm versus a primary acquired abnormality affecting cardiac conduction. Hyperkalemia can present with a wide, bizarre QRS as can tricyclic antidepressant overdose and overdose of Class I antiarrhythmic agents such as flecainide and propafenone. Both tricyclic antidepressants and the Class I antiarrhythmic agents inhibit cardiac sodium channels prolonging phase 0 of the cardiac action potential resulting in a broad, bizarre QRS complex. Classically, tricyclic antidepressant toxicity presents with signs of anticholinergic poisoning (flushed, dry skin, dilated pupils, and altered mental status) coupled with an ECG demonstrating a wide QRS with an extreme rightward axis and a broad terminal R wave in lead aVR. Tricyclic poisoning was suspected in this patient. The treatment of choice is bicarbonate which displaces the drug molecule from the cardiac sodium channel. The next tracing is taken after an infusion of sodium bicarbonate: the QRS is still slightly wide, there is sinus rhythm at 100 beats/min, and the QT interval remains prolonged.

ANSWERS (Cont.)

ECG after sodium bicarbonate:

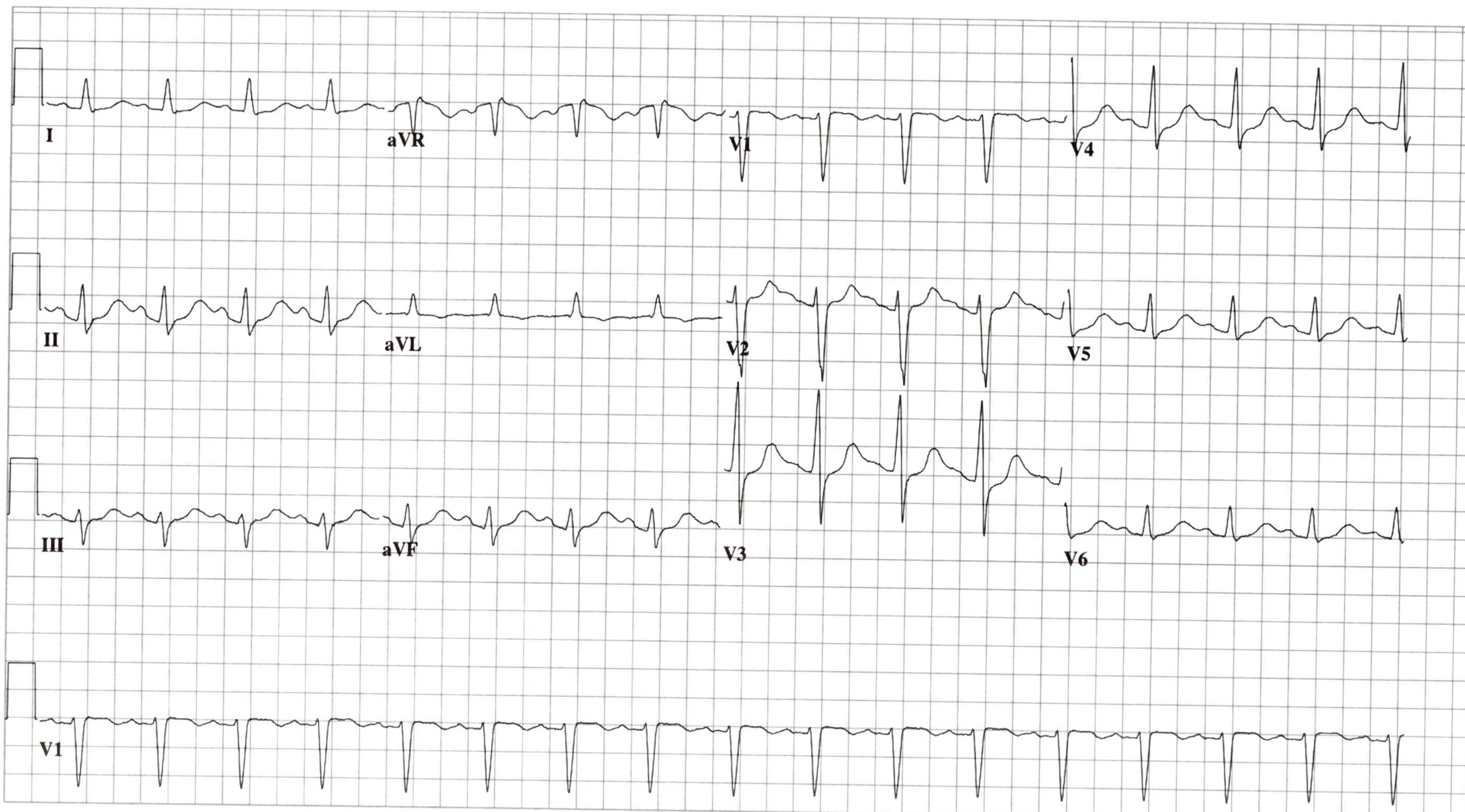

Case #145. A 64-year-old woman presents with dizziness.

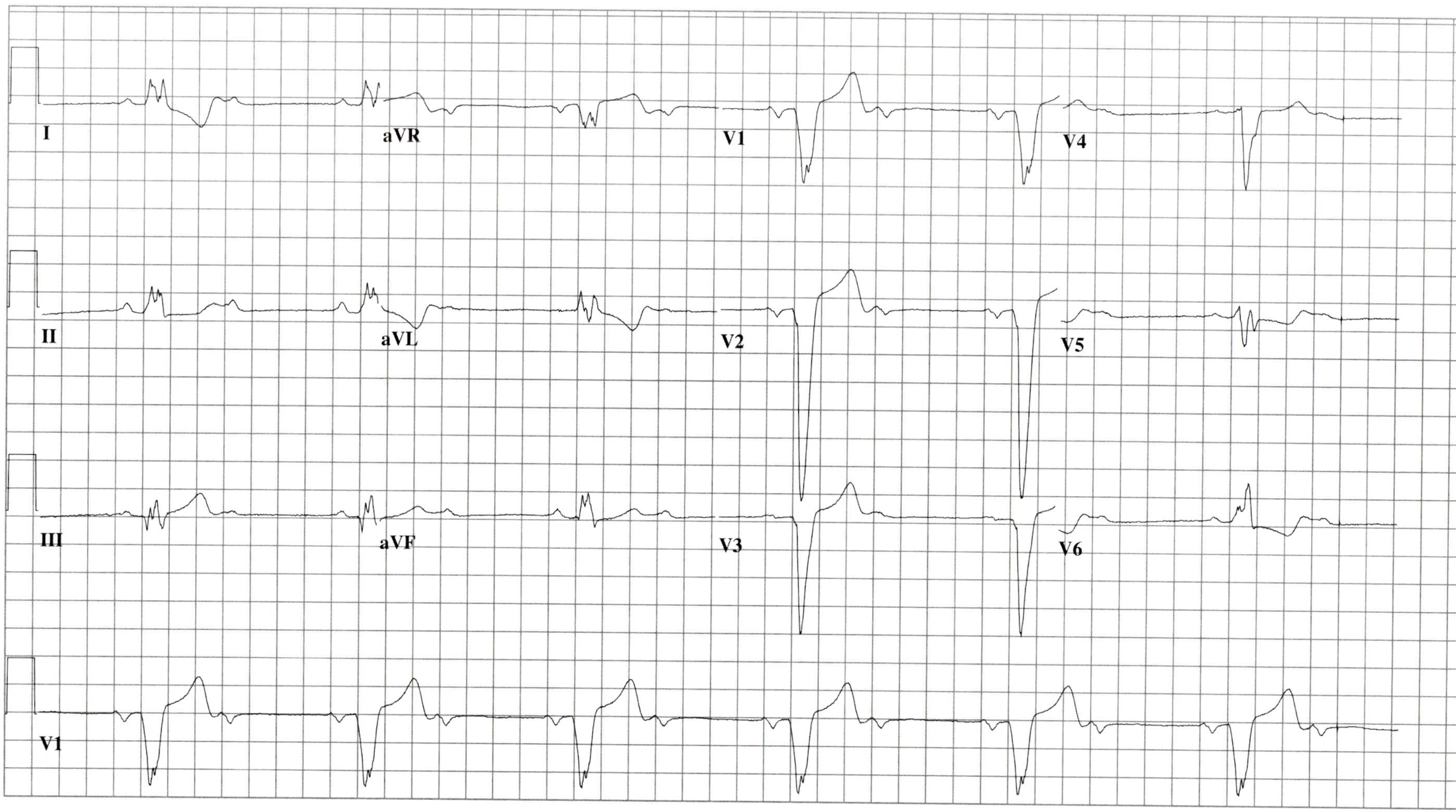

QUESTIONS

145-1. Interpret this ECG.

145-2. Is there AV block? If so, where in the conduction system is the block *most likely* located?

83
15.0 cm MI 0.9
P2-4AC
Gen TIs 1.1
[2d] G78/71 d
FA4/P90
HAR/FS|0
[C] G50/0.80 kHz
FA5/F1/8
TDI
S-T
interval
2.5
3
Time (s)
3.5

ANSWERS

145-1. Interpret this ECG.

The atrial rate is approximately 75 beats/min. The P waves are upright in lead II and biphasic in lead V1 consistent with a sinus origin. Every other P wave is not conducted, and the ventricular rate is therefore approximately 36 beats/min (6 ventricular impulses in the 10-second rhythm strip is 36 beats/min). The conducted QRS complexes demonstrate left bundle branch block, with a broad notched R wave in leads I and V6, and deep QS waves in the anterior precordial leads. There are no ischemic changes, and the ST segments and T waves are appropriately oriented opposite to the direction of the QRS complex. In summary, there is sinus rhythm with 2-to-1 AV block and left bundle branch block.

145-2. Is there AV block? If so, where in the conduction system is the block *most likely* located?

When there is 2-to-1 AV block, one cannot state with certainty whether the block is Mobitz type I (with progressive PR prolongation followed by a nonconducted P wave) or Mobitz type II (with a constant PR interval followed by a nonconducted P wave). When every other complex is nonconducted, there is no opportunity to observe progressive PR-interval prolongation. Although we cannot state for certain where this patient's block is located, the coexistence of left bundle branch block suggests that the block is located below the level of the AV node, or "infra-Hisian." An invasive electrophysiology study would be needed to definitively determine the site of block. Pacemaker placement would be indicated given her symptomatic bradycardia.

Case #146. A 75-year-old man presents with crushing substernal chest pain, syncope, and a sense of impending doom.

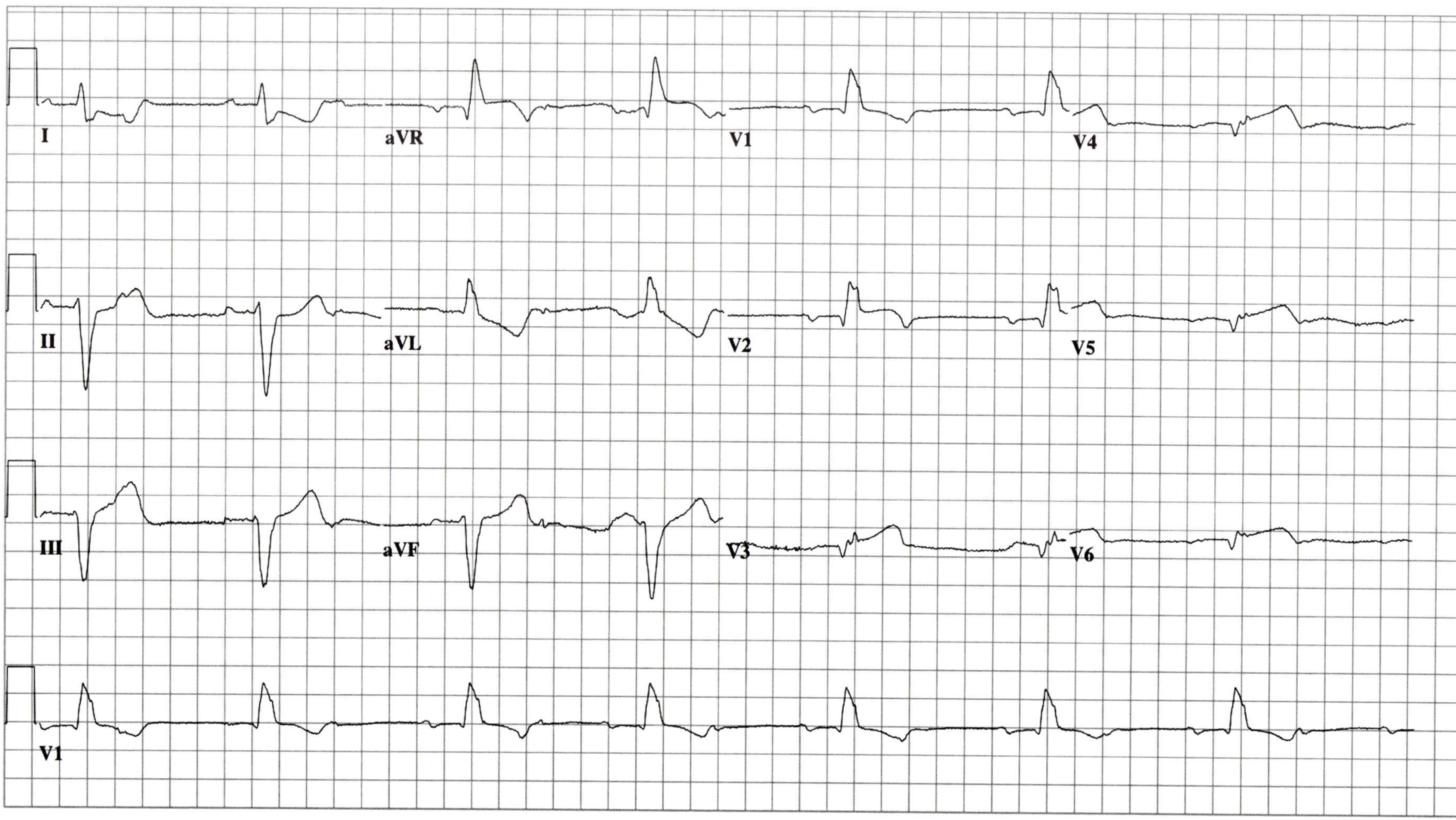

QUESTIONS

146-1. Interpret this ECG.

146-2. What would you do next?

146-3. Explain the conduction abnormalities.

83
P2-4AC
15.0 cm MI 0.9
Gen TIs 1.1
[2d] G78/71 d
FA4/P90
HAR/FS0
[C] G50/0.80 kHz
FA5/F1/8
TDI
Amplitude (V)
S-T
interval
2.5
3
Time (s)
3.5

ANSWERS

146-1. Interpret this ECG.

The atrial rhythm is sinus, and the atrial rate is 75 beats/min. There is 2-to-1 heart block present with every other atrial impulse nonconducted (see the figure with P waves denoted by asterisks). Conducted beats have a leftward axis consistent with left anterior fascicular block and a widened appearance with right bundle branch block morphology. The combination of right bundle branch block and left anterior fascicular block can be called bifascicular block. There are ST-segment elevations across the anterior precordial leads with pathologic Q waves seen. There are reciprocal ST-segment depressions in leads I and aVL.

2 to 1 AV block with P waves denoted by asterisks.

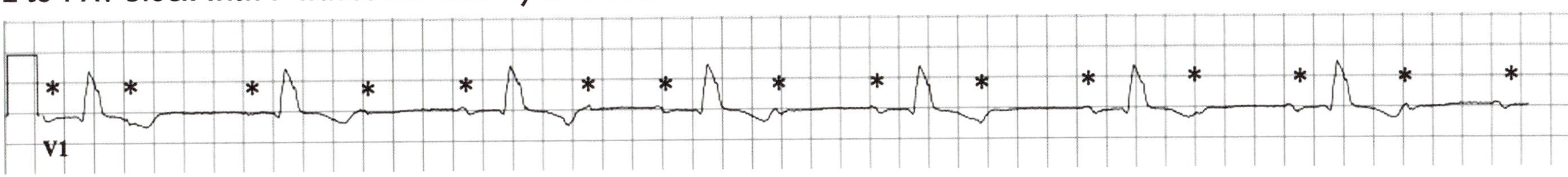

ANSWERS (Cont.)

146-2. What would you do next?

Urgent reperfusion therapy is indicated for this patient with evidence of ST-segment elevation myocardial infarction. Placement of a temporary pacemaker should be considered as discussed in the next answer.

146-3. Explain the conduction abnormalities.

Recall the blood supply to the cardiac conduction system: the AV node is supplied by the posterior descending artery, which is a branch of the right coronary artery in a majority of individuals and a branch of the circumflex coronary in a minority. The left anterior fascicle and right bundle are supplied by septal perforator arteries arising from the left anterior descending coronary artery. The left posterior fascicle usually has a dual blood supply. In the setting of inferior myocardial infarction, AV block is typically due to AV nodal ischemia and is well tolerated, rarely requiring pacemaker placement. In the setting of anterior infarction, as in this case, right bundle branch block and left anterior fascicular block signify significant ischemia and necrosis of the septum and His–Purkinje tissue. The presence of bifascicular block with AV block in the setting of anterior infarction, as seen here, confers a high risk of progression to complete heart block, and a temporary pacemaker should be considered as prophylaxis.

Case #147. A 42-year-old woman with a history of rheumatic mitral stenosis presents with palpitations.

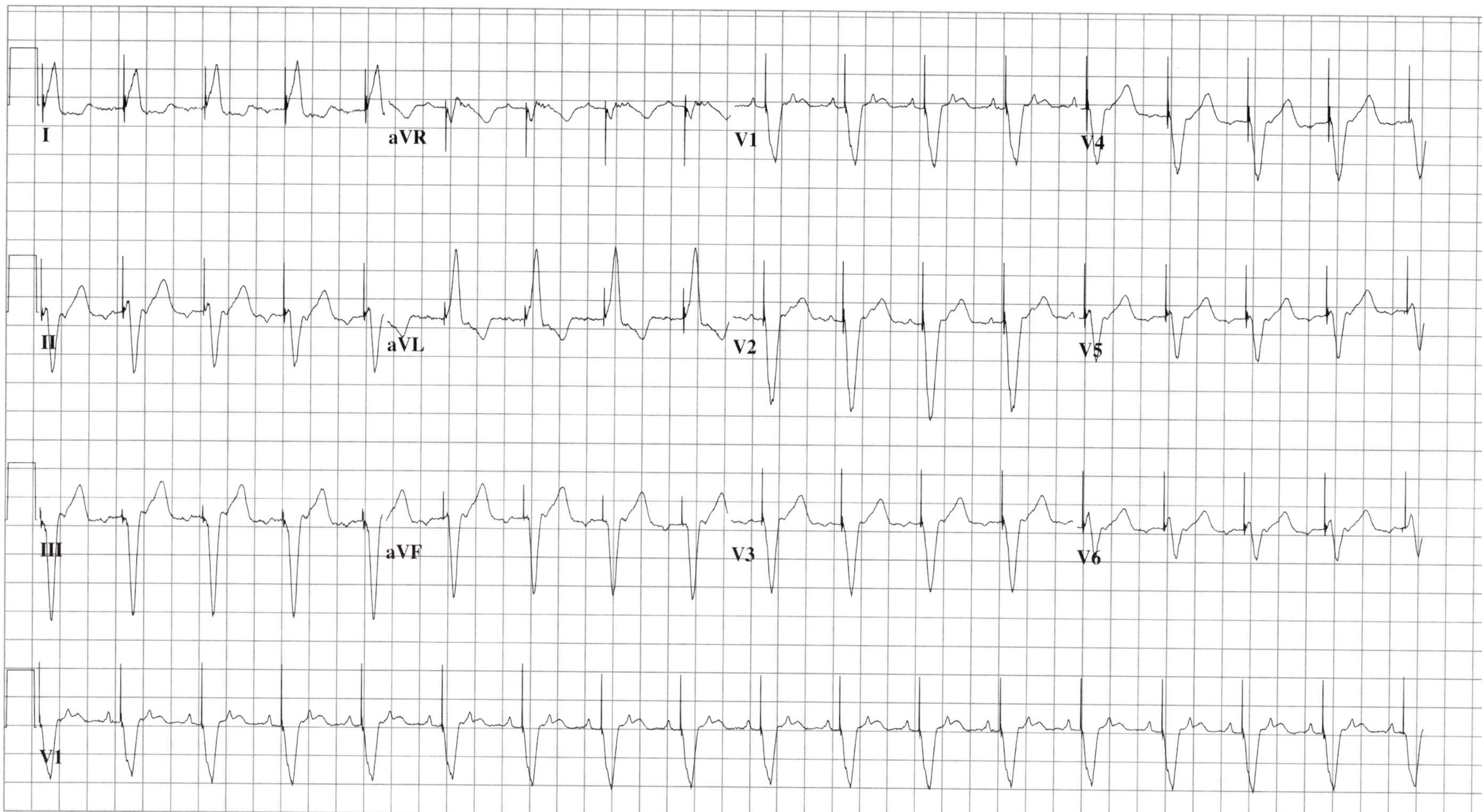

QUESTION

147-1. What is the rhythm? Describe the behavior of the pacemaker; is there malfunction?

83
P2-4AC
15.0 cm MI 0.9
Gen TIs 1.1
[2d] G78/71 d
FA4/P90
HAR/FSI0
[C] G50/0.80 kHz
FA5/F1/B
TDI
Amplitude (V)

ANSWER

147-1. What is the rhythm? Describe the behavior of the pacemaker; is there malfunction?

The ventricular rate is slightly faster than 100 beats/min. Ventricular pacemaker spikes are evident. The QRS complex has a left bundle branch block morphology with a leftward axis, consistent with right ventricular apical pacing. Preceding each QRS complex is a P wave with a consistent PR interval. This indicates sensing of atrial activity by an atrial lead with subsequent triggering of a ventricular lead. The P waves themselves are negative in leads II, III, and aVF indicating a nonsinus origin. Looking closely, a second atrial deflection is buried in the T wave, best seen in lead V1, but this P wave does not trigger a ventricular impulse. Thus, the rhythm is best described as an ectopic atrial tachycardia with ventricular pacing associated with every other atrial beat.

This finding does not represent pacer malfunction, since the pacemaker is usually programmed to "ignore" atrial activity occurring faster than an "upper rate limit" set by the pacemaker programmer. If that safeguard were not in place, the ventricular rate would be 200 beats/min in this case, which could be deleterious. The "ignored" P wave is occurring during the so-called postventricular atrial refractory period (PVARP). The PVARP is an interval set by the programmer during which the atrial lead "ignores" any impulses following a ventricular depolarization. This is typically set at a length so as to encompass the T wave and is meant to avoid the phenomenon of the atrial lead erroneously sensing the T wave and triggering the ventricular lead again.

Case #148. **A 56-year-old gentleman presented with chest pain and ST-segment elevation myocardial infarction and is now status post successful treatment with thrombolytic medications. As his chest pain is resolving, he has this arrhythmia.**

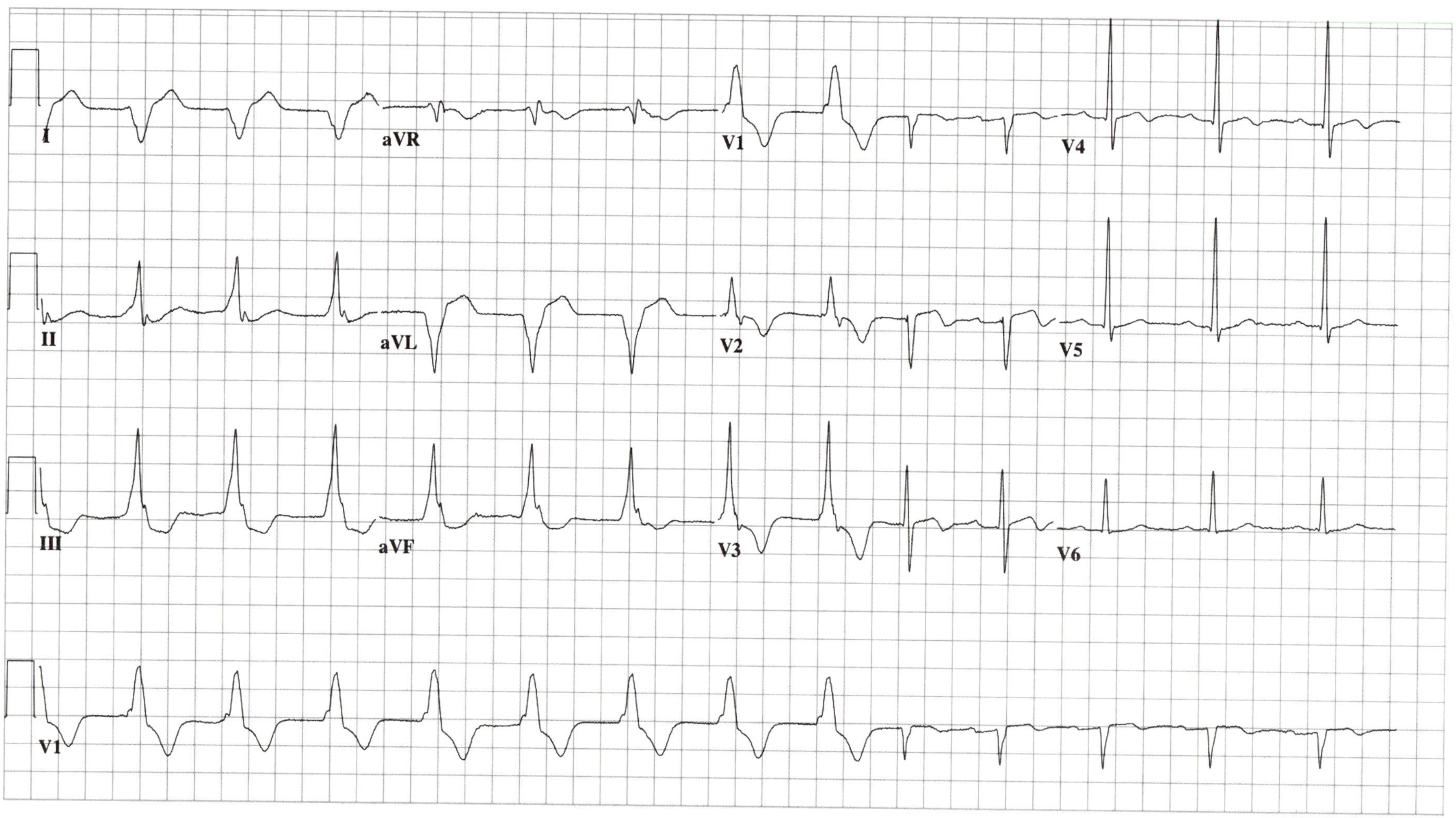

QUESTIONS

148-1. What is the diagnosis?

148-2. Does this arrhythmia have any prognostic connotations?

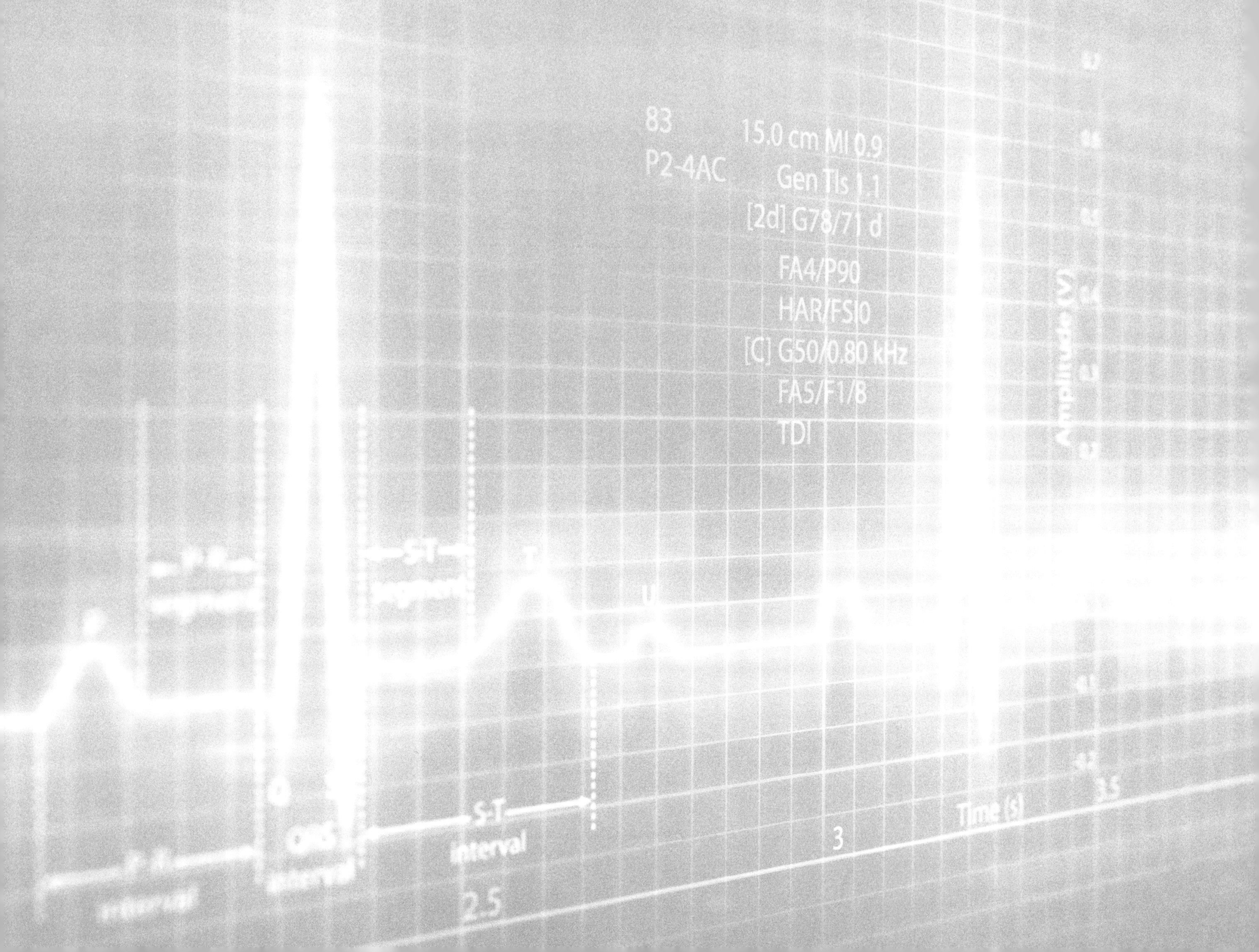
83
P2-4AC
15.0 cm MI 0.9
Gen TIs 1.1
[2d] G78/71 d
FA4/P90
HAR/FSI0
[C] G50/0.80 kHz
FA5/F1/8
TDI
Amplitude (V)
S-T
interval
3
2.5
3.5
Time (s)

ANSWERS

148-1. What is the diagnosis?

The second half of the tracing demonstrates sinus rhythm with a narrow QRS. There are inverted T waves and slight ST-segment elevation seen in the precordial leads, particularly in lead V2. The first half of the tracing is composed of a wide complex ventricular rhythm at a rate of approximately 80 beats/min. The QRS complex has positive polarity in lead V1 and hence is classified as "right bundle branch morphology" (whereas a wide complex rhythm with a negative polarity in lead V1 would be classified as having a "left bundle branch morphology). Ventricular rhythms with a left bundle branch morphology are originating from the right ventricle and ventricular rhythms with a right bundle branch block morphology are originating from the left ventricle. The rate of this rhythm is much faster than the usual rate of ventricular pacemaker cells (30-40 beats/min) but slower than ventricular tachycardia. This is best classified as an accelerated idioventricular rhythm or AIVR.

148-2. Does this arrhythmia have any prognostic connotations?

In the setting of reperfusion therapy for acute myocardial infarction, the presence of AIVR has been shown to be associated with successful reperfusion and has a good prognosis. It is usually transient, abates with time, and rarely causes symptoms. Treatment is not needed.

Case #149. A 36-year-old woman presents with syncope.

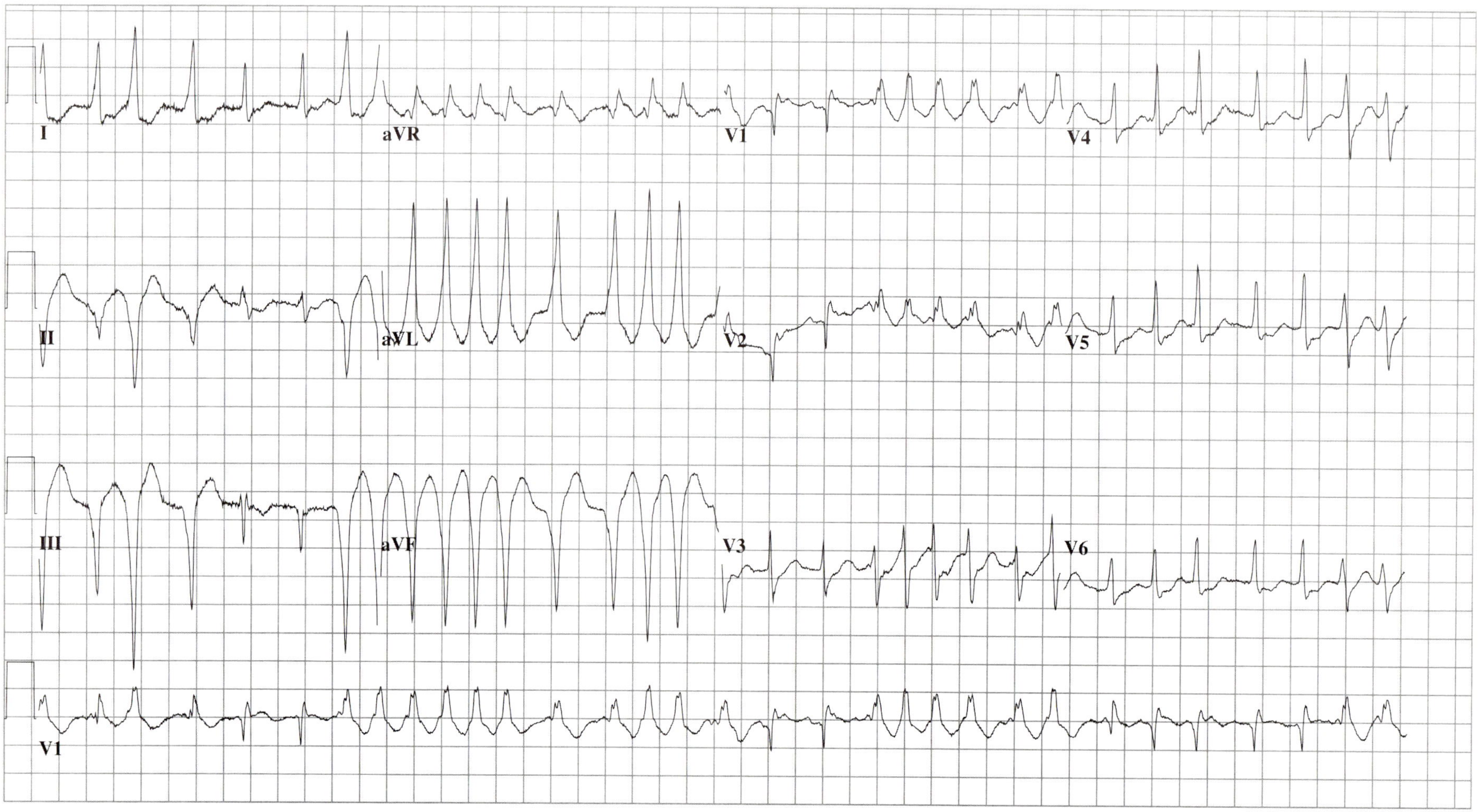

QUESTIONS

149-1. What is the diagnosis?

149-2. What is the next step in management?

83
15.0 cm MI 0.9
P2-4AC
Gen TIs 1.1
[2d] G78/71 d
FA4/P90
HAR/FS10
[C] G50/0.80 kHz
FA5/F1/B
TDI
Amplitude (V)
S-T
interval
3
Time (s)
3.5
2.5

ANSWERS

149-1. What is the diagnosis?

There is an irregularly irregular rhythm with both wide and narrow QRS complexes. The rate is very rapid; on average, the rate is 180 to 190 beats/min, with some beats conducting as fast as 300 beats/min. The axis is leftward and the QRS has a right bundle branch block morphology. There are no signs of ischemia. The differential diagnosis of a wide complex irregularly irregular tachycardia includes atrial fibrillation with preexisting bundle branch block or rate-related aberrant conduction, polymorphic ventricular tachycardia, or atrial fibrillation in the presence of an A-V bypass tract/Wolff-Parkinson-White (WPW) syndrome. The morphology of this tracing is not consistent with polymorphic ventricular tachycardia. One may be tempted to call this atrial fibrillation with aberrancy, but note that some narrow QRS complexes occur at faster rates and some wide QRS complexes occur at slower rates. If aberrant conduction were present, broad QRS complexes should occur predictably with faster rates, narrowing at slower rates. The combination of irregularly irregular rhythm with varying QRS width unrelated to the rate is diagnostic of the WPW syndrome in the presence of atrial fibrillation. Recall that the WPW syndrome involves simultaneous conduction down the AV node (which conducts slowly but recovers quickly) and down an extranodal bypass tract (which conducts quickly but recovers slowly). In sinus rhythm, this results in the typical appearance of a short PR interval with a delta wave. In atrial fibrillation, rapid chaotic atrial impulses bombard the AV node and the bypass tract and each QRS complex will consist of some combination of summed conduction down the bypass tract and the AV node. The relative conduction properties of these 2 tissues determine the resulting rhythm, and, as in this case, it can result in varying QRS widths and rapid rates.

149-2. What is the next step in management?

Agents that block the AV node should be avoided, as blocking the AV node can lead to rapid conduction down the bypass tract and cardiovascular collapse. If there is any clinical instability, the patient should receive DC cardioversion. Otherwise, procainamide intravenously is the agent of choice.

The same patient after DC cardioversion:

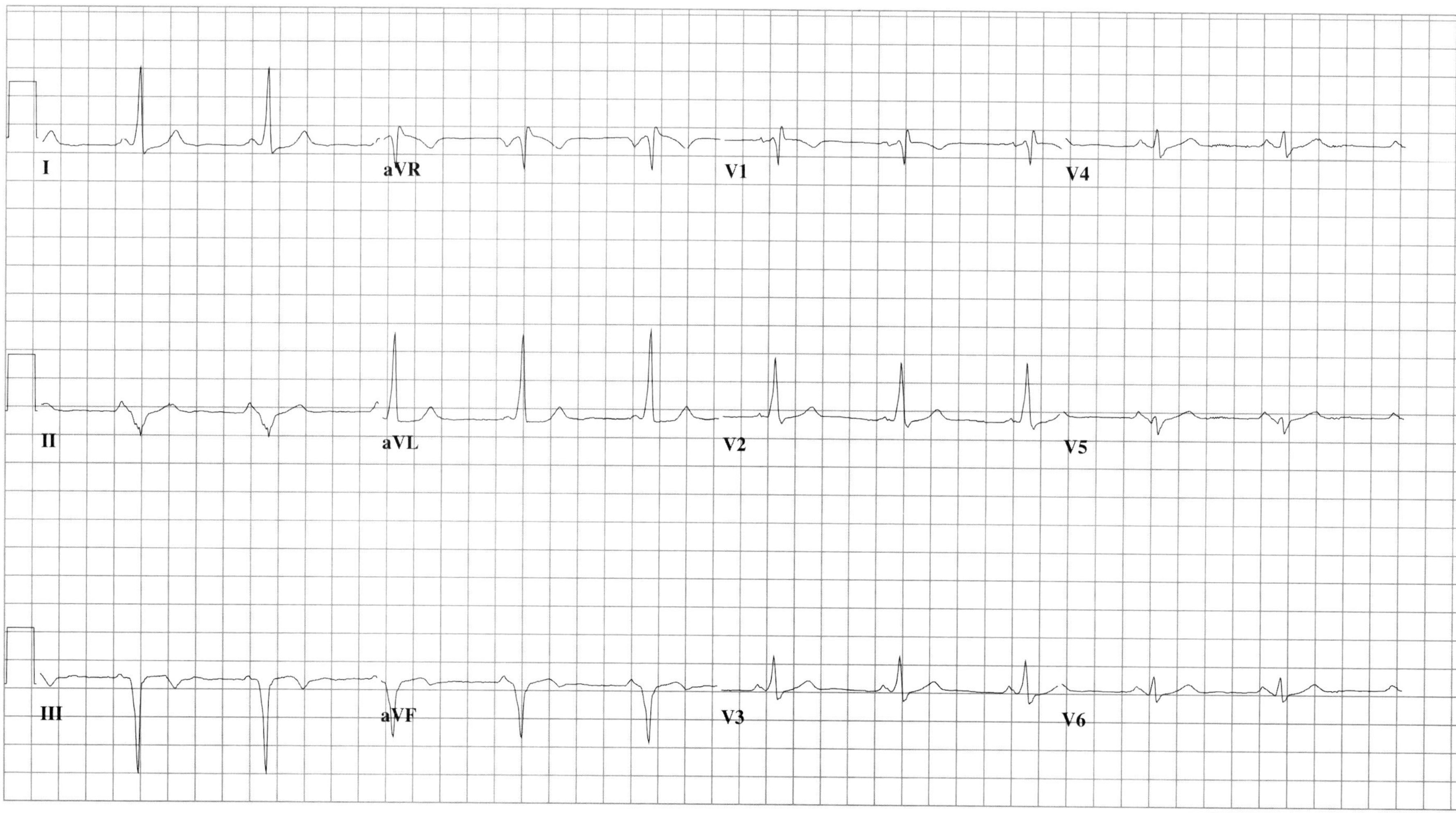

QUESTIONS

149-3. What is the diagnosis?

149-4. What is the next step in management?

83
P2-4AC
15.0 cm MI 0.9
Gen TIs 1.1
[2d] G78/71 d
FA4/P90
HAR/FSI0
[C] G50/0.80 kHz
FA5/F1/B
TDI
Amplitude (V)
S-T
interval
2.5
3

ANSWERS

149-3. What is the diagnosis?

This ECG reveals the typical findings of WPW syndrome: a short PR interval less than 120 milliseconds in duration and a broad, slurred initial portion of the QRS called a delta wave. The delta wave is the result of conduction down the bypass tract directly depolarizing ventricular myocardium. In this case, the delta wave results in inferior Q waves in a "pseudo-infarct pattern." The axis and orientation of the delta wave can give clues to the location of the bypass tract; in this case, the delta wave is negative in the inferior leads and lead VI, positive in V2 through V4, and isoelectric in the lateral precordial leads.

149-4. What is the next step in management?

Catheter ablation of the bypass tract is the treatment of choice for the WPW syndrome, particularly in this case where the bypass tract has been documented to conduct rapidly in the setting of atrial fibrillation causing syncope. Cure rates with catheter ablation exceed 90%.

Case #150. A 55-year-old gentleman presents with 10 minutes of crushing substernal chest pressure.

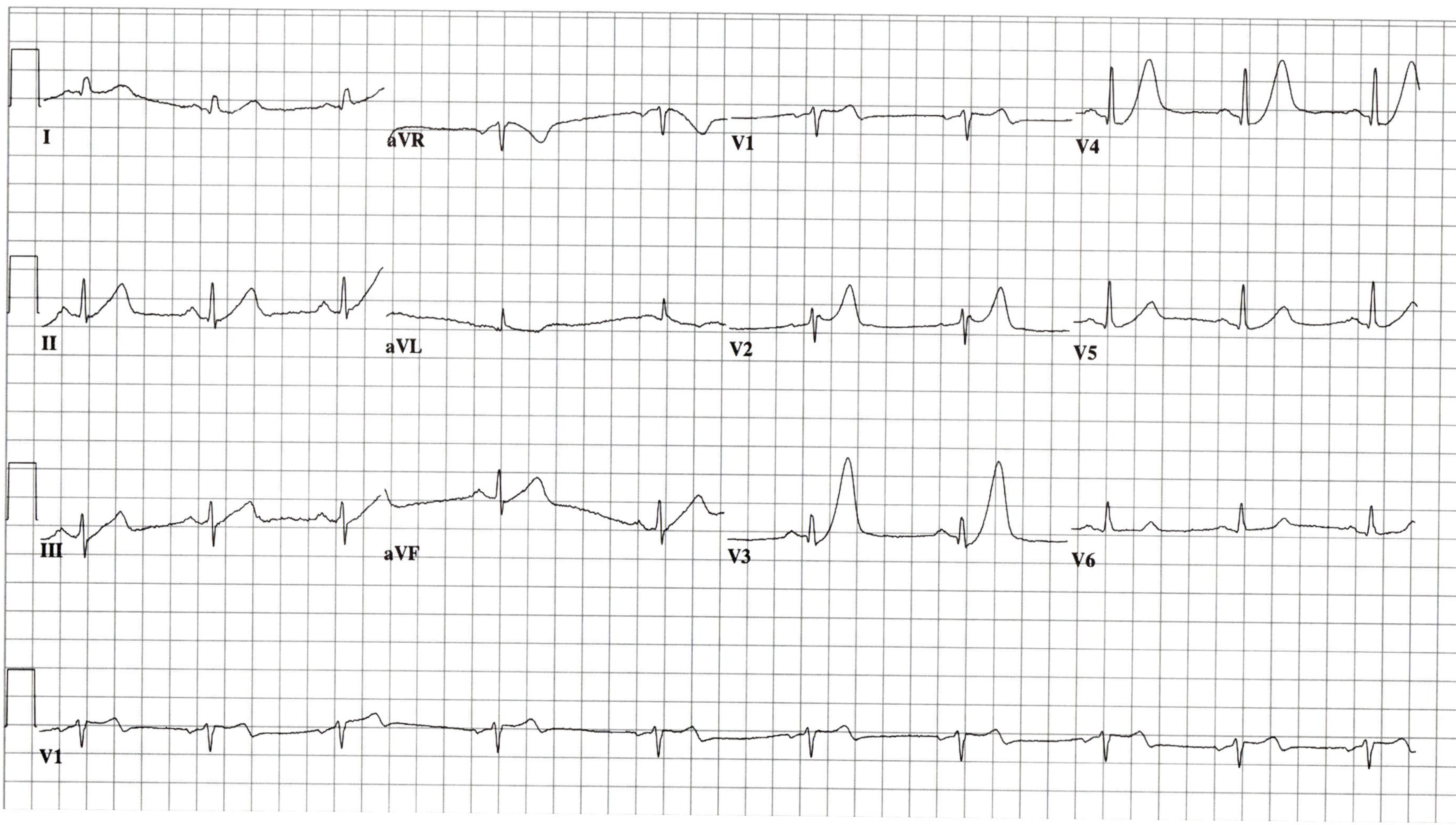

QUESTIONS

150-1. What findings are present on this ECG?

150-2. Is ischemia present on this tracing?

150-3. What would you do next?

83
P2-4AC
15.0 cm MI 0.9
Gen TIs 1.1
[2d] G78/71 d
FA4/P90
HAR/FS10
[C] G50/0.80 kHz
FA5/F1/8
TDI
2.5
3

ANSWERS

150-1. What findings are present on this ECG?

The rhythm is sinus bradycardia. Axis and intervals are normal. The T waves in leads V2, V3, and V4 appear tall and broad based, towering over the QRS complexes. Very slight ST elevation is present in leads V1 and V2. The ST segments in leads II, III, and aVF, although isoelectric, have an abnormal morphology with subtle straightening in contrast to the normal concave appearance. There is an inverted T wave in lead aVL.

150-2. Is ischemia present on this tracing?

Yes! This is an example of a very early presentation of ST-segment elevation myocardial infarction (STEMI). The first ECG changes associated with occlusion of an epicardial coronary artery are hyperacute T waves, seen here in the anterior T waves. These occur within the first minutes and are followed thereafter by elevation of the ST segment. The slight ST elevations in V1 and V2 seen in this tracing are likely the beginning of this evolution. The hyperacute T waves of early myocardial infarction should be distinguished from the peaked T waves seen in hyperkalemia, which are narrow based, tall, and pointed. The T waves seen in this case are broad based and tall, present in a defined coronary distribution.

150-3. What would you do next?

Treatment for this patient should be the same treatment for any patient with STEMI, despite the fact that ST segments have yet to elevate. Medical therapy may include nitrates, aspirin, morphine, and oxygen along with other antiplatelet and antithrombin therapies. Urgent reperfusion should be explored, either with thrombolytics or cardiac catheterization.

INDEX

D

E

F

H

O

P

Q

R

S